MW01097111

OBAGI
SKIN HEALTH
RESTORATION
AND
REJUVENATION

Springer
New York
Berlin
Heidelberg
Barcelona
Hong Kong
London
Milan
Paris
Singapore
Tokyo

OBAGI SKIN HEALTH RESTORATION AND REJUVENATION

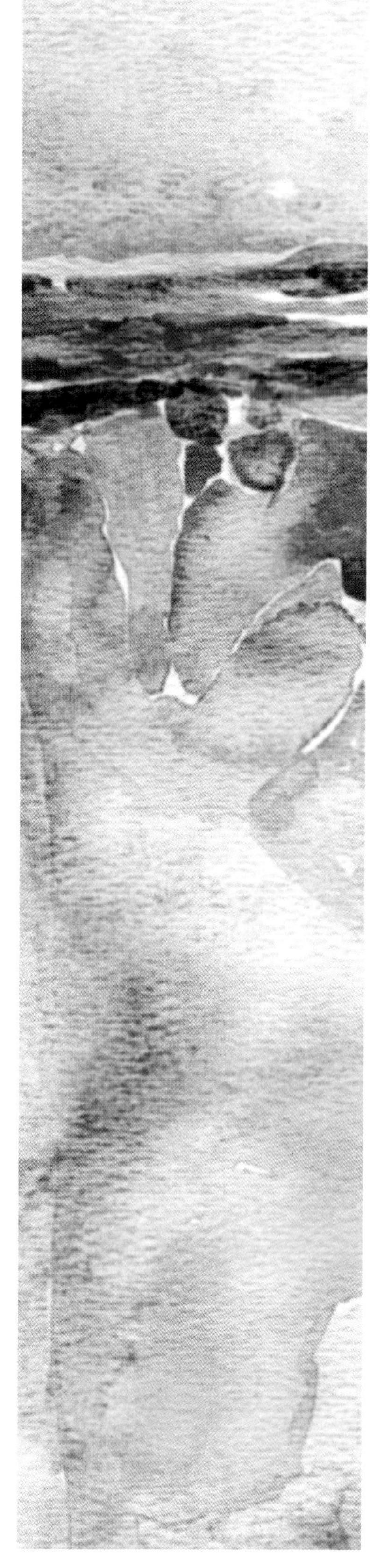

ZEIN E. OBAGI, M.D.

Obagi Dermatology Medical Clinics
Beverly Hills, California

With 196 Illustrations

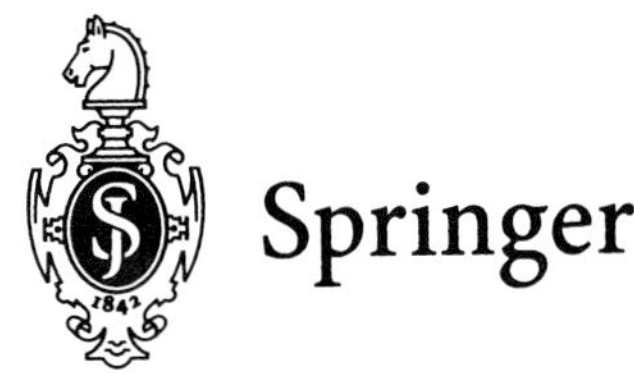

Springer

Zein E. Obagi, M.D.
Obagi Dermatology Medical Clinics
Beverly Hills, CA 90211
USA

Library of Congress Cataloging-in-Publication Data
Obagi, Zein E.
Obagi skin health restoration and rejuvenation / Zein E. Obagi.
p. cm.
Includes bibliographical references and index.
ISBN 0-387-98469-0 (hardcover : alk. paper)
1. Chemical peel. 2. Skin—Care and hygiene. I. Title.
RD520 .023 1998
617.4'770592—ddc21 98-46307

Printed on acid-free paper.

Production coordinated by Matrix Publishing Services, Inc., and managed by Lesley Poliner; manufacturing supervised by Rhea Talbert.
Typeset by Matrix Publishing Services, Inc., York, PA.
Printed and bound by Friesens, Altona, Manitoba, Canada.
Printed in Canada.

9 8 7 6 5 4 3 2 1

ISBN 0-387-98469-0 Springer-Verlag New York Berlin Heidelberg SPIN 10664741

To my most loving and supportive wife,
Samar

PREFACE

THE OBAGI APPROACH TO SKIN HEALTH

Dermatologists, cosmetic and plastic surgeons, and other physicians involved in skin care have the responsibility of providing the best available professional treatment to people who desire improvement in their appearance. To this end, the Obagi Skin Health Restoration programs were developed, and they are destined to become the "gold standard" in skin rejuvenation. Unlike existing procedure-oriented approaches, Obagi Skin Health Restoration programs address prevention, skin function, and maintenance to keep skin healthy, young-appearing, and free of deteriorative signs of aging and skin disease. Procedures may be used, but they are not the main focus. My approach to skin rejuvenation is comprehensive, and procedures constitute a part of the whole. My objective is to help physicians use a systematic approach to restore skin to its natural, healthy, youthful state. When procedures are involved, I wish to share my knowledge on proper selection, the factors that increase a procedure's safety margin, how to maximize and maintain results, and how to manage the skin properly before and after procedures.

Performing skin rejuvenation through procedures alone is like building a house on a weak foundation or without the follow-up touches of interior design. The final result usually is suboptimal. While most books published on skin rejuvenation neglect to address skin properly, this book focuses on skin rejuvenation in general and skin health and tolerance in particular. Prior to any procedure, proper conditioning is necessary to bring the skin to a normal, tolerant state, which optimizes results and decreases the chance of adverse reactions. Postoperative care is just as necessary, so that healing is rapid and uneventful, the benefits of the procedure are maintained, and skin functions are kept at optimal levels, thus maintaining the state of healthy skin indefinitely.

Healthy, youthful, attractive skin is the goal physicians and patients strive for, and it should be possible for persons of all skin types and colors to achieve, whether through the Skin Health Restoration program alone or in conjunction with a procedure. In this book, I share my knowledge and experience to show how this goal can be accomplished. Understanding the comprehensive skin classification system presented in this book is essential.

The concepts presented here are based on scientific principles as well as clinical observations. I have attempted to remove the confusion, mystery, and effects of popularity associated with skin rejuvenation processes and present information based only on merit. The field of skin rejuvenation is constantly changing, and our body of knowledge on the molecular, histological, and clinical levels is growing rapidly. We must keep our minds open to the new and be prepared to abandon that which is no longer valid.

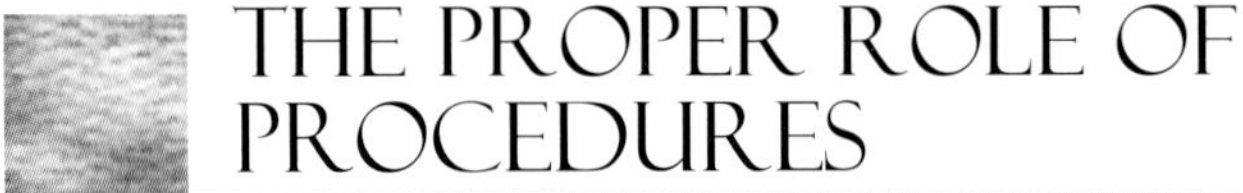

THE PROPER ROLE OF PROCEDURES

At present, physicians are wrongly focused on learning to perform skin rejuvenation procedures, and most journal publications share this focus, as if a procedure were all that is needed to treat skin. Furthermore, physicians usually become skilled in one procedure, be it chemical peeling, laser resurfacing, or dermabrasion, and then use that procedure for all patients indiscriminately. This is much like the toss of a coin—the results may or may not be good. When the results are not the best, the physician, not the procedure is usually at fault. This is due to 1) selection of an improper procedure or depth, 2) failure to take into consideration the patient's skin type, or 3) failure to perform the proper preconditioning.

The indiscriminate use of the same procedure for every patient—whether it is laser resurfacing, chemical peeling, or incisional surgery such as facelifts—should end. Expensive, deep, and invasive procedures are not necessarily better and may be worse than more limited procedures. Procedure selection should be based on the necessary depth for the particular patient's problem, the level of safety, the length of healing time, and the consistency of results that can be obtained. In any ethical medical practice, the well-being of patients should be the first priority; striving for monetary gain through use of unnecessary procedures that may harm the patient is disgraceful.

Many rejuvenation procedures are discussed in this book, each associated with a particular mechanism of action. I strongly recommend that physicians learn the various mechanisms of action associated with each type of rejuvenation procedure and master at least one procedure for each mechanism. Of great importance is an understanding of the interaction between skin type, the particular mechanism of action, the steps to be taken to prepare skin before the procedure, and the management of the return to normalcy afterwards.

In short, by tying together skin classification; regulation of skin-cell functions; proper procedure selection based on mechanism of action; and measures to prevent, detect, and properly treat complications, I hope to make skin rejuvenation easier to comprehend and practice. Both physicians and patients around the world will benefit from this knowledge.

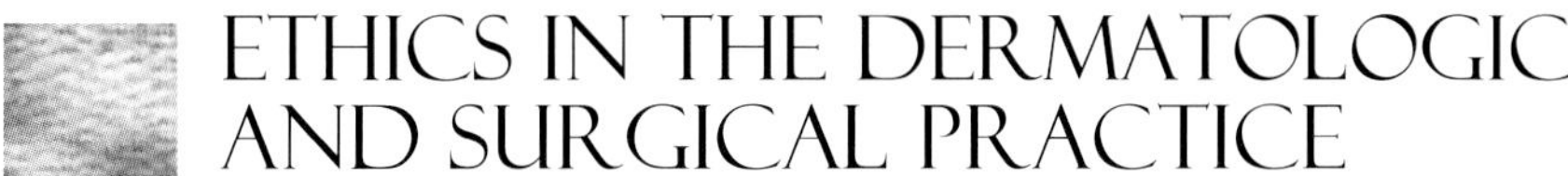

ETHICS IN THE DERMATOLOGIC AND SURGICAL PRACTICE

The issue of ethics in the practice of dermatology and cosmetic surgery has recently come to the forefront. Various practices have been criticized, and multiple definitions of ethical standards have been proposed. As a practicing clinical dermatologist, researcher, and teacher, I would like to give my input on several of these issues. In my mind, the components essential to an ethical practice are: 1) being truthful to the patient about outcomes; 2) presenting all available treatment options to the patient; 3) performing only those procedures in which the physician has sufficient training and competence; 4) placing the patient's welfare ahead of other considerations; 5) treating patients with respect and without discrimination based on sex, race, ethnicity, or religion; and 6) when unable to provide the necessary level of care, referring patients to the proper caregiver.

Discourses concerning the ethics of physician advertising are only marginally significant. Except for a few holdouts, most physicians today agree that advertising that is informative, in good taste, and not misleading is perfectly acceptable. Indeed, good advertising performs a valuable public service in that it educates consumers on medical products and services.

One area of medical ethics getting scant attention is what I refer to as the tyranny of some medical societies or academies. Although the problem is not obvious, it is potentially detrimental to the advancement of the medical profession. Practitioners of almost every medical specialty or subspecialty have formed medical societies. A review of the typical by-laws of these societies reveals that they are established for the principal purposes of fostering and promoting investigative knowledge in the specialty, promoting standards in practice and patient care, providing continuing medical education, and providing a forum for the exchange of ideas.

Like almost any other voluntary organization with many members, these medical societies, their sister societies, and certain committees tend to be dominated at certain intervals by a few individuals. A review of their records will reveal, for example, that the person who is president one year is a board member another year, a committee member in yet another year, and a member of the editorial board of the society's journal in another year. Although members join and leave this governing elite, a consistent core of members remain who determine the society's activities.

This governing elite quite often has the power to exercise tremendous control over the dissemination of information to the members. For example, the governing body decides who speaks at forums and annual meetings and determines which articles are accepted for publication. Thus, it is readily foreseeable that the ideas of the governing elite will be promoted by the medical society while competing ideas will be relegated to a secondary status or ignored altogether. Such censorship of experimental medical treatments or methodologies can have great impact on the consuming public.

In addition to control of dissemination of information, many physicians use their affiliations and offices within these societies for monetary gain. This is usually in the form of consultation for pharmaceutical, cosmetic, or technology companies. These society-affiliated physicians also may sponsor studies to promote companies for whom they consult. There is no easy remedy for these situations; however, more active involvement by all members of professional societies may cut down on the domination of the governing elite. Furthermore, a requirement for financial disclosure and term limits within the societies may ensure constant renewal and do much to foster new ideas and concepts.

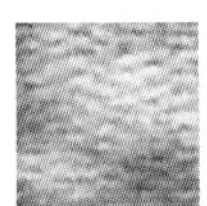

ROLE OF UNIVERSITIES

We must not forget that innovation in skin care has come from several sources, including the private practitioner who was guided by the needs of patients for effectiveness and safety, as well as from the efforts of academics. However, those of us who expected the university sector to exhibit leadership in the development of new products and procedures, provide unbiased opinions, and generally serve as a fountain of knowledge have been disappointed. University faculties have in the past been averse to affiliating themselves with products or procedures that are construed as "cosmetic." Therefore, the publication of valid studies (subjected to review by the institutional review boards) in a nonbiased setting and with a large patient population is hampered. Valuable research in this field has been left up to community physicians, who may have fewer resources, smaller patient populations, or a conflict of interest in the procedure or product being evaluated.

For the field of skin rejuvenation to move forward, universities must abandon the notion that rejuvenation is strictly cosmetic and view it as a means for restoring healthier skin. Keeping skin healthy and preventing its deterioration is as important as the prevention of illnesses such as diabetes, high blood pressure, or hypercholesterolemia.

In addition, while the responsibility of learning to perform the procedures lies with the physician, access to training should be available so that the practitioner can learn the best techniques and become aware of ways to prevent problems and complications. I enjoy sharing my discoveries and welcome opportunities to teach my programs to others.

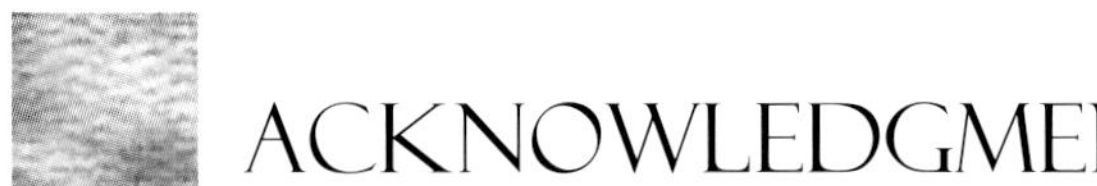

ACKNOWLEDGMENTS

I have dreamed of writing this book for many years. My dream has been realized as a result of the valuable help provided by Dr. Vartan Libaridian, Dr. Yelena Michelle, Mr. Leonard Steiner, Dr. Suzan Obagi, Dr. Samer Alaiti, my office staff, my consultant writer, Julia Petrauskas, and the constant support and encouragement of my wife, Samar.

Zein E. Obagi, M.D
Beverly Hills, California
May 1999

ABOUT THE AUTHOR

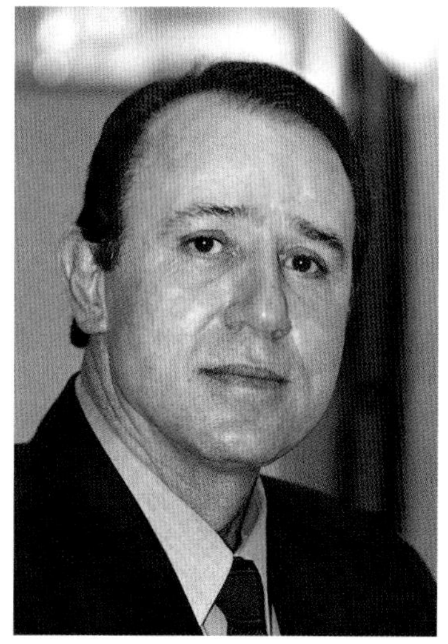

Zein E. Obagi, M.D.

Researcher, innovator, scientist, and board-certified dermatologist, Dr. Obagi has dedicated his career to the concepts of skin health, skin health restoration, and the development of facial rejuvenation techniques and formulations that help in restoring skin to its original health and beauty.

Dr. Obagi is the originator of various programs and procedures including the Skin Conditioning and Skin Health Restoration Programs, the Blue Peel, and the Obagi Controlled-Depth TCA Peel. He also developed a novel method of skin classification, defined the mechanism of action of several procedures, and developed the approach of regulating skin cell functions in order to treat pigmentation problems and rejuvenate aging skin. He has lectured and conducted courses all over the world and has taught his technique and philosophy to hundreds of physicians.

Dr. Obagi graduated from Damascus Medical School in 1972 and emigrated to the United States, where he interned in general medicine and completed a 2-year anatomic pathology residency in Michigan. He then joined the United States Navy, where he did his residency in dermatology and served for 6 years. He began his private practice in San Diego in 1981 and moved to Beverly Hills in 1989. Father of 9 children, he has worked and lived in Beverly Hills with his wife Samar and 6 of his children since that time.

CONTENTS

PART ONE

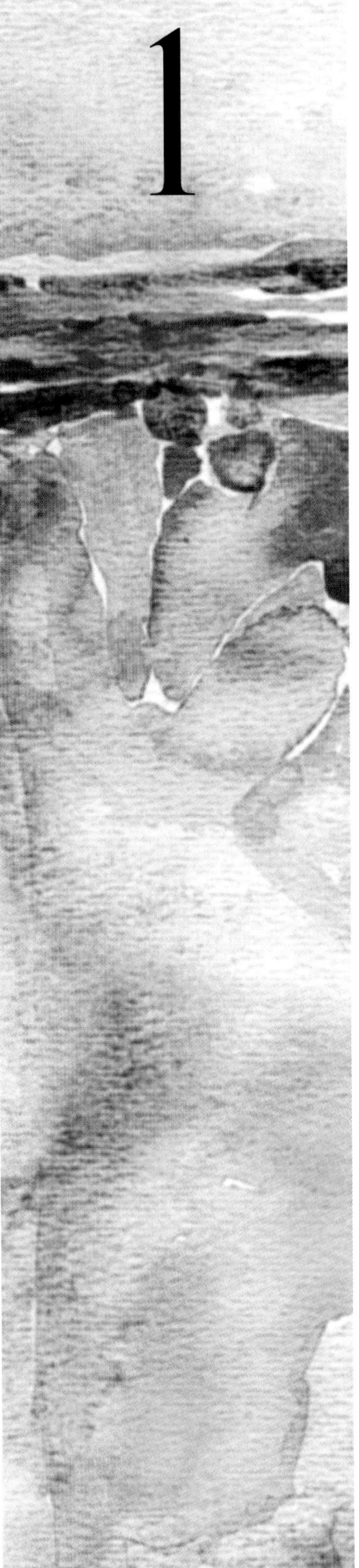

SKIN ANATOMY AND PHYSIOLOGY

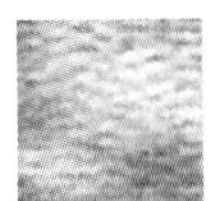

HUMAN SKIN

The skin is the body's largest organ, occupying over a square meter of surface area and accounting for about 20% of body weight. Architecturally, it is a complex organ, stratified horizontally into three compartments, the epidermis, dermis, and the subcutis, and penetrated vertically by appendages, such as hair follicles, sweat glands, and sebaceous glands. As the boundary between the body and its environment, the skin performs several functions (Table 1-1).

During a lifetime, the skin undergoes numerous changes: adapting to the change from a water to air environment at birth, adapting to hormonal influences at puberty; and, in the female, adapting to the effects of hormonal changes seen during menstruation, pregnancy, and

TABLE 1.1	
FUNCTIONS OF THE SKIN	
Function	***Activity***
Fluid barrier	■ Keeps internal fluids within the body and excludes the penetration of external fluids
Temperature control	■ Heat conservation • constriction of blood vessels • insulating properties ■ Cooling • vasodilation • evaporation of sweat
Melanin and keratin	■ Decreases damage to cellular DNA from ultraviolet light penetration
Source of sensory input	■ Sensory nerve endings that terminate at the junction of the epidermis and dermis carry information to the brain regarding the external environment
Site of metabolism	■ Example: epithelial cells synthesize vitamin D
Role in immune system	■ Langerhans cells are macrophages involved in antigen processing and immune surveillance

while taking contraceptive pills during the reproductive years. Additional profound changes can occur during illness, trauma, environmental exposures, and the process of aging.[1,2]

Some of the factors leading to deteriorative changes in the skin are controllable, while others, with our present state of knowledge, are not. This chapter will examine the structure and function of the skin at the cellular level with an emphasis on defining the controllable factors of skin health. This will assure scientific justification for clinical treatments and procedures described in the remainder of the book.

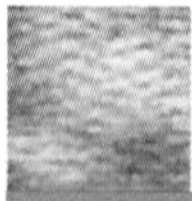

LAYERS OF THE SKIN

The skin can be divided into three main components: the epidermis, the dermis and its appendages, and the subcutaneous layer. Figure 1-1 illustrates the cell layers that comprise the adult skin.

The basement membrane is an undulating structure that attaches the epidermis to the papillary dermis and helps to support the shape of the plasma membrane of the basal cells.

The basal layer is a heterogenous mixture of cells, some of which divide and produce differentiating keratinocytes while others function as anchoring cells. Interspersed among the basal keratinocytes, melanocytes

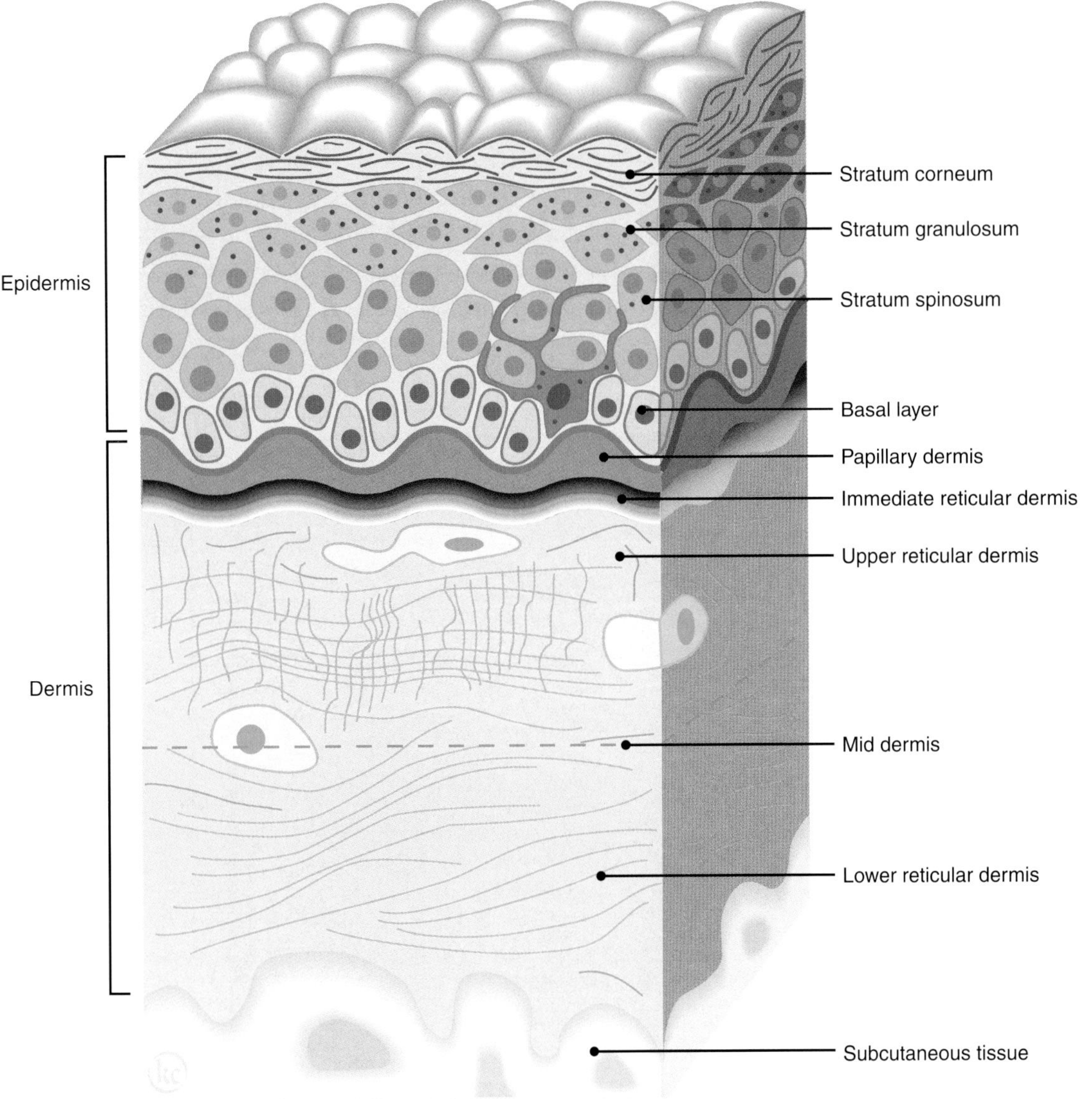

FIGURE 1-1. *The layers of the skin (blood vessels omitted for clarity).*

appear as clear cells. They have a pale cytoplasm, round nucleus, and dendrites that extend between the keratinocytes.

The granular layer is identified by densely staining granules of keratohyalin. In this layer, the epidermal cell is converted from a nucleated dividing cell into a flattened cell remnant lacking a nucleus and composed almost entirely of a tough, pliable protein called keratin.

The stratum corneum, the topmost layer, has flat, nonnucleated cells.

THE EPIDERMIS

The outer region of the skin, the epidermis, is completely cellular, typically composed of a stratified, squamous epithelium that contains 5 histologically distinct cell types (Figure 1-2). These cells are organized into layers from superficial to deep: horny layer (stratum corneum), clear or transitional layer (stratum lucidum), granular layer (stratum granulosum), prickle-cell (spinous) layer (stratum spinosum), and basal layer (stratum basale). Although there is great variation in thickness based on anatomical site, the epidermis can be said to be approximately 100 μm thick.

Approximately 80% to 90% of the cells in the epidermis are keratinocytes in different stages of differentiation[3] with lymphocytes, melanocytes, Langerhans cells, and Merkel cells interspersed among the keratinocytes. Langerhans cells constitute approximately 5% of the cells of the epidermis,

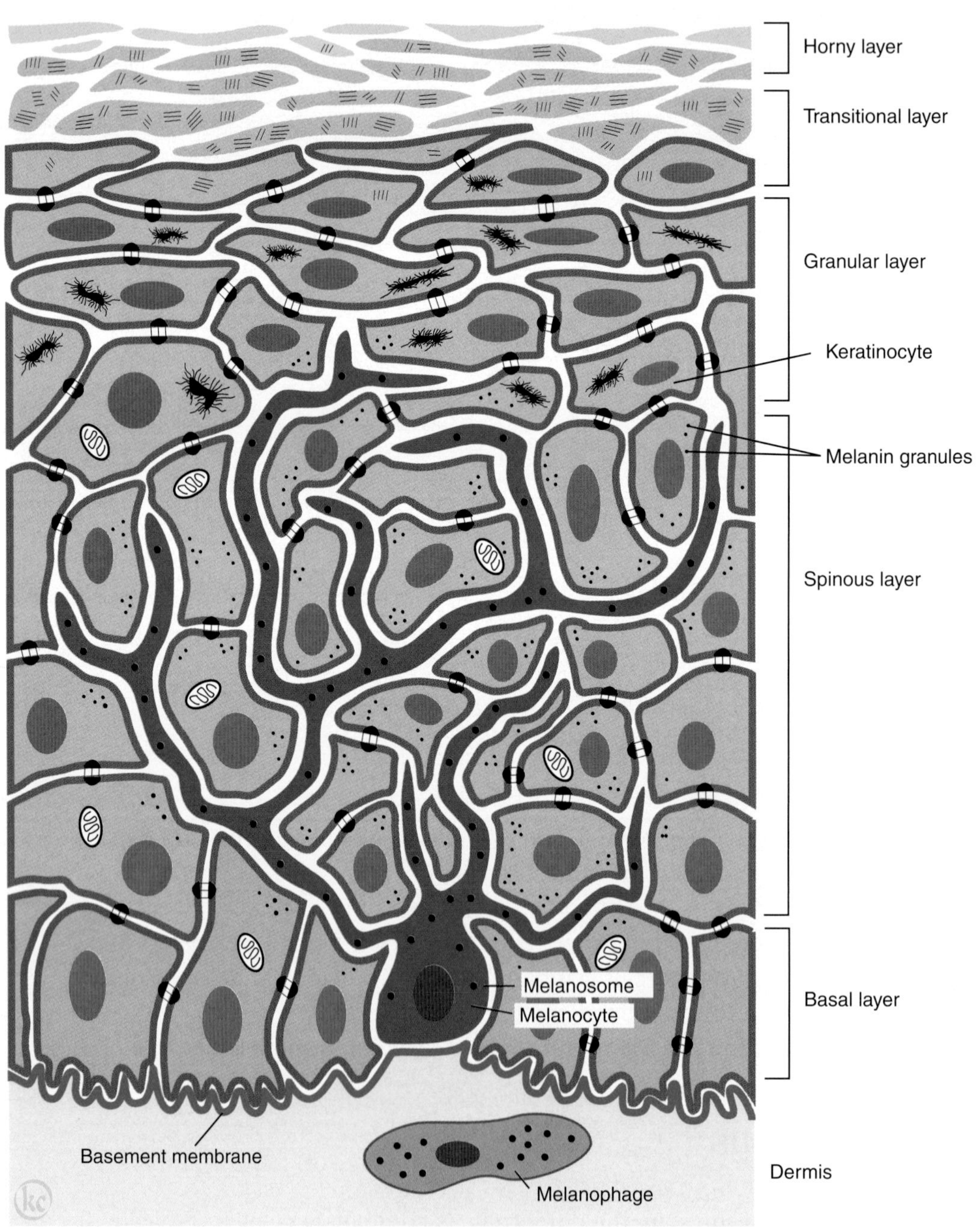

FIGURE 1-2. *The layers of the epidermis (bottom to top).*

but with aging this proportion decreases. These cells are macrophages and play a role in antigen processing and immune surveillance.

Keratinocyes are involved in a steady state of cell production and cell loss. Mitotically active cells in the basal layer of the epidermis move upward, differentiate, and die. The transit time from the basal layer to the horny layer is about one month in normal skin, but is considerably shortened after mild injury or major trauma.[4] Some of the factors that participate in the regulation of this process are the dermis, hormones, vitamin A and its derivatives, epidermal growth factor, and cyclic nucleotides. The thickness of the epidermis varies according to body site, age, sex, and racial origin but, in general, it can be viewed as being no thicker than 3 or 4 book pages.

Keratinocytes above the basal layer of the epidermis produce large amounts of the fibrous protein keratin. The high concentration of keratin in the epidermis restricts the movement of fluid across the barrier zone at the junction of living and nonliving keratinocytes and thus makes the skin impermeable. Keratin in epidermal cells also helps to reduce the penetration of ultraviolet light into deeper levels of the skin.

There are no blood vessels in the epidermis, and nutrients and removal of waste products must come by diffusion from the highly vascular dermal papillae. The skin is richly supplied with nerve endings, some of which are free and respond to heat and trauma. Others terminate in Merkel cells or special end organs, such as Paccinian and Meissner corpuscles, which are mechano-receptors and lie just beneath the epidermis.

Keratinocytes

Keratinocytes are generated in the deepest layer of the epidermis, the basal or germinative cell layer. Approximately half of the generated cells remain in place as anchoring cells, while the other half undergo differentiation. In this process, the keratinocytes change from nucleated, dividing cells to non-nucleated, nonviable cells as they travel toward the skin surface where they are exfoliated. It normally takes 4 to 6 weeks from the time a newly formed cell leaves the basal layer until it is shed.[5,6] Disease states like psoriasis and the process of aging change this amount of time considerably.

The basal layer of cells is a heterogeneous mixture, with some cells that divide and produce keratinocytes and others, mainly distributed along the sides of the rete ridges, that serve the specialized function of anchoring the epidermis onto the dermis.

Basal cells are attached to one another and to the underlying basement membrane by points of attachment known as hemidesmosomes. These cell wall connections hold the epidermal cells together while allowing the passage of nutrients and other materials through the epidermis. The tonofilaments (tonofibrils), which are aggregates of keratin, insert into the desmosomes to form a complex that minimizes the effects of mechanical stress in the epidermis. Above the basal layer, the keratinocytes have differentiated to become spinous or prickle cells. These are polygonal cells with basophilic cytoplasm and a round nucleus, and they form the bulk of the epidermis. Spot "welds" between cells are accomplished by desmosomes.

The granular layer, superficial to the prickle cell layer, is composed of only one or two layers of flattened, horizontally elongated cells. Two types of granules are present in these cells: 1) keratohyalin granules that contain the protein fillagrin, which help to form the aggregates of keratin fibrils, and 2) the smaller lamellar granules or Odland bodies that contain acid hydrolases and may act as lysosomes.

At the transition layer, the keratinocytes flatten, lose their keratohyalin granules, and, as they die, lose their nuclei. This process ends in the formation of the horny layer, the stratum corneum. This layer provides a durable, pliable, and effective barrier of tightly packed dead cells called corneocytes. The mixture of keratins in the corneocytes provides an excellent covering for the underlying tissues, as it is chemically unreactive, hard, and waterproof (in both directions), yet elastic and resistant to abrasions and physical insult. Thus water loss and the penetration of external substances are mostly prevented by the horny layer.

Above the stratum corneum, in the thick skin of the palm and soles only, a fifth layer, the stratum lucidum, may be seen. It has overlapping keratin scales constructed somewhat like a shingled roof.

Epidermal proliferation is tightly controlled so that the production of keratinocytes in the basal layer balances the loss from the horny layer. If the skin is injured, however, the production of keratinocytes increases and more cell divisions occur within a set time. When the wound has been repaired, the kinetics of keratinocyte proliferation return to a resting state.

Interspersed among the basal keratinocytes are melanocytes or melanin-synthesizing cells, which interact with a specific number of keratinocytes in an "epidermal-melanocyte unit."

Melanocytes

In normal skin, melanocytes are found only in the basal layer where they are interspersed among the basal keratinocytes. Through its fingerlike dendritic processes, each melanocyte is in contact with 30 to 40 keratinocytes. Melanocytes have no tonofibrils and do not have desmosomal junctions with adjacent cells.

Inside the melanocyte, organelles known as melanosomes produce melanin pigment. These pigment granules move from the cytoplasm into the dendrites and are transferred from there to the surrounding keratinocytes where they form a protective cap over the keratinocyte nucleus, protecting the nuclear DNA from mutation as a result of ultraviolet radiation.

Variation in normal skin color, including that due to racial differences or from the process of tanning, is not determined by the number of melanocytes but by the number, size, and distribution of melanosomes, the distribution of the pigment granules in the melanosomes, and the quantity of melanin produced. Melanosomes in black skin are large, single, and individually bound by a membrane. Also, dendrites are thicker, branched, and long. In white skin melanosomes are smaller and grouped together in complexes enclosed by a membrane.

Box 1-1

Color of skin depends on the pigment in the melanosomes and not on the density of the melanocytes.

Solar radiation reaching the earth's surface can be divided into UVB (290–320 nm), UVA (320–380 nm), visible light (380–760 nm), and near-infrared light (>760 nm). Wavelengths in the visible region have been shown to induce photobiological effects, but it is the UVB spectrum that causes the tanning response. Two reactions are involved: the immediate reaction (occurs within a few minutes and lasts up to 4 hours) in which preformed melanin is photooxidized, and the delayed reaction (apparent only after 2 to 3 days of repeated exposure). The delayed reaction occurs in response to both UVA and UVB and involves an increase in active melanocytes, enhanced melanosome production, and an increase in melanogenesis. There is also an increase in keratinocyte proliferation and transfer of melanosomes into the keratinocytes from the melanocytes.[7]

The skin can also darken in response to hormonal stimulation, such as increased synthesis of melanocyte-stimulating hormone (MSH) or adrenocorticotropic hormone, or during the poorly understood process of postinflammatory hyperpigmentation.

Box 1-2

Ultraviolet light darkens the skin through:

- **immediate oxidation of preformed melanin**
- **new melanin production during tanning**

Persons with lentigines show increased numbers of melanocytes at the dermal/epidermal junction. These lesions are believed to result from an increase in metabolically active melanocytes. Ephelides or freckles, on the other hand, are not due to an increase in melanocytes but represent areas of increased melanin synthesis. Freckles appear in childhood, and their pigmentation usually increases during the summer, indicating that melanocytes respond to ultraviolet light.

Other Epidermal Cells

Two other cells, the Langerhans cell and the Merkel cell, join the keratinocytes and melanocytes in the normal epidermis. Langerhans cells are dendritic cells that superficially resemble melanocytes, and they comprise 3% to 5% of the cells in the epidermis. Langerhans cells lack melanin and contain a characteristic ultrastructural organelle resembling a tennis racket. They originate in the bone marrow and move in and out of the epidermis as required by their role as the antigen-processing cells of the epidermis. Langerhans cells may be important in the pathogenesis of skin malignancy because they are unusually susceptible to destruction by ultraviolet light.

Merkel cells are dendritic cells found in the basal layer of the epidermis. The function of these cells is not definitely known, but they are believed to play a role in skin sensation.

THE DERMIS

The dermis is a layer of connective tissue 500 to 1,000 μm thick, composed mainly of collagen fibers and about 5% elastin. It lies beneath the epidermis and gives it structural support. It also provides all nutrition and waste product removal since the epidermis lacks blood vessels of its own. A basement membrane lies between the basal cells of the epidermis and the connective tissue of the dermis and attaches the 2 tissues to each other by means of hemidesmosomes.

The plane of contact between the epidermis and dermis is not straight but is an undulating surface, more so in some locations than in others. Upward projections of the dermis, the papillae, fit into the epidermal depressions, the rete ridges. This kind of arrangement provides a greater interface between the epidermis and the dermis than would result from contact between 2 flat surfaces.

The dermis is subdivided into 2 layers: the more superficial papillary dermis and the reticular dermis. The papillary dermis is a thin layer of loose, connective tissue in and around the rete ridges of the epidermis. Its connective tissue fibers are oriented vertically. The papillary dermis contains a rich supply of blood vessels that penetrate from the deeper layers as well as numerous nerve endings, thermoreceptors, and cryoreceptors. Below the papillary dermis is the thicker, major layer of the dermis, the reticular dermis. Its collagen and elastic fibers are densely packed and oriented horizontally.

Collagen

Collagen and elastic fibers are the main types of fibers in the dermis. Collagen is an insoluble protein (due to chemically stabilizing intermolecular cross-linking) that constitutes 75% of the dry weight of the skin. In young skin that has not been exposed to sun, mature collagen is cross-linked into collagen fibrils that come together into small groups of fibers, which are then organized into thin, wavy, fiber bundles. The collagen fiber bundles are arranged in a matlike orthogonal pattern, i.e., each layer is at right angles to the one above and the one below. Fibroblasts lie among collagen fibers and are known to synthesize collagen and the ground substance of the dermis. Newly formed collagen fibrils become less soluble and more stable as they mature. Fully mature collagen fibers have a very low turnover compared with other body proteins.[8]

Box 1-3

Collagen provides the skin with both tensile strength and elasticity

All collagens are composed of three polypeptide chains known as alpha chains which take on the configuration of a helix in a collagen molecule. The alpha chains can combine to form 8 different types of collagen in the human skin. Of these 8 types, type I is the predominant form (60% to 80%) in adult skin; type III constitutes 15% to 20%. The papillary dermis has a high content of type III collagen, which consists of large-diameter fibrils woven into large fiber bundles. The ratio of type I to type III collagen in the dermis and the size of collagen fibers and fiber bundles increase progressively as the dermis deepens. In the lower reticular dermis, the fiber bundles are mostly of type I, 40 μm or more in width, and the meshwork is elaborate.[8–11]

In elderly persons, the dermal collagen fibers become more heterogeneous and the dermis become thinner. Skin exposed to sunlight shows similar but more severe changes than normally aged skin, although actinically damaged skin has less insoluble collagen than normal skin.[8] Reports on the changes in the amount of collagen in unexposed human skin over time have been contradictory, but it appears that the absolute amount of skin collagen decreases with age as skin becomes thinner but that the relative amount of collagen does not undergo a very significant change.

Elastic Fibers

The integrity of the elastic fiber network in skin is very important because wrinkling, looseness, sagging, and other structural and mechanical changes in aging skin appear to be due to alterations in this network. Elastic fibers make up 2% to 4% of the total volume of the dermis and form a network that borders on collagen bundles. Some elastic fibers are associated with blood vessels, lymph vessels, hair follicles, eccrine sweat glands, and apocrine glands.

The elastic fiber network is composed mostly of the protein elastin, which has unusual elasticity and tensile strength, and a small amount of microfibrils.[10] The strength of the elastic fibrils arises from the cross-linking amino acids desmosine and isodesmosine, not found in other mammalian proteins.

Elastic fibers in the papillary dermis, known as elaunin, are thin and oriented mostly perpendicularly to the epidermis in an arcadelike pattern. Rising almost vertically from the papillary dermis are even thinner elastic fibers that end just below the dermal-epidermal junction. In the reticular dermis, elastic fibers, here known as oxtalan fibers, are thicker and greater in number. Elastic fibers maintain normal skin tension and provide extensibility. In young skin, elastic fibers snap back quickly after stretching. The metabolic turnover of the skin's elastic structure is slow; however, elastic

Box 1-4

Alterations in the elastic fiber network are responsible for the looseness and sagging of aged skin.

fibers are continuously degraded and replaced by newly synthesized fibers in normal situations.[12]

Extracellular Matrix

The insoluble fibers of collagen and elastin are imbedded in the ground substance of the extracellular matrix of the dermis. This matrix contains soluble polysaccharides, glycosaminoglycans, and polysaccharides covalently bonded to a protein, proteoglycans (glycoproteins).[13] Although the glycosaminoglycans are less than 1% of the dry weight of the skin, they have a dramatic effect on its hydration since they are able to bind up to 1,000 times their own weight in water.[9] Hyaluronic acid and dermatan sulfate are the major glycosaminoglycans in adult skin. Fibronectin, a filamentous glycoprotein in the ground substance, is associated with collagen and elastic fibers and the basal lamina.[14]

The roles of the ground substance in addition to water-binding have not been completely defined, but it known to form a pathway for the diffusion of nutrients through dermal spaces and to bind collagen fibers into bundles. It is believed to contribute to the skin's rheological properties, especially in stretching. Other possible functions are the regulation of cell growth, adhesion, migration, and differentiation.[9]

The subcutaneous tissue lies below the reticular dermis. This tissue contains a variety of cells: adipocytes, fibroblasts, histiocytes, plasma cells, lymphocytes, and mast cells. Many of these cells are involved in the processing of foreign antigens that may be introduced into the skin by trauma. Dendritic cells of the dermis have a similar function. The thickness of the subdermal layer is highly variable, decreasing markedly during starvation and increasing greatly in obesity. It serves as thermal insulation, as protection from mechanical trauma, and as a storage site for energy.

Box 1-5

- **Collagen provides tensile strength and prevents tearing**
- **Elastic fiber network provides resiliency and elasticity (the "snap-back" of skin)**
- **Extracellular matrix controls the tone and turgor of the tissue and helps to resist compression**

Box 1-6

- **Skin becomes thinner with age because of decreased dermal thickness.**
- **The amount of collagen decreases proportionately with the decrease in skin thickness.**

Fibroblasts

Fibroblasts, the "master" cells of the dermis, are spindle-shaped cells responsible for producing collagen, reticulin, elastic fibers, and the ground substance of the dermis. In addition, they can remove fibers by secreting enzymes such as collagenase and elastase. They are more numerous and larger in the papillary dermis than in the reticular dermis. Fibroblasts also control the turnover of connective tissue by producing enzymes that degrade collagens (collagenases), elastin (elastases), and proteoglycans and glycosaminoglycans (stromelysin and lysosomal hydrolases). With advancing age, fibroblasts generally become smaller and less active. In photodamaged skin, however, they are often hypertrophied.

Mast Cells

The second cell type of the dermis is the mast cell, which contains large cytoplasmic granules. These granules contain histamine, enzymes, and other mediators, which are discharged during an inflammatory response. Binding of mast cells to immunoglobulin type E occurs during an allergic reaction. Mast cells are frequently seen lying close to fibroblasts, which may indicate cell-to-cell communication. The amount of collagen produced by fibroblasts has been shown to be influenced by mast cells.[10,14]

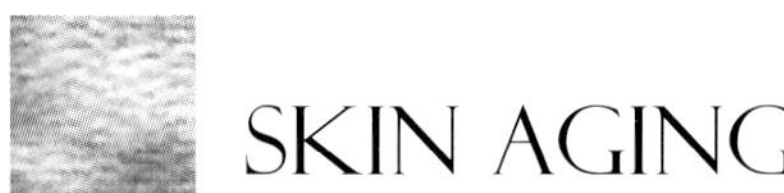

SKIN AGING

BIOLOGICAL CUTANEOUS AGING

In a discussion of skin aging, it is important to differentiate between biological aging and aging that is the result of exposure to sunlight. Clinically, photoaged skin is distinctly different from biologically aged but sun-protected skin (Table 1-2). Biologic aging is characterized by a decrease in functional capacity and increased susceptibility to certain diseases and environmental insults. The most obvious visible changes include laxity, deepening of expression lines, dryness, general thinning, and a flatter dermal/epidermal interface.

TABLE 1.2

CLINICAL CHARACTERISTICS OF INTRINSICALLY AGED AND PHOTOAGED SKIN

Intrinsic Aging	*Photoaging*
laxity	leatheriness
deepening of expression lines	dryness
dryness	nodularity and hypertrophy
overall thinning	yellowness
	telangiectasia
	deep wrinkles
	accentuated skin furrows
	sags and bags
	variety of benign, premalignant, and malignant neoplasms

Epidermis

Although it has been frequently stated that the epidermis thins and becomes atrophic in old age, this finding was the result of tissue shrinkage in laboratory specimens and was thus a study artifact.[10] While the dermal layer does become thinner with age, the epidermis decreases only 20% in height over the human lifespan.[5,15] What leads to the appearance of a diminished epidermal area in a histological section is that the rete pegs disappear with age and the lower surface of the epidermis loses its undulating contour. Thus the epidermis flattens and has less surface contact with the dermis, leading to more likelihood of peeling off of the epidermis following a shearing force.

Elastic Fibers

One of the most prominent changes occurring in biological aging is the decrease, fragmentation, and increasingly abnormal structure of the elastic fibers, which may cause skin laxity and the loss of resiliency after stretching.[10] Loss of elastic microfibrils and the appearance of cavities are also highly characteristic of biologic aging.[16] Sun-exposed skin, on the other hand, has massive levels of elastic material with a disorganized fiber network and clinically appears thick, leathery, and inelastic.

Collagen

Collagen is a tougher, more stable material, and does not show the well-defined aging changes of elastic fibers. However, there is less collagen per surface area and it is less dense and stiffer, probably due to progressive cross-linking.[8,16] In aging skin, the fibers of collagen appear thickened and stain differently. These changes are accelerated in sun-exposed skin. It has been proposed that the 3-dimensional meshwork of collagen may become distorted from many years of mechanical stress and could contribute to the laxity of older skin. Men have a thicker dermis than women, and this may explain why facial skin of women appears to show greater deterioration with age.[10]

Cells

During the biological aging process, the dermis becomes thinner and the dermal-epidermal junction flattens. Fibroblasts become smaller and show decreased metabolic activity and a decreased proliferation rate. Compared with the case in young adults, the papillary dermis in aging adults has fewer mast cells, which may result in decreased levels of mast cell–derived heparin that may be involved in angiogenesis.

Extracellular Matrix

Turnover of the ground substance decreases in the aged dermis. The decrease of glycosaminoglycans with increasing age is only slight,[10] but it has been reported to be significant after 67 years of age and to be due to decreased synthesis.[8] One study showed that glycosaminoglycan concentrations drop markedly from newborn to infancy, are stable until approximately age 40, and then fall continuously.[17] A decrease in soluble glycosaminoglycans could explain the dried and wrinkled appearance of aged skin if such skin showed a decrease of water content, but the water content of aged skin has not been shown to be decreased.[10] The moisture content of the skin has been shown to be 80% in the fetus, 68% in the newborn, and 62% in adolescents and adults. In old age, however, the pattern changes and an increase in moisture content is seen.[18]

Other Changes

The androgen-dependent production of sebum by the sebaceous glands begins to decrease in postmenopausal women and declines steadily thereafter. The clinical consequences are a 40% to 50% decrease in sebum output, which may account for the prevalence of dry skin in older women. Excessive use of soaps, cosmetics, and actinic damage may be even more important. In men, the output of sebum does not begin to decline until about the early seventies.

There is a loss of small blood vessels in aged skin, and many capillaries and vessels disappear altogether. With resorption of the dermal papillae, the capillary loops disappear. The degeneration of small blood vessels is an intrinsic age change, even in protected skin, but unlike sun damaged skin, these vessels are not dilated or deranged.[19] In actinically damaged skin, however, the microvasculature collapses, showing only a few dilated, thickened, tortuous vessels.[8,19] Although free nerve endings remain constant with age, the elderly have less acuity in the perception of pain.[20,21]

PHOTOAGING

Ongoing photoaging is characterized by hypertrophy, while in intrinsic aging "less is usually the rule."[22] In nonphotodamaged aging skin, the dermal/epidermal junction flattens and dermal thickness decreases. With photoaging, on the other hand, the dermis thickens because of massive elastosis, and the elastotic material accumulates.[9] Sebaceous glands become enlarged, and neoplastic growths are frequent. Seborrheic and actinic keratoses, solar lentigos, keratoacanthomas, basal cell epitheliomas, and squamous cell carcinomas develop almost exclusively in sun-exposed areas.[23]

The amount of elastic fibers, ground substance, and new collagen is initially increased as repair and destruction are simultaneously at work. The skin of hairless mice exposed to UV radiation shows thickened elastic fibers, a loss of collagen, and increased amounts of glycosaminoglycan.[24] Other photoaging changes include injury to basal keratinocytes, which results in a scaly stratum corneum and actinic keratoses. Changes in collagen and elastin fibers and possibly in glycosaminoglycans cause prominent wrinkling.

Epidermal Sun Damage

Excessive sun exposure causes profound changes in the epidermis. Melanocytes increase, enlarge, and become more branched. Keratinocytes may become vacuolated, atrophy, become necrotic, or show variation in size, shape, and staining properties. The stratum lucidum may be thick and swollen, with vesicles that stain atypically. Intercellular edema may be present. There is also a decrease in the number of functional Langerhans cells. The subepidermal grenz zone appears in actinic skin, representing a repair zone in which new, healthy collagen is laid down by hypersecretory fibroblasts.

Solar lentigines, also known as liver spots, are benign lesions that occur on photodamaged skin. Most lightly pigmented persons develop solar lentigines on sun-exposed hands, wrists, arms, neck, and face in middle age. The hyperpigmented, flat spots are a result of hyperplastic melanocytes that produce great amounts of pigment.

Dermal Damage

Many of the visible signs of deterioration in photoaged skin reflect major structural changes in the dermis.[22] The dominant change of photoaged skin is hyperplasia of the elastic tissue, ending in complete disorganization. Histologically, large quantities of thickened, tangled, and degraded elastic fibers are seen, and with extreme damage, an amorphous mass of what once was elastic tissue is present. In sun-protected skin, elastosis this extensive is never seen, even in people of advanced aged.

Collagen bundles dissolve and disappear in sun-damaged skin. Ultraviolet B radiation is believed to produce chronic inflammatory products that degrade collagen.[25] In intrinsic aging, however, mature collagen appears to become more stable and resistant to enzymatic degradation. The bundles appear larger and form ropelike structures. There is an increase in glycosaminoglycan in actinically damaged skin, while there is little or no change in protected skin.[10]

Box 1-7

Skin elasticity is one of the best biological indicators of chronological age.

PART TWO

CHAPTER

1

SKIN ANATOMY AND PHYSIOLOGY: A PERSONAL VIEW

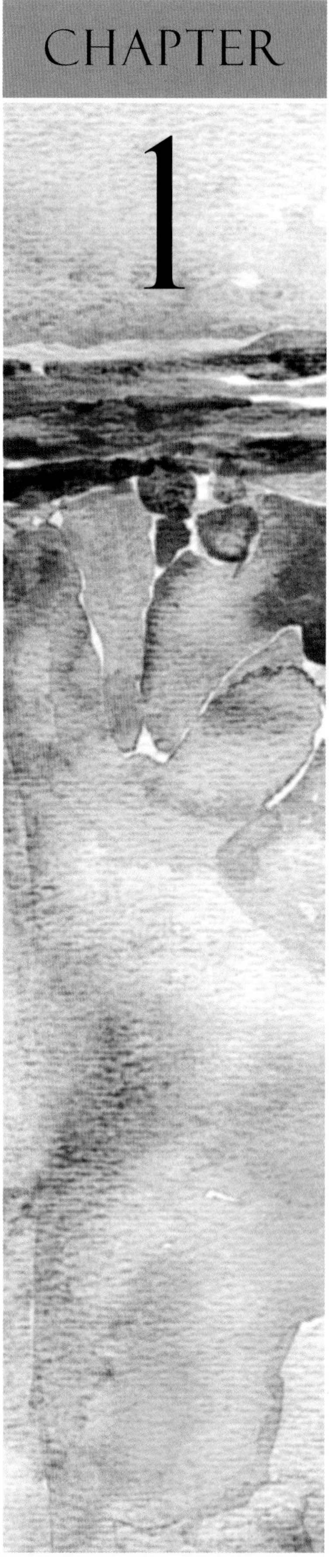

Many textbooks are available on the structure and the physiology of the skin, and reading of these is recommended for a firm grounding in dermatologic science. The purpose of this chapter is to connect the author's approach to skin rejuvenation to the anatomical and physiological properties of the skin.

The skin has many specific functions: thermal regulation, detection of sensation, immune responsiveness, energy storage, vitamin D production, and protection against environmental insults. This last function, known as the barrier function, is one of the most important. It prevents most, but not all, external substances from entering the body and also prevents body fluids from leaving. This barrier function is carried out by the layers of a healthy epidermis.

Box 1-8

Despite the effects of aging, it is theoretically possible to keep the skin functioning properly throughout life so that it overcomes damage from the environment and stays in a healthy state.

Box 1-9

Restoring the skin barrier function is one of the main goals of the Skin Health Restoration program.

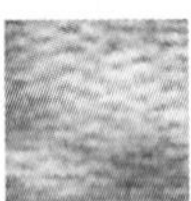

THE LAYERS OF THE SKIN

THE EPIDERMIS

The skin has 3 layers: the epidermis, the dermis, and the subcutaneous layer. The layers interact with each other such that changes to one layer have profound effects on the other two. The epidermis, the outermost sheath, shows the genetic expression of skin color and reveals dryness, softness, or roughness. It can be clear or diseased, as is the case with acne, precancerous or cancerous lesions, pigmentation problems, and psoriasis. The stratum corneum, the semipermeable membrane at the uppermost part of the epidermis, exfoliates naturally on a daily basis, while the entire epidermis renews itself usually in cycles of 30 to 40 days.

THE DERMIS

The dermis determines skin thickness and elasticity. To correct wrinkles and scars with any rejuvenation procedure, the dermal layer must be reached; exfoliation procedures that penetrate only to the epidermis will not work. Bleaching and blending, which effectively correct hyperpigmentation at the level of the epidermis, will not be effective if the pigment deposition is at the dermal level. In such cases, chemical peels or specific lasers are the best treament. Vascular skin lesions, such as telangiectasias and port-wine stains, are mainly dermal, but may involve the subcutaneous layer.

Dermal regeneration of new epidermis following procedures, such as chemical peels, dermabrasion, and laser resurfacing, depends on the integrity and function of adnexal structures of the dermis (pilosebaceous units and sweat glands). Skin can stay firm and young after these procedures if the dermis is capable of renewing and repairing itself.

THE SUBCUTANEOUS LAYER

The subcutaneous layer, composed of lobules of fatty tissue, functions as a buffer against blunt trauma and gives the skin its appealing full and plump appearance. It also provides "gliding ability" to both the dermis and epidermis, which helps to make skin more flexible. Areas with abundant subcutaneous tissue heal better and have less severe scarring than areas with a very thin or no subcutaneous layer. This can explain why certain areas of the face, such as the upper lip, jawline, and neck, where the dermis is in contact with the underlying muscles with little or no fat in between, have an increased tendency for fibrosis and scarring after procedures. It is very important to avoid deep dermal penetration in these areas.

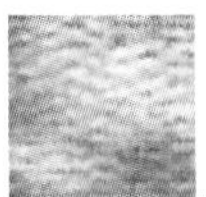

IMPORTANT SKIN CELLS

Several types of cells are vital for maintaining the properties of the skin. In the Obagi Skin Conditioning and Skin Health Restoration programs, the focus is on regulating the function of 4 cell types—keratinocytes, melanocytes, fibroblasts, and angioblasts—before and after rejuvenation procedures, especially when the goal is to slow down the aging process.

KERATINOCYTES

Keratinocytes are the major cells of the epidermis. They originate at the basal layer, mature, lose their nucleus, and flatten as they move upward. At the uppermost level, they form a strong, flexible, dry surface known as the stratum corneum. This layer, composed of cells firmly attached to one another, continually loosens, detaches, and falls away in the natural process of exfoliation. The entire cycle takes 30 to 40 days in normally maturing skin. Throughout the body, the epidermis is uniform in thickness, except for certain thickened areas, such as the palms and soles.

Keratin, the major protein of the epidermis, reacts with chemical peel acids, such as phenol (carbolic acid) or trichloroacetic acid (TCA), precipitating the protein and forming a frost. During this precipitation process, keratin acts as the first line of defense to neutralize the acid. Glycolic acid, however, does not precipitate keratin to form a frost, and skin must be washed after it has been in contact with this acid for a certain amount time to prevent necrosis. CO_2 laser resurfacing evaporates the epidermis and a certain amount of dermis using water as the chromophore. If the epidermis and dermis are well hydrated, a more even and uniform response is obtained for both CO_2 laser resurfacing and chemical peeling.

Keratinocytes are very sensitive to ultraviolet light exposure, and repeated exposure tends to damage their DNA, leading to mutated precancerous cells. This sensitivity is more apparent in fair-skinned individuals. Only intracellular agents such as tretinoin are capable of repairing DNA and correcting photodamage. Extracellular agents such as glycolic acid are not effective.

At any given time, 40% of skin basal cells are undergoing mitosis. This continuous process generates healthy keratinocytes to renew the epidermis so that its barrier function is maintained. Inducing exfoliation with alpha hydroxy acids

Box 1-10

Tretinoin:

- **increases the rate of keratinocyte mitosis**
- **produces a thicker epidermis**
- **creates a soft, compact stratum corneum**
- **restores epidermal hydration**
- **strengthens skin barrier function**

(AHAs) increases the rate of mitosis in the basal layer and leads to increased epidermal thickness. Tretinoin, however, is more potent than any of the AHAs. It produces a higher rate of mitosis and a thicker epidermis; clinically, it creates a soft, compact stratum corneum, restores epidermal hydration, and strengthens the barrier function, thereby returning natural skin tolerance.

The barrier function depends greatly on epidermal thickness and quality of the stratum corneum. Ideally, deeper layers of the stratum corneum are gelatinous and compact, with minimal surface basketweaving seen histologically. This correlates with the texture of healthy skin, which is soft, silky, and moist compared with the dry and rough texture of damaged skin.

MELANOCYTES

Melanocytes, the second major group of cells in the epidermis, lay side by side along the basal cells. They produce melanin, the substance that determines skin color in racial groups. Melanin is protective against ultraviolet light during limited sun exposure but is not fully effective with long-term exposure. Long-term exposure leads to photodamage, especially in light-skinned persons, although it can occur in all skin color groups. The melanocyte is a very sensitive cell whose function can be affected by UV light exposure, hormones, skin injury, medications, inflammation, genetic factors, immunological disorders, autoimmune diseases, and others. In response to these factors, the melanocyte reacts by overproducing melanin, becoming inactive, or dying, as is seen after phenol peels and other deep skin rejuvenation procedures.

Postinflammatory hyperpigmentation (PIH) after a skin rejuvenation procedure is partly due to the overproduction of melanin as a result of the inflammatory process caused by the procedure. Skin Conditioning before any procedure (as described in Chapter 5) can reduce such melanocyte hyperactivity. The main objective of Skin Conditioning is to restore or increase skin tolerance to external factors, including the tolerance of melanocytes. Also, the blending process in Skin Conditioning enhances the even transfer of melanin to adjacent keratinocytes, resulting in a more even even skin color tone. Figures 1-3a,b show a patient with melasma before and after using the Obagi Skin Conditioning program; Figures 1-4a,b show a patient with a skin pigmentation problem before and after Skin Health Restoration topical treatment program.

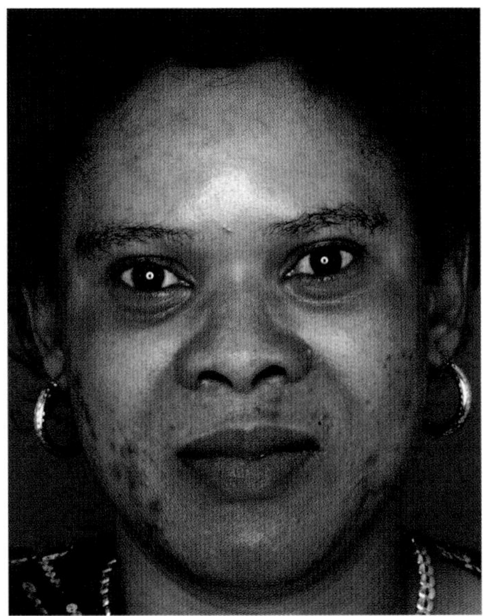
a

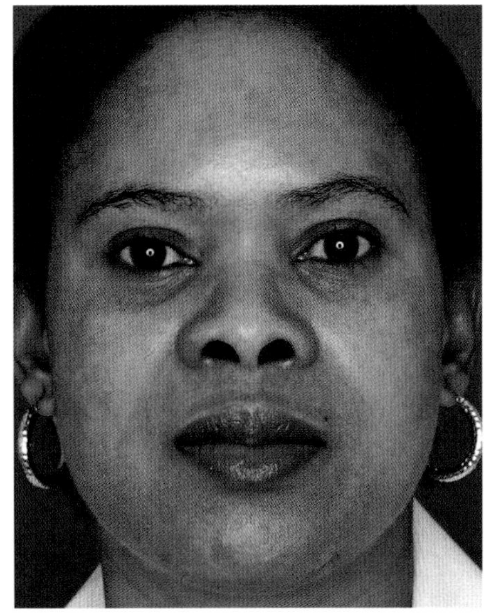
b

FIGURE 1-3. *(a) Before. Patient with melasma before topical skin treatment (regulating cellular functions and Skin Health Restoration program). (b) After. Patient with melasma after undergoing Obagi Skin Health Restoration topical treatment program (no procedure).*

THE EFFECTS OF COMMONLY USED TOPICAL AGENTS

The "feel" of an individual's skin depends on the quality of the stratum corneum and the condition of the pores. Skin feels rough to the touch when there is an accumulation of partially attached surface stratum corneum cells. This can occur in normal conditions as well as in medical conditions such as asteatosis.

AHAS (ALPHA HYDROXY ACIDS)

Forced exfoliation with topical agents, such as the AHAs, can restore a smoother texture, but the concentration of the agent is critical. At low concentrations of 2% to 8%, only a few layers of stratum corneum are removed, and enough cells remain to keep the skin's barrier function intact. Concentrations higher than 12%, on the other hand, may lead to a total loss of stratum corneum and irritate the skin, especially if they are used more than once daily. AHA effects are temporary because they do not regulate the process of keratinization or produce softer keratin as tretinoin does. Thus when their use is discontinued, the condition being treated often returns in 2 to 3 weeks.

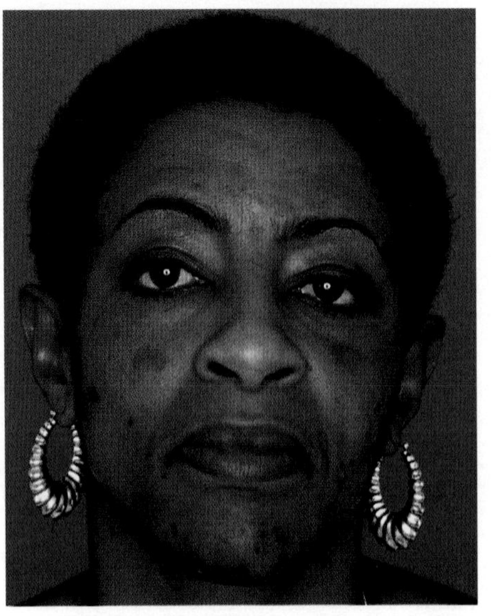

a

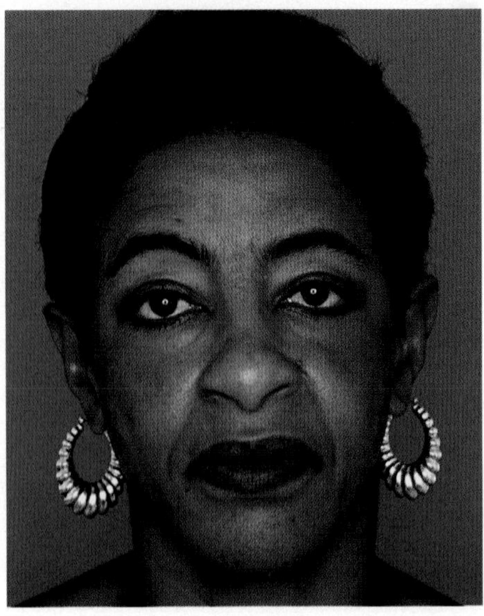

b

FIGURE 1-4. *(a) Before. Patient who had CO_2 laser treatment for lentigo by another physician. Condition worsened. Postinflammatory hyperpigmentation, acne rosacea, and excoriations are present. (b) After treatment with Skin Health Restoration topical treatment program, (no procedure).*

Box 1-11

Alpha hydroxy acids, used in concentrations of 2% to 8%, can make skin texture smoother, but their effects are temporary, and the treated condition reappears rapidly after discontinuation of AHAs.

BETA HYDROXY ACIDS (SALICYLIC ACID)

This agent is keratolytic and induces smoothness of the stratum corneum surface. However, salicyclic acid is irritating, increases skin sensitivity, and is not recommended for daily use on normal skin because of the potential for allergic reactions. Usually it is used to increase the effectiveness of some chemical peels, to treat warts or acne, or as a salicylic acid "peel." Calling the exfoliation that this agent induces a "peel" is incorrect since it has no dermal effects and is not recommended for treating wrinkles or scars.

KINERASE (BRAND OF KINETIN)

Kinetin is chemically known as N-6 furfuryl adenine. The molecule was orginally isolated in the 1960s and is known to be part of the biological plant growth process. It is claimed, in some of the literature describing the molecule's activity, to be a plant growth hormone or plant growth factor.

The molecule was recently studied under the same protocol as was used for the analysis of the efficacy and safety of the retinoic acid that is FDA approved for fine lines and wrinkles. It is important to note that this was not a comparative (double blinded, randomized) trial; therefore it is impossible to compare the products clinically or scientifically. The study did not measure any dermal effects or any cellular regulatory effects of kinetin.

The current data on kinetin point out the side effect benefits of kinetin over retinoids, but they do not address the efficacy benefits of retinoids. If the goal of the treatment is to illustrate the dermal or cellular regulatory benefits of retinoids, kinetin clearly is not a choice. This is probably why the makers of kinetin do not compare the products on a head-to-head basis.

The benefits of retinoic acid, which are extensively documented, are preceded with certain side effects such as redness, dryness, and exfoliation. These reactions usually disappear once skin tolerance is restored. It is in these processes that the anti-aging effect of retinoids is achieved. Kinetin, illustrated well by the TEWL values, acts primarily as a skin moisturizer by surface hydration. It is by this skin hydration processs that kinetin achieves the apparent improvement in fine wrinkles and surface skin roughness, as seen in the only study performed on the product.

In my opinion, kinetin is best ulilized as a supportive agent, as opposed to an active agent, in the skin rejuvenation process. The product should be categorized as a moisturizer, and clinicians should expect the same benefits and risks from it as they would from any other moisturizing product. Please reference the section in this publication on the appropriate selection and use of moisturizers.

TRETINOIN

This agent has profound beneficial effects on the stratum corneum as well as other layers of the skin. By making keratin softer and more gelatinous, the stratum corneum becomes soft and compact. These effects last up to four months, even after application has been discontinued, in contrast to the short-lasting, mechanically smoothing effects of AHAs. Initially, tretinoin dehydrates the outer surface of the stratum corneum and causes a rapid, coarse exfoliation (shedding of attached groups of cells) instead of the individual cell shedding seen with the AHAs. Tretinoin is the preferrred agent for treating the stratum corneum as well as deeper epidermal disorders because it repairs damaged keratinocytes, increases mitosis, and restores proper hydration.

MOISTURIZERS

The cosmetic industry mistakenly equates skin roughness with skin dryness, although oily skin can also be rough. Although dryness may induce roughness to some extent, the main cause of roughness is abnormal keratinization. Occasional use of moisturizers when the stratum corneum is truly dry from prolonged exposure to wind, cold, or heat can help reduce temporary skin dryness and irritability, but habitual use is detrimental.

The notion that facial skin needs external moisturizers is firmly entrenched in people's minds throughout the world. Following aggressive promotion by cosmetic companies, women everywhere have accepted the notion that the daily use of moisturizers is necessary. Extravagant, scientifically invalid claims of effects obtained from the use of moisturizers are made routinely: restoration of youthful skin; elimination or improvement of wrinkles; vibrant, silky, smooth skin, etc. Each product has its own twist: some contain collagen, elastin, AHAs, aloe, placenta, or herbs; others are specifically for use on the lips, neck, eyelids, etc. Some are to be used in the daytime, others at night. There are even oil-free moisturizers for oily skin!

The value of moisturizers can be assessed by asking the following questions:

1. Why do children have well-hydrated skin without the use of moisturizers?
2. Why do men who rarely use mosturizers not complain of dry skin?
3. Can long-term use of moisturizers cause damage?

The answers lie in the ability of the skin to function properly. When all skin functions at the cellular level are intact, skin does not feel dry and moisturizers are not needed. (The exception is with the dry-skin type, which can benefit from moisturizers. See Chapter 4 on Obagi Skin Classification.)

In children, every skin cell performs its function: epidermal cells divide at a normal rate and generate healthy keratinocytes within a 40-day cycle, epidermal glycoproteins are abundant, the stratum corneum is soft and the cells are firmly attached, the skin exfoliates naturally at the proper rate, and the dermis has good circulation and proper hydration. The barrier function is intact, tolerance is normal, and moisturizers are neither necessary nor recommended. In men, skin changes that come with aging are generally more accepted. Skin roughness is not usually a concern since daily shaving mechanically reduces roughness. Tolerance is usually normal and moisturizers are rarely used on a regular basis.

With the exception of persons with certain medical conditions, neither men nor children report skin sensitivity or intolerance to various external products or conditions. Women in general are more concerned with appearance and looking youthful and are thus more susceptible to media in-

Box 1-12

Intensive advertising has convinced the public that an aged appearance is the result of skin dryness and that externally applied over-the-counter products (moisturizers) will hydrate dry skin and restore a youthful appearance.

fluence in the "dry-skin" area. Clever advertising has convinced many women that their skin needs to be nourished and pampered with moisturizing products to prevent dryness, which will in turn prevent aging. According to the claims, "dry, thirsty skin" is the major offender in aging or problematic skin. Moisture must be "restored" through external means—moisturizers, special "hydrating cleansers," moisturizing foundations, moisturizers to complement the foundations, and so on—or a woman's youth and beauty will be lost forever. The acceptance of these marketing claims has been so widespread that even dermatologists and plastic surgeons often recommend use of facial moisturizers to their patients.

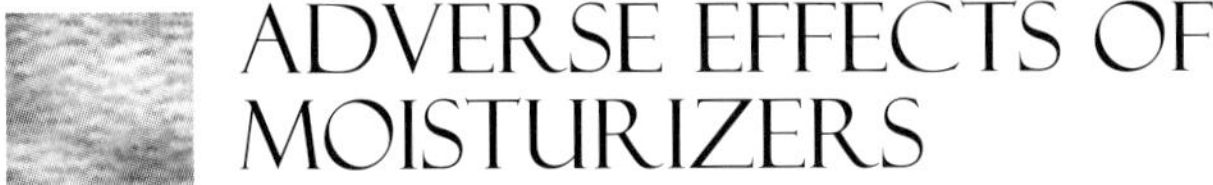

ADVERSE EFFECTS OF MOISTURIZERS

ADDICTION

The habitual daily use of facial moisturizers can create a number of problems, such as moisturizer addiction, increased skin sensitivity, and possibly accelerated aging. Initially moisturizers may give skin a smooth, silky feeling and reduce the appearance of fine lines by increasing hydration in the stratum corneum. After a few months, however, the skin becomes dependent on the moisturizers to combat the false sensation of dryness and constant use is required. In a sense, an addiction develops, with a need for more frequently applied and more potent moisturizers and other "hydrating" products. This addiction in women may result from intolerance of the temporary sensation of dryness after washing and from an actual reduction in skin tolerance, due to the use of moisturizing products, to this dryness. Children and men, on the other hand, wash their faces, perhaps experience some dryness for a few minutes afterwards, but do not turn to moisturizers to alleviate this temporary sensation.

SENSITIVITY

By keeping the stratum corneum at a high level of moisture saturation, moisturizers slow down the rate of stratum corneum exfoliation. This may lead to a reduction of the population of keratinocytes, due to a reduced rate of mitosis in the basal layer, and possibly to a reduction in the release of growth factors needed for these processes. Clinically, an overly moisturized epidermis (following 2 to 3 years of steady moisturizer use) is dull, dry, and sensitive, e.g., easily irritated by factors that reduce the moisture saturation level, such as wind, cold, topical agents containing alcohol, etc. After moisturizers have been discontinued and the moisture saturation level has been reduced, exfoliation of the stratum corneum accelerates and creates the roughness and dryness that initiated the use of moisturizers. The individual then feels the need to resume moisturizer use, with even greater dependence.

Box 1-13

Use of moisturizers makes the skin less tolerant of any substance that lowers the stratum corneum moisture saturation level.

Box 1-14

Misleading advertising has led to the widespread belief that moisturizers have a beneficial effect on wrinkles.

Complaints of skin sensitivities are increasingly heard in clinical practice that, in the author's opinion, are attributable to the widespread use of moisturizers. (Note: These are personal clinical observations by the author that have not been confirmed by histological correlation studies). Although most physicians recognize that moisturizers do not prevent wrinkles, laxity, and other signs of aging, they need to recognize that the unwise use of moisturizers can be detrimental to skin health.

ACCELERATED AGING

In addition to increased skin sensitivity, moisturizer use may accelerate skin aging. Through many years of clinical experience, the author has observed that women who are dependent on moisturizers have more sensitive skin and a more aged and wrinkled appearance than women who have not depended on moisturizers. The questions that come to mind are whether these products slow down the ability of the skin to regenerate, suppress collagen production, and decrease the resistance of skin to external factors, such as sunlight, that accelerate the aging process. It is the author's belief that women who use moisturizers may also show more profound wrinkling and seek out cosmetic and plastic surgery at an earlier age than those who have not used moisturizers habitually.

THE CLINICAL BASIS FOR DRYNESS

True skin dryness does exist, and the cause is not known. Physiological studies have shown that the epidermis of persons who complain of dry skin has the same water content as the epidermis of normal skin. Dryness is believed to originate in the dermis with a reduction in the production of or an alteration in the structure of glycosaminoglycan that decreases the water-binding capacity of the dermis. This may explain the existence of a group of people who truly have dry skin, possibly as a result of a certain genetic deficiency at the molecular level. Moisturizers will temporarily relieve, but not fundamentally change, the dry condition of such patients. The author has found that agents, such as tretinoin, that increase the production of glycosaminoglycan in the dermis are effective in correcting dryness in these patients.

Box 1-15

Moisturizers can exacerbate dermatological problems, such as acne vulgaris, acne rosacea, seborrhea, and clogged pores. They also tend to reduce skin tolerance to agents such as tretinoin, AHAs, and benzoyl peroxide.

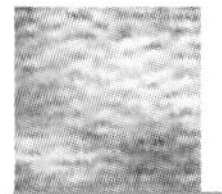

REFERENCES

1. Priestley G. An introduction to skin and its diseases. In: Priestley GC, ed. *Molecular Aspects of Dermatology*. Chichester, England: John Wiley & Sons; 1993:1–17.
2. Goldsmith LA, ed. *Physiology, Biochemistry, and Molecular Biology of the Skin*. 2nd ed. Oxford, England: Oxford University Press; 1981:432–452.
3. Gilchrest BA. Aging of differentiated cells (excluding the fibroblast) in skin: In vitro studies. In: Kligman AM, Balin AK, eds. *Aging and the Skin*. New York, NY: Raven Press; 1993:77–92.
4. Mast BA. The skin. In: Cohen IK, Diegelmann RI, Lindblad WJ, eds. *Wound Healing: Biochemical and Physical Aspects*. Philadelphia, Pa: W.B. Saunders; 1992:344–355.
5. Balin AK, Lin AN. Skin changes as a biological marker for measuring the rate of human aging. In: Kligman AM, Balin AK, eds. *Aging and the Skin*. New York, NY: Raven Press; 1993:43–75.
6. Grove GL. Age-associated changes in human epidermal cell renewal and repair. In: Kligman AM, Balin AK, eds. *Aging and the Skin*. New York, NY: Raven Press; 1993:193–204.
7. Thody AJ. Skin pigmentation and its regulation. In: Priestley GC, ed. *Molecular Aspects of Dermatology*. Chichester, England: John Wiley & Sons; 1993:55–73.
8. Kohn RR, Schnider SL. Collagen changes in aging skin. In: Kligman AM, Balin AK, eds. *Aging and the Skin*. New York, NY: Raven Press; 1993: 121–139.
9. Edward M. Proteoglycans and glycosoaminoglycans. In: Priestley GC, ed.

Molecular Aspects of Dermatology. Chichester, England: John Wiley & Sons; 1993:89–110.

10. Kligman AM, Balin AK. Aging of human skin. In: Kligman AM, Balin AK, eds. *Aging and the Skin.* New York, NY: Raven Press; 1993:1–42.
11. Weiss JB. Dermal proteins and their degradative enzymes. In: Priestley GC, ed. *Molecular Aspects of Dermatology.* Chichester, England: John Wiley & Sons; 1993:111–122.
12. Matsuoka LY, Uitto J. Alterations in the elastic fibers in cutaneous aging and solar elastosis. In: Kligman AM, Balin AK, eds. *Aging and the Skin.* New York, NY: Raven Press; 1993:141–151.
13. Weitzhandler M, Bernfield MR. Proteoglycan conjugates. In: Cohen IK, Diegelmann RI, Lindblad WJ, eds. *Wound Healing: Biochemical and Physical aspects.* Philadelphia, Pa: W.B. Saunders; 1992:195–208.
14. Montagna W, Kligman AM, Carlisle KS. *Atlas of Normal Human Skin.* New York, NY: Springer-Verlag; 1992.
15. Whitton J, Everall JD. The thickness of the epidermis. *Br J Dermatol.* 1973;89:467–476.
16. Miller EJ, Gay S. Collagen structure and function. In: Cohen IK, Diegelmann RI, Lindblad WJ, eds. *Wound Healing: Biochemical and Physical aspects.* Philadelphia, Pa: W.B. Saunders; 1992;130–151.
17. Fleischmajer R, Perlish JS, Bashey RI. Human dermal glycosoaminoglycans and aging. *Biochim Biophys Acta.* 1972;279:265–275.
18. Perlish JS, Longas MO, Fleischmajer R. The role of glycosoaminoglycans in aging of the skin. In: Kligman AM, Balin AK, eds. *Aging and the Skin.* New York, NY: Raven Press; 1993:153–165.
19. Kligman AM. Perspectives and problems in cutaneous gerontology. *J Invest Dermatol.* 1979;73:39–46.
20. Procacci P, Bozza G, Buzzelli G, Cortz MD. The cutaneous pricking pain threshold in old age. *Gerontology Clinics.* 1970;12:213–218.
21. Salavisto E, Orma E, Tawast M. Aging and relation between stimulus intensity and duration in corneal sensibility. *Acta Physiol Scand.* 1951;23:224–230.
22. Kligman L. Skin changes in photoaging: Characteristics, prevention, and repair. In: Kligman AM, Balin AK, eds. *Aging and the Skin.* New York, NY: Raven Press; 1993:331–346.
23. Urbach F. Geographic pathology of skin cancers. In: Urbach F, ed. *The Biologic Effects of Ultraviolet Radiation.* Oxford, England: Pergamon Press; 1969:635–650.
24. Schwartz E. Connective tissue alterations in the skin of ultraviolet irradiated hairless mice. *J Invest Dermatol.* 1988;91:158–161.
25. Kligman LH, Akin FJ, Kligman AM. The contribution of UVA and UVB to connective tissue damage in hairless mice. *J Invest Dermatol.* 1985; 84:272–276.

CHAPTER

2

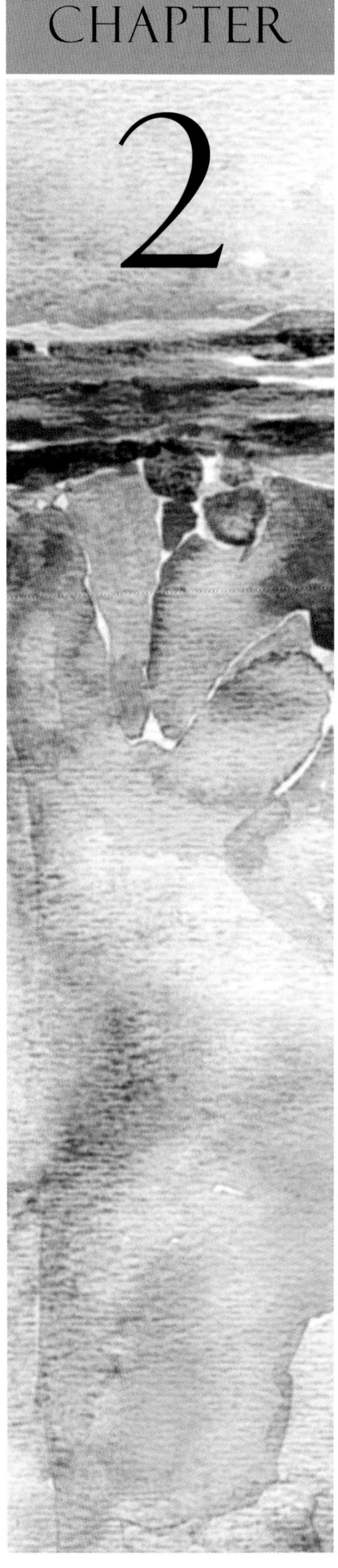

SKIN HEALTH: THE CONCEPTS

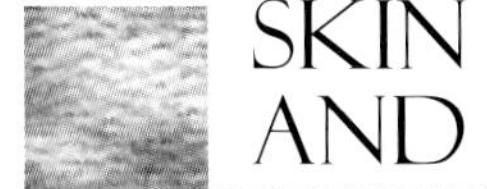

SKIN HEALTH DEFINITION AND MODEL

CATEGORIES OF SKIN HEALTH

Current dermatological treatment does not address or recognize the presence of skin health as an entity and focuses instead on the treatment of skin diseases. Neither prevention of deterioration nor maintenance of skin in a healthy state are recognized, and thus there is no model for healthy skin. Procedures (skin rejuvenation with chemical peels, CO_2 laser resurfacing, dermabrasion, or plastic surgery) are considered essential to correct some of the changes seen in the deteriorated state, but little emphasis is placed on prevention of skin deterioration and enabling skin to repair itself before and after such procedures through the regulation of

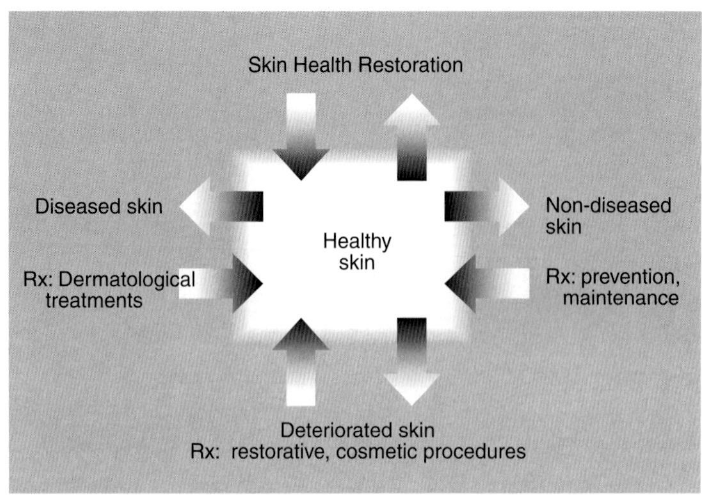

FIGURE 2-1. *Skin in the deteriorating, diseased, and healthy states.*

its functions. For that reason, improvement following procedures is often temporary and the deterioration continues following the procedure. Thus I found it necessary to categorize skin with regard to its state of health (Figure 2-1) and to define and create a model for healthy skin:

Deteriorating—No skin disease exists, but intrinsic aging and/or photoaging have caused anatomical, physiological, and clinical changes. These range from a sensation of dryness and dull, weathered skin to wrinkling, jowling, laxity, hypertrophy, and easy bruising.

Box 2-1

CHARACTERISTICS OF HEALTHY BABY SKIN

- **smooth because of production of soft keratin, normal keratinization, and minimal basketweaving**
- **firm with abundant, functioning collagen and elastin**
- **evenly colored due to properly functioning melanocytes**
- **properly hydrated (rich in glycosaminoglycan); moist without the use of moisturizers**
- **not damaged from medical conditions or the environment (no photodamage, large pores, acne)**
- **functions properly with efficient and continuous renewal (new cells regularly come up to replace the old, has good circulation)**
- **tolerant of external factors (repairs itself quickly when scratched, scraped, or otherwise injured) because of an intact barrier function**

Diseased—Acne, seborrhea, actinic keratoses, solar elastosis, photodamage with skin cancer, secondary pigmentation problems, etc. are present.

Healthy—Skin has normal functions and is free of environmental and medical changes and deterioration. The opposite condition is skin in the deteriorated state.

DEFINITION AND MODEL

Clinical, histological, and appearance aspects of skin must be taken into consideration in defining healthy skin. The definition is greatly aided by observing the features of the Obagi healthy skin model—the skin of a baby—which is smooth, firm, unwrinkled, evenly colored, and blemish free (Box 2-1). Most of us begin life with unflawed skin (Figure 2-2; Table 2-1); however, environmental, internal, and hereditary factors and the normal process of aging proceed to undo what was ours at birth. Deterioration proceeds in most skin due to changes in skin function. Sallowness, fine and coarse wrinkles, rough texture, blotches, broken blood vessels, and lentigines or "age spots" to a greater or lesser extent are the result.

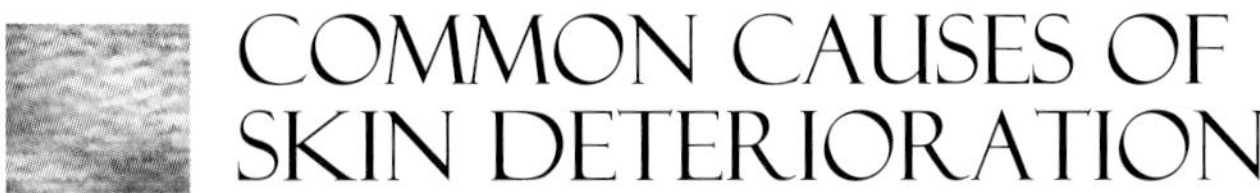

COMMON CAUSES OF SKIN DETERIORATION

Before practicing skin restoration, it is important to understand the changes that cause skin deterioration and a loss of skin health over an individual's lifetime (in Box 2-2).

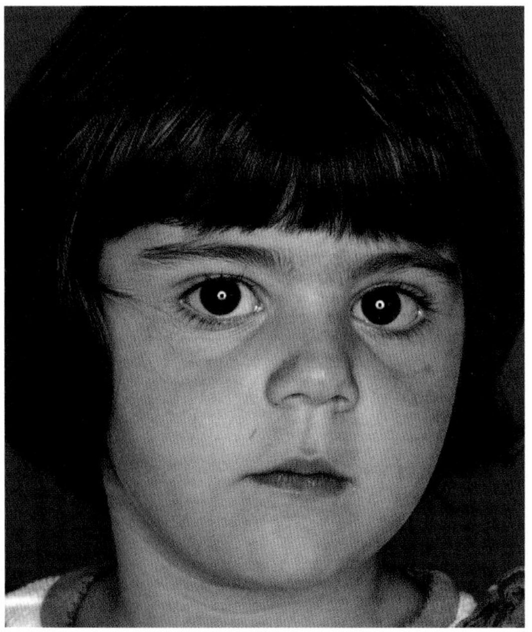

FIGURE 2-2. *The skin of a baby is a model of healthy skin. Such skin is smooth, firm, unwrinkled, evenly colored, and blemish-free.*

TABLE 2.1

DEFINITION OF HEALTHY SKIN

Clinical Aspects		
■ smooth, firm, evenly colored ■ free of medically and environmentally induced deterioration or diseases ■ functioning properly ■ optimal skin tolerance ■ good hydration		
Histological Aspects		
Epidermis ■ soft, compact stratum corneum ■ healthy keratinocytes ■ normal-sized melanocytes that function properly with melanosomes evenly distributed throughout	*Dermis* ■ normal vasculature (circulation) ■ intact collagen fibers in tridimensional pattern (firmness) ■ intact elastin fibers (tightness) ■ rich in glycosaminoglycan (hydration)	*Subcutaneous layer* ■ lipocytes, lipoblasts with well-defined lobules ■ elastic and firm septae encapsulating and dividing the lobules
Appearance Aspects		
■ silky to the touch ■ rosy, radiant, glowing, vibrant ■ tight	■ moist ■ clear	

Box 2-2

COMMON CAUSES OF SKIN DETERIORATION*

- **Abnormalities in pilosebaceous units**
- **Dysfunction of melanocyte/keratinocyte units**
- **Intrinsic aging**
- **Photoaging**
- **Alteration of the barrier function through use of topical agents (make-up, moisturizers, etc.)**

*excluding trauma and disease states

ABNORMALITIES IN PILOSEBACEOUS UNITS

Conditions arising from abnormalities in pilosebaceous units include various types of acne and sebaceous gland hyperplasia or increased sebum production with pore enlargement. Acne in youth may start as early as 8 to 11 years of age with clinical manifestations such as comedones, papules, and inflammatory cysts. This dysfunction is mainly caused by abnormal keratinization, androgen hormones, clogged pores, bacteria, and other factors. As many as 80% to 90% of all adolescents have some type of acne and more than 30% require medical treatment.[1] Resolution of inflammatory cystic acne often leaves behind scars, uneven coloring, and uneven skin texture.

DYSFUNCTION OF MELANOCYTE/ KERATINOCYTE UNITS

In adulthood, melasma and dermal melanosis may be associated with pregnancy, hormonal imbalances, use of oral contraceptives, and certain medications in susceptible individuals and may cause hyperpigmentation, usually on cheeks, forehead, upper lip, and chin. Genetic influences and exposure to ultraviolet radiation are the main factors contributing to its development and severity. Skin pigmentary problems occur more often in individuals with a darker complexion (Fitzpatrick skin types IV to VI), especially women of Hispanic, Asian, or Afro-American origin.[2,3]

Based on Wood's light examination or stretching of the skin, skin hyperpigmentation conditions can be divided into four types: 1) epidermal, 2) dermal, 3) epidermal/dermal, and 4) total, involving the subcutaneous layer. The epidermal variety is characterized by increased melanin in the basal, suprabasal, and stratum corneum layers. Pigmentation is intensified by Wood's light and becomes lighter when skin is stretched. In dermal melanosis, there is a preponderance of melanophages in the superficial dermis and possibly the deeper dermis, which is not enhanced by Wood's light and remains at the same intensity when the skin is stretched. Epidermal and dermal pigment alterations may exist in different variations and at different depths. Dermal pigmentation is often present in individuals with Fitzpatrick skin type V or VI[3] and may be attributed to genetic influences. Histologically, the patterns of increased pigmentation in melasma and other types of hyperpigmentation are described as epidermal, epidermal/dermal, or dermal. The total type of skin hyperpigmentation involves the subcutaneous layer, as is seen in nevus of Ota and congenital hairy nevus.

INTRINSIC AGING

A comparison of the features of photoaged and intrinsically aged skin is shown in Table 2-2. Skin changes from intrinsic (chronological) aging are inevitable, but changes from exposure to sunlight can be prevented.[4–8] Intrinsically aged skin shows a process I call "mummification," in which atrophic changes predominate (Figure 2-3). There is thinning of the epidermis, a flatter dermal/epidermal interface, and loss of dermal collagen, elastin, anchoring fibrils, cellular components, elastic fibers, blood vessels, glycosaminoglycan, and fat. There is also a reduction in the density of sebaceous glands, hair follicles, and sweat ducts; reduced skin circulation leading to decreased functional capacity; and an increased susceptibility to certain diseases and environmental insults. Immunocompetence is decreased in elderly persons, but this does not increase the risk of malignant skin tumors. However, the risk of nonmelanoma skin cancer is directly proportional to the amount of sunlight exposure.

Clinically there may be laxity, deepening of expression lines, dryness, general thinning, easy bruising, and slower healing. Often chronologically aged skin is dull and lusterless, with roughness, uneven color tone, and loss of elasticity. However, persons with intrinsically aged but photoprotected skin generally appears years younger than those with photodamaged skin at the same chronological age.

PHOTOAGING

Photoaging or damage from light exposure is a quite distinct form of skin deterioration, and the notion that light exposure simply accelerates chrono-

TABLE 2.2

FEATURES OF PHOTOAGED AND INTRINSICALLY AGED SKIN

Feature	*Photoaging*	*Intrinsic Aging*
Clinical Appearance	Nodular, leathery surface, fine and coarse wrinkles, blotches and yellowing, dryness, telangiectasias	Fine wrinkling, dryness, deepening of expression lines, laxity, slower wound healing, easier bruising
Epidermis	Marked acanthosis, cellular atypia, irregular pigmentation	Thin and viable, flattening of dermal/epidermal junction
Papillary dermis	Solar elastosis	No elastosis
Reticular dermis	Hyperactive fibroblasts, increased mast cells, mixed inflammatory infiltrate	Inactive fibroblasts, normal mast cells, no inflammation
Elastic tissue	Massive deposition of thickened, tangled, degraded elastic fibers	Decreased, cystic spaces associated with loss of elasticity
Collagen	Decrease of bundles and fibers, homogenization	Loss of dermal collagen, thick bundles, disorientation
Microvasculature	Significant loss and collapse of small vessels, telangiectasias	Loss and generation of small vessels, decreased overall circulation
Appendage Structures	Similar to changes in intrinsical aging plus additional decreases related to damaged microvasculture	Decrease in sweat and sebaceous gland activity, decrease in hair growth
Neoplasms	Variety of benign, premalignant, and malignant growths	Decreased immunocompetence of elderly increases risk of malignant skin tumors; however, the risk of nonmelanoma skin cancer is directly proportional to amount of sunlight exposure

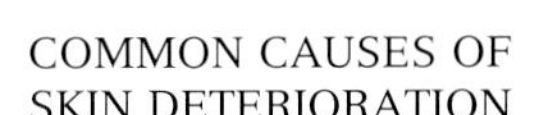

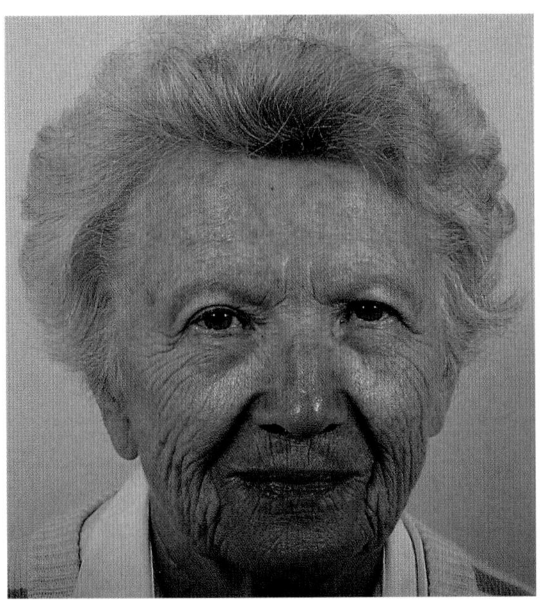

FIGURE 2-3. *Patient with thin, intrinsically aged skin and muscle laxity showing deep nasolabial folds and the extension of wrinkles characteristic of thin skin.*

logical aging signs is too simplistic. In chronological aging, most skin functions are slowed and there is atrophy, while in photoaging, there is an increase in irregular activity with hypertrophy of certain tissues, which may be a result of a chronic inflammatory process.[9]

Photodamaged skin shows more extensive microscopic as well as clinical degeneration than is seen with chronological aging (Figure 2-4). Histologically, the photodamaged epidermis shows atypical keratinocytes and variability in thickness, with alternating areas of atrophy and hyperplasia. The atrophy may be a result of the depletion of competent cells from the basal layer, while the areas of hyperplasia may reflect compensatory overgrowth by ultraviolet light-damaged tissue. Melanocyte hyperplasia is also seen, causing areas of irregular pigmentation interspersed with more severely damaged areas in which melanocytes are depleted or unable to transfer pigment normally to keratinocytes.[10]

The most profound changes in photodamaged skin, however, occur in the dermis, where it is characterized by solar elastosis, a massive deposition of thickened, tangled, and degraded elastic fibers (Figures 2-4 to 2-8). The subepidermal Grenz zone is evident (while it is not apparent in intrinsically aged skin) and has collagen fibers in a densely packed linear arrangement. This zone may represent newly synthesized collagen[11] or be the result of a crowding-out phenomenon due to the accumulation of elastotic material in the dermis. Because the architecture of the Grenz zone is consistent with that of a healing wound, it might be considered a "solar scar" resulting from decades of repair of ultraviolet damage.[12]

The degree of elastosis correlates with the amount of exposure to ultraviolet light in general and infrared light in particular. The earliest histopathological change is elastic fiber hyperplasia. Subsequently, elastic fibers become coarse, twisted, and highly branched. The origin of the elastotic material remains controversial, and questions remain whether the material is formed from degradation, abnormal synthesis, or both.[13]

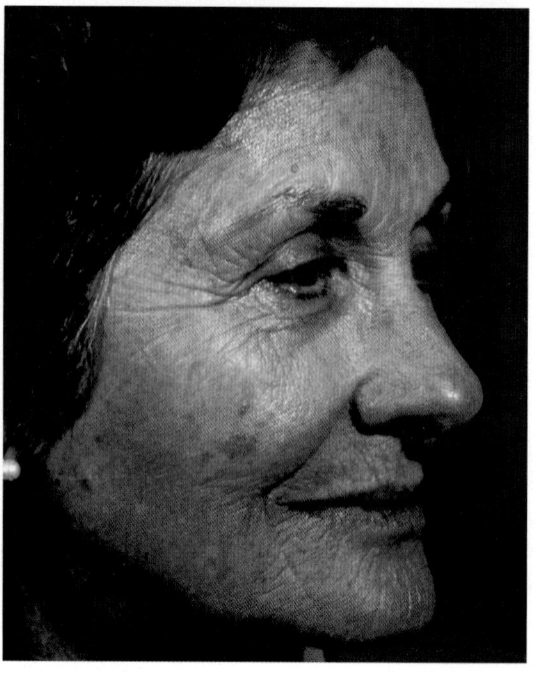

FIGURE 2-4. *Patient with classical signs of photoaging and solar elastosis.*

Fibroblasts, which play an important role in the production of elastin, collagen, and ground substance (glycosaminoglycan), undergo changes during photoaging. Normally these cells proliferate at a low rate and synthesize low levels of proteolytic enzymes. Following ultraviolet irradiation, however, fibroblasts may reenter the cell cycle and up-regulate the expression of proteolytic enzymes. This may contribute to the degener-

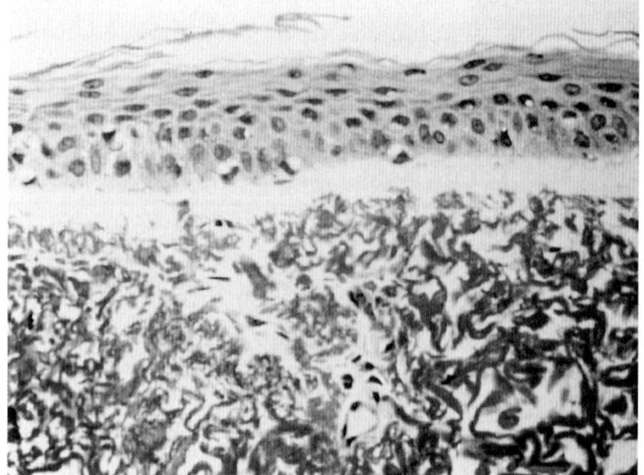

FIGURE 2-5. *Photoaged epidermis (histological view). The epidermis of a photoaged face shows effacement of rete ridges and melanocytic hyperplasia with mild atypia. Focal mild to moderate keratinocytic atypia is also seen. From Gilchrest B.* Aging Skin: Clinical Challenges *[slide-lecture kit]. Boston, Ma: Boston University School of Medicine; 1996.*

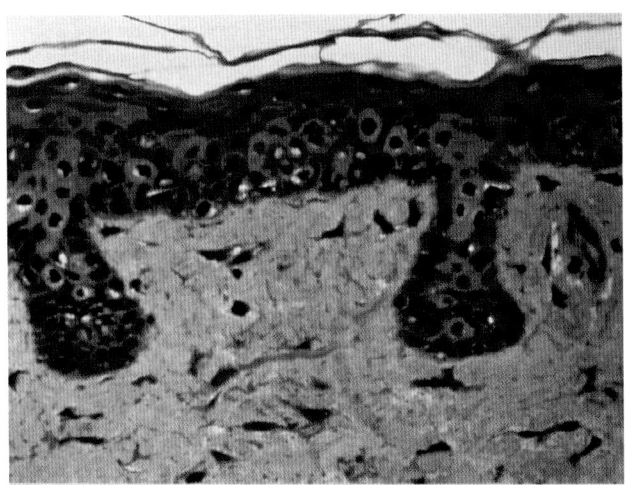

FIGURE 2-6. *Intrinsically aged epidermis (histological view). Intrinsically aged postauricular skin of the same patient as in Figure 2-5. A normal rete ridge pattern of the epidermis is maintained and there is less epidermal atrophy. No epidermal melanocytic hyperplasia or atypia is seen. From Gilchrest B.* Aging Skin: Clinical Challenges *[slide-lecture kit]. Boston, Ma: Boston University School of Medicine; 1996.*

ation of elastic fibers and collagen. Furthermore, collagen type I levels are reduced and collagen type III levels are increased in sun-exposed sites, and the fibers show abnormal basophilic degeneration and homogenization. The mechanism for these changes has not yet been explained.[10]

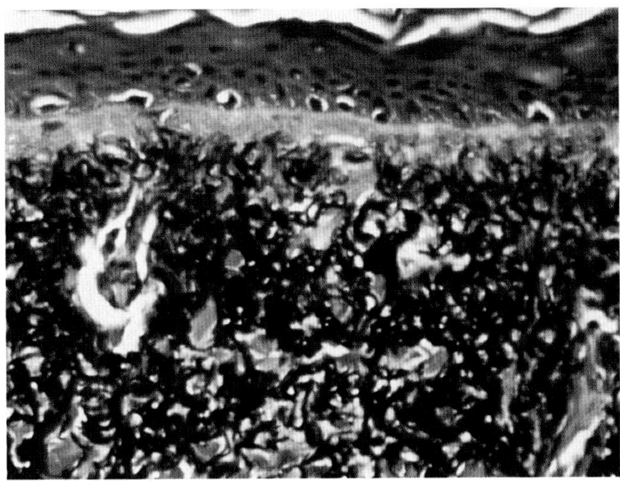

FIGURE 2-7. *Photoaged skin—solar elastosis (histological view). A hallmark of photoaged skin is solar elastosis. A massive deposition of thickened, tangled, and degraded elastic fibers can be seen. From Gilchrest B.* Aging Skin: Clinical Challenges *[slide-lecture kit]. Boston, Ma: Boston University School of Medicine; 1996.*

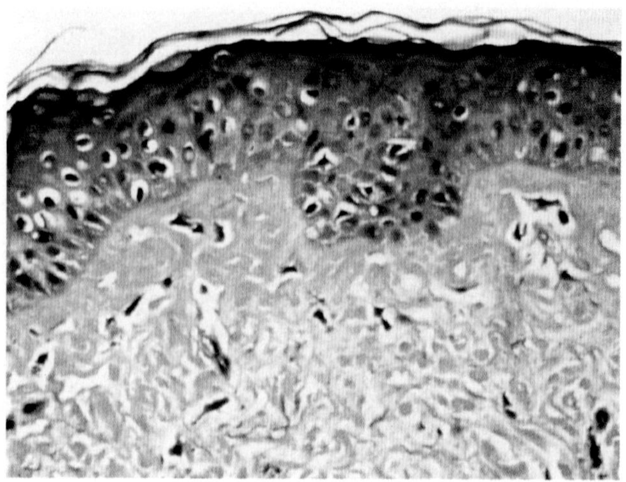

FIGURE 2-8. *Intrinsically aged skin—solar elastosis absent (histological view). Solar elastosis is absent in intrinsically aged skin. Only scant elastic fibers are seen. From Gilchrest B.* Aging Skin: Clinical Challenges *[slide-lecture kit]. Boston, Ma: Boston University School of Medicine; 1996.*

In clinical appearance, photodamaged skin is more deeply wrinkled, shows irregular pigmentation (patches, blotches, hyperpigmentation, hypopigmentation, freckles, lentigines) and rough or nodular texture, appears yellow and sallow, is dry, and has many broken or enlarged blood vessels (Figures 2-9, 2-10). Actinic keratoses and basal and squamous cell carcinomas are common (Figure 2-11). Photodamage is believed to be responsible for more than 90% of the changes that occur in the areas of the body

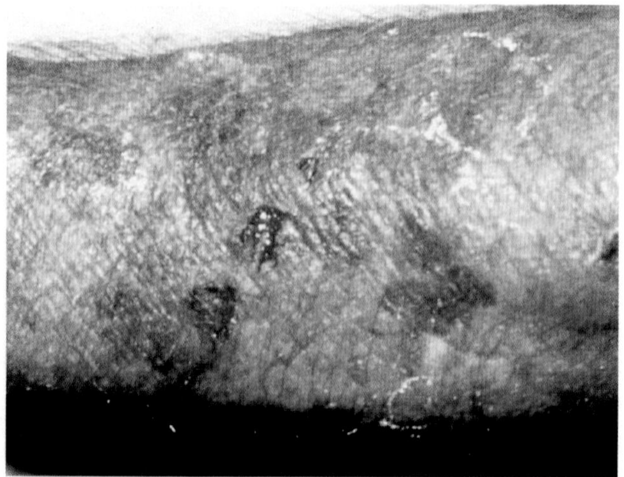

FIGURE 2-9. *Photoaged forearm. Forearm of elderly man with many years of sun exposure. The collagen and elastic fibers have been profoundly damaged, resulting in skin that bleeds and tears easily. From Gilchrest B.* Aging Skin: Clinical Challenges *[slide-lecture kit]. Boston, Ma: Boston University School of Medicine; 1996.*

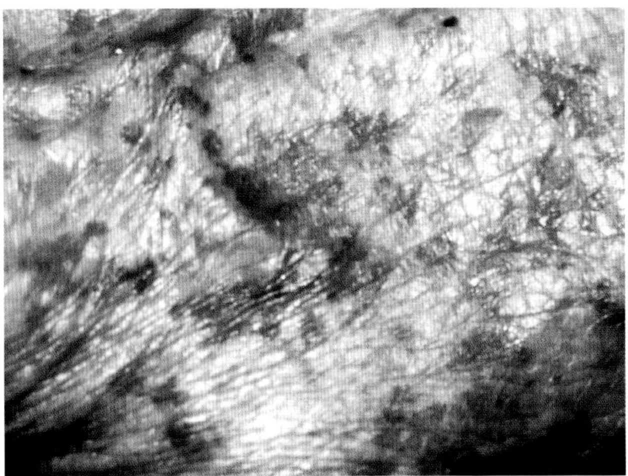

FIGURE 2-10. *Solar lentigines. Back of the hand of an elderly woman showing areas of hyperpigmentation. These solar lentigines are composed of increased numbers of melanocytes capable of producing large quantities of melanin. From Gilchrest B.* Aging Skin: Clinical Challenges *[slide-lecture kit]. Boston, Ma: Boston University School of Medicine; 1996.*

exposed to the sun, including the face, V of the neckline, the back of the neck, and the back of the hands.[14] Furthermore, 50% of photodamage has already occurred by age 18 but does not become apparent until middle age, so sun protection in children is very important in preventing later changes.[15] Photodamage is more severe in fair-skinned individuals both histologically and clinically, but dark-skinned individuals are not spared.

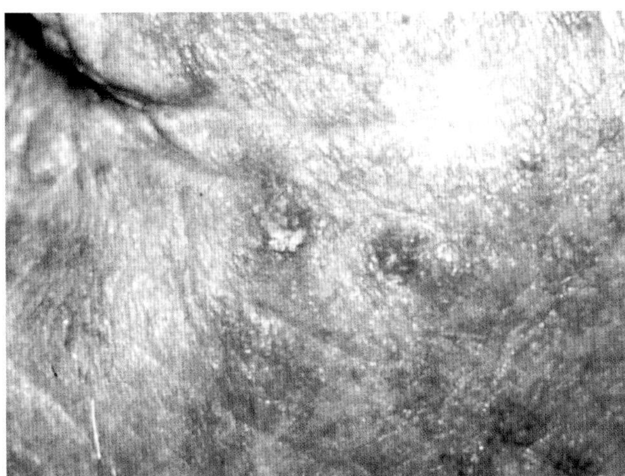

FIGURE 2-11. *Actinic keratoses. Face of middle-aged man showing two subtle, slightly inflamed scaly patches of actinic keratoses. These are precursors of squamous cell carcinoma. From Gilchrest B.* Aging Skin: Clinical Challenges *[slide-lecture kit]. Boston, Ma: Boston University School of Medicine; 1996.*

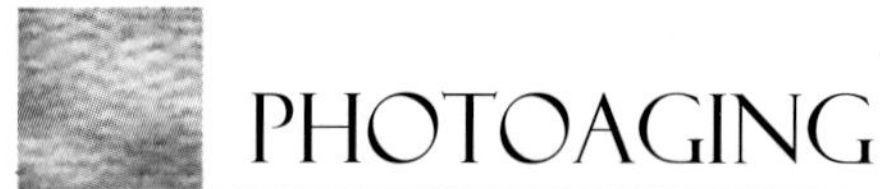

PHOTOAGING

MECHANISMS AND EFFECTS OF ULTRAVIOLET RADIATION EXPOSURE

Ultraviolet radiation (UVR) is a spectrum of light wavelengths from 200 to 400 nm that is generated by the sun but can also be produced by artificial sources such as lamps used in phototherapy or tanning salons. Ultraviolet B (UVB) at 290 to 320 nm is the most potent ultraviolet light wavelength that reaches the earth's surface and is the most efficient wavelength for producing skin erythema. Ultraviolet A (UVA), at 320 to 400 nm, is less potent in producing erythema but is 10 to 100 times more abundant on the earth's surface than UVB.

The effects of sun exposure on the skin are directly related to the wavelengths and total dose of UVR. Factors such as clothing, occupation, lifestyle, and age affect individual exposure to sunlight. Geography is also important: UVR exposure increases with decreasing latitude, and every 1,000 feet above sea level produces a 4% compounded increase in exposure.[16]

Onset of erythema occurs within 2 to 8 hours after UVB exposure, and the maximum is reached in 15 to 24 hours. A typical MED (Minimal Erythemal Dose—the time in minutes that it takes for an individual's skin to become red) value for an individual who burns easily and tans slightly (skin type 2) is 20 minutes at midday in midsummer in southern California. In most people, 4 to 5 MED will produce a painful sunburn. While the MED from UVA exposure for a fair-skinned person is higher, UVA can also produce a sunburn and degenerative dermal changes.[8,10] Chronic UVR exposure is associated with an increased incidence of skin cancer, especially basal and squamous cell carcinomas.

Ultraviolet light darkens (tans) the skin through two pathways: immediate oxidation of preformed melanin and delayed new melanin formation resulting from the stimulation of melanogenesis in the epidermis. An increased amount of melanin in the epidermis acts as a photoprotective mechanism, decreasing the amount of ultraviolet light that can pass through the epidermis and damage the DNA in the nucleus and cause mutations and malignancy. However, the protection given by increased melanin alone without thickening of the stratum corneum is moderate, approximately equal to a sun protection factor of 2 to 4. The spectrum of skin damage due to sun exposure is shown in Figure 2-12.

Individuals with darker skin usually have a stable form of melanin (eumelanin), and variable amounts of the unstable subtype, pheomelanin. Light-skinned persons, on the other hand, have predominantly pheomelanin, which produces larger amounts of free radicals upon UV exposure and may damage DNA and contribute to tumor formation.[17]

In response to chronic UVB exposure, the stratum corneum can increase to 6 times its original thickness. As a result, it absorbs or reflects up to 95% of UVB and increases skin tolerance to subsequent radiation.

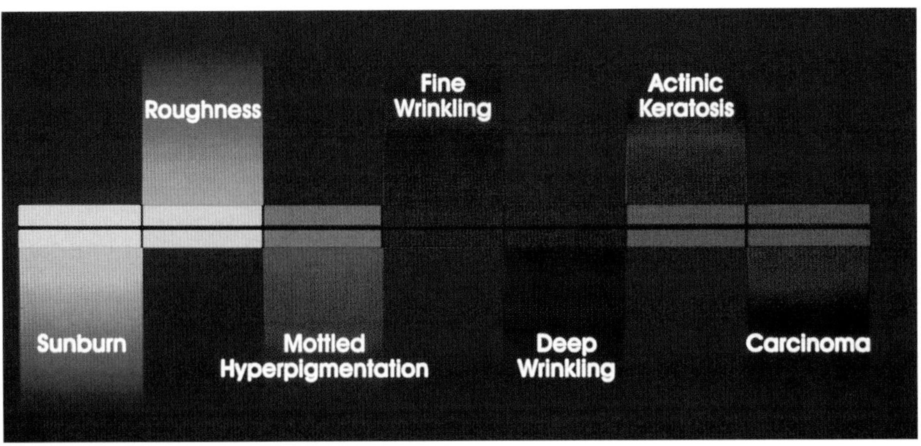

FIGURE 2-12. *Spectrum of skin damage due to sun exposure. From Gilchrest B.* Aging Skin: Clinical Challenges *[slide-lecture kit]. Boston, Ma: Boston University School of Medicine; 1996.*

Tanning with UVA alone (as in tanning parlors) provides less sunburn protection than a naturally acquired UVB suntan. This is due to 2 factors: 1) UVA does not induce thickening of the stratum corneum, and 2) the stimulation of melanogenesis occurs primarily in the basal layer, while with UVB the oxidation of melanin occurs throughout the entire epidermis.

PHOTODAMAGE PREVENTION

Skin damage due to ultraviolet light exposure can be reduced by adopting a comprehensive program of skin care to maintain healthy skin and by proper sun protection, such as use of a sunscreen with a sun protection factor (SPF) of 15 or higher and protective clothing, if needed.

The efficacy of sunscreen products is indicated by the SPF. This factor is calculated as the ratio of minutes of sunlight necessary to produce minimal redness (the MED) in sun-protected skin versus that for unprotected skin. Thus if redness appears in 15 minutes without sunscreen, but does not appear until after 150 minutes with sunscreen, the sunscreen product is said to have an SPF of 10. Some sunscreens protect against UVB, others against UVA and UVB. Agents that physically block UV light, such as zinc oxide or titanium dioxide, are also available for use in prolonged sun exposure. The importance of sunscreens in a skin health program will be discussed further in the next section.

Box 2-3

$$\text{SPF} = \frac{\textbf{Time for redness to appear with sunscreen}}{\textbf{Time for redness to appear without sunscreen}}$$

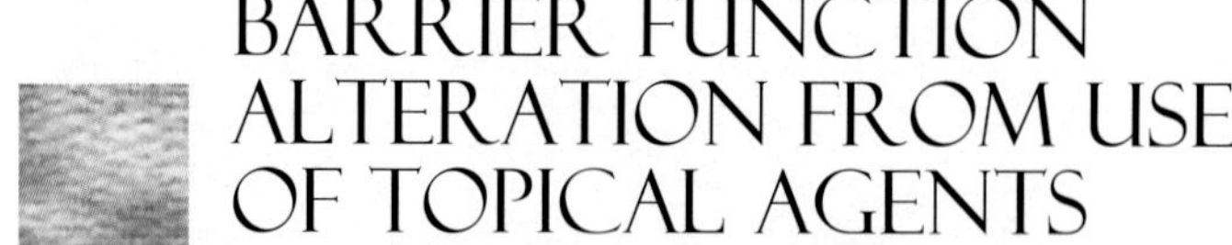

BARRIER FUNCTION ALTERATION FROM USE OF TOPICAL AGENTS

The health of our skin, like the health of our bodies, is affected internally by nutrition, exercise, and the functioning of body organs as well as by external factors. Among the external factors are numerous topical agents that are used and abused without any consideration given to their possible harmful effects. These include soaps, make-up, perfumes, moisturizers, chemical depilatory products, waxes, and many other products, all of which tend to alter the barrier function of the skin.

Soap is created by combining fat with an alkali to produce a fatty acid salt with detergent properties. The alkalinity of soaps can make skin feel dry and uncomfortable, and surfactant-induced irritation can occur in susceptible individuals. Synthetic detergent bars have been developed that contain less than 10% soap and have a pH of 5.5 to 7.0, which may be less irritating.[18]

Make-up, especially heavy foundation products applied to oily skin, can cause a variety of clinical problems, including large pores, contact dermatitis and other irritation reactions, allergic sensitivities, aggravation of acne, and infection. Most allergic or irritant contact dermatitis reactions are due to the fragrance or preservative in the product.[19]

Moisturizers are cosmetic companies' best-selling products. In the long run, they can damage skin by slowing epidermal renewal and increasing skin sensitivity to external factors. Use of moisturizers can also lead to an artificial sense of dryness when their use is terminated, which can be called "moisturizer addiction." The effects of moisturizer use were discussed in Chapter 1.

Chemical depilatory hair removal products can cause allergic and irritant contact dermatitis.

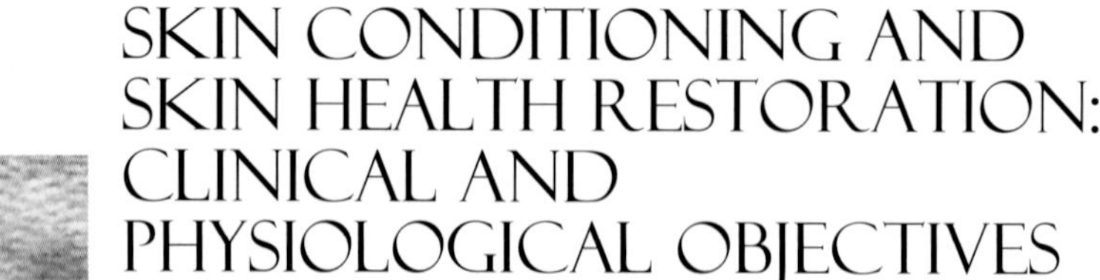

SKIN CONDITIONING AND SKIN HEALTH RESTORATION: CLINICAL AND PHYSIOLOGICAL OBJECTIVES

THE DEVELOPMENT OF OBAGI SKIN CONDITIONING AND SKIN HEALTH RESTORATION PROGRAMS

Eighteen years ago the author observed that skin treated with retinoic acid and hydroquinone for melasma or acne healed faster and with better results after a dermabrasion or chemical peel procedure, and the concept of skin conditioning was born. Later results confirmed the author's early observations and it became clear that retinoic acid, hydroquinone, and hydrocortisone, used before and after a procedure, may have some beneficial effects early in their usage. Unfortunately the concept of skin conditioning was not widely adapted and its science has not advanced for many years. Skin conditioning is still viewed only as a program to prepare skin for a procedure, and it is not applied for the purpose of improving skin for normal daily life when a procedure is not planned. How conditioning is carried out is usually left to the patient, and emphasis is given to comfort rather than efficacy.

When dermatologists, plastic surgeons, and cosmetic surgeons do practice a form of skin conditioning, it is often used ineffectively and does not benefit the patient. Approaches are often haphazard, and agents such as tretinoin, AHAs, and hydroquinone are prescribed without a treatment plan, objective, or standards. The patient is told to use an agent for 2 to 4 weeks before a procedure but is not told the purpose, how much to use, or what to expect from the agent. Instructions after the procedure tend to be even more ambiguous, with the physician unclear about when to start, what to use, and how long to use it. This author maintains that the high incidence of complications and dissatisfied patients may be attributed to poor physician understanding and utilization of skin conditioning.

Box 2-4

Current approaches to skin conditioning are haphazard, and agents such as tretinoin, AHAs, and hydroquinone are prescribed without a treatment plan, objective, or standards.

In the Obagi approach, skin conditioning is not limited to use as a preparation before a procedure. The skin conditioning program Skin Health Restoration can quantitatively and qualitatively improve skin, prevent deterioration, and delay or eliminate the need for later procedures. If a procedure has been carried out, the Skin Health Restoration program can maintain the results much longer.

REGULATION OF THE FUNCTION OF SKIN CELLS

The main objectives of skin health restoration and skin conditioning are the regulation of the functions of the four skin cell types:

1. keratinocytes, to obtain a soft, compact stratum corneum and a thick epidermis with proper keratinization (for barrier function)
2. melanocytes, to obtain even and normal melanization (for skin color)
3. fibroblasts, for collagen, elastin, and glycosaminoglycan production (for firmness, tightness, and proper hydration)
4. angioblasts, for normal angiogenesis (improved skin circulation).

To control and regulate the function of these cells, the author has developed the concepts of 1) correction, 2) stimulation, and 3) bleaching and blending. These are discussed in depth in Chapter 5.

THE KERATINOCYTE MATURATION CYCLE

A major objective of Skin Health Restoration is continued and constant renewal of the epidermis. To meet this objective, a normal skin maturation cycle (the amount of time it takes for a keratinocyte to mature, reach the stratum corneum, and exfoliate) should be restored in each patient's skin (Figure 2-13). A normal skin maturation cycle takes approximately 40 days, with a range of 28–60 days.[20] It can be shortened by factors such as psoriasis, malignant growth, and verrucae (warts) and lengthened by factors such as intrinsic aging, photoaging, and use of hydrocortisone. To restore the cycle to normal, the Obagi programs of Skin Health Restoration and Skin Conditioning provide specific instructions for the use of tretinoin and AHAs (Chapters 3 & 5).

In general, 3 maturation cycles ($4^1/_2$ to 5 months) are needed to renew most of the epidermis, and 1 to 2 maturation cycles are necessary to attain a good level of tolerance. Tolerance usually can be perceived after 1 cycle (6 weeks) of an aggressive conditioning has been completed. With less aggressive approaches, tolerance takes longer to build up: 2 to 3 months with a moderately aggressive approach, 4 to 6 months with a standard approach, and up to 8 months with a weak approach. To treat postinflammatory hyperpigmentation (PIH) after a procedure, one half to 1 cycle of aggressive to moderately aggressive skin conditioning is needed. Tolerance is important because rejuvenation procedures should not be performed until it has been attained. For example, in treating melasma, 2 to 3 cycles of aggressive or moderately aggressive skin conditioning may be needed before and after a procedure for the best results, followed by 3 to 6 cycles of the standard approach to maintain the correction. Details of each type of approach are presented in Chapter 5.

Clinical Benefits of Cycle Regulation

Completion of 2 to 3 cycles in the Skin Health Restoration program will establish sufficient skin tolerance and produce a number of clinical benefits.

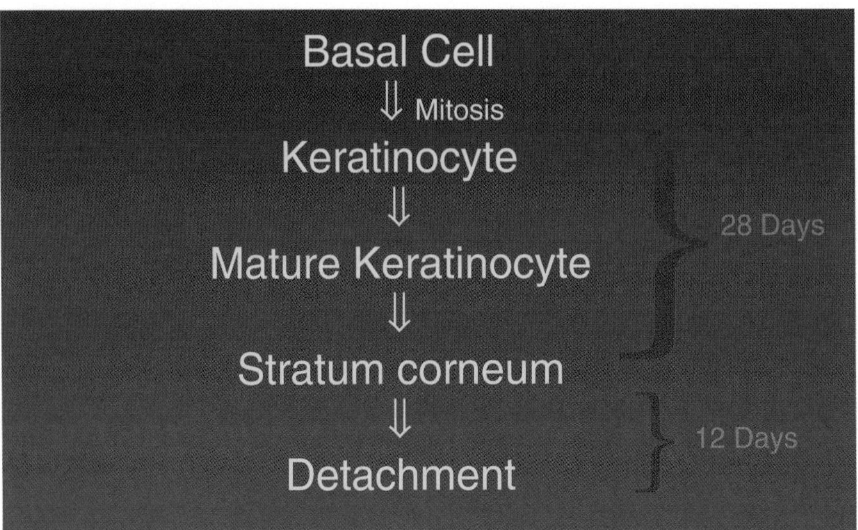

FIGURE 2-13. *Skin maturation cycle.*

The stratum corneum becomes smooth, soft, and compact, with a minimal basket-weave pattern. Mitosis in the basal layer and adnexal structures proceeds at an optimal rate, producing a population of healthy keratinocytes and a thicker epidermis. Bacterial flora are reduced and acne, comedones, and large pores diminish. Skin becomes properly hydrated and moisturizers may not be necessary. With restoration of the skin's barrier function, skin tolerance to cosmetics, dermatological treatments, and changes in the environment increases. Finally, with control of the pigmentary system, melanocytes are regulated, melanin is evenly dispersed, and skin tone evens out.

CLINICAL OBJECTIVES

Skin Conditioning and Skin Health Restoration are similar programs with similar objectives toward skin health. Their major difference is in their relationship to a skin rejuvenation procedure, such as a chemical peel, laser resurfacing, or face-lift. Skin Health Restoration is performed to improve the quality, appearance, and tolerance of the skin and to slow down the signs of aging. It is not intended to be performed in conjunction with a procedure but is meant to delay the need for a procedure. Skin Conditioning, on the other hand, has 2 clinical objectives: 1) to improve skin quality, appearance, and 2) to restore tolerance so that skin is prepared for a rejuvenation procedure.

Patients with very young and healthy skin may follow the Skin Health Restoration program to improve and maintain the quality of their skin, while patients with more deteriorated and aged skin may follow the Skin Conditioning program to prepare for a procedure. Studies have shown that skin preconditioning can enhance wound healing after a procedure and lengthen the effects of a rejuvenation procedure.[21–23] In other words, it can help the surgeon get more out of the procedure.

A comparison of the objectives of the Skin Conditioning and Skin Health Restoration programs is shown in Table 2-3 and the desirable effects of skin conditioning in Table 2-4.

TABLE 2.3

SKIN CONDITIONING AND SKIN HEALTH RESTORATION: OBJECTIVES

Objective	*Skin Health Restoration*	*Skin Conditioning*
Physiological	• Regulate skin cell function • Improve circulation and hydration	• Regulate skin cell function • Improve circulation and hydration
Clinical	• Slow down skin aging process • Improve skin appearance and quality • Daily skin care program indefinitely	• Restore skin tolerance • Improve skin appearance and quality • Shorten the postprocedure healing phase • One cycle before, one cycle after a procedure
Relationship with Skin Rejuvenation Procedures	• Delay need for rejuvenation procedures	• Prepare skin for rejuvenation procedures • Enhance procedure results

Table 2.4	
DESIRABLE EFFECTS OF SKIN CONDITIONING	
Epidermis	
Cellular Level	***Clinical Level***
■ Increased mitosis in the basal layer of the epidermis and adnexal structures; population of healthy keratinocytes are increased ■ More even melanin distribution and control of melanocyte function ■ Up-regulation of immunological function (restored Langerhans cell population and healthy keratinocytes), growth factors release ■ Decreased inflammatory response	■ Increased speed of re-epithelialization, skin tolerance to external factors, barrier function ■ Improved hydration ■ Decreased incidence PIH, melasma, and other dyspigmentations ■ Decreased sensitivity; faster healing after injury; lower risk of sun-damage–induced skin cancer and other cutaneous diseases ■ Shorter period of erythema
Dermis	
Cellular Level	***Clinical Level***
■ Increased formation of glycosaminoglycan ■ New collagen and elastin deposition ■ Increased angiogenesis	■ Proper skin hydration ■ Increased skin firmness and elasticity ■ Increased skin circulation, less sallowness, more pink tone to skin; faster wound healing; better clearance of potentially toxic substances

Box 2-5

- **Skin Conditioning:**

  improves skin quality, circulation, hydration, and tolerance

  prepares skin for a skin rejuvenation procedure, such as a chemical peel or laser resurfacing

  short-term approach; 1 cycle before and 1 cycle after a procedure; no long-term emphasis.

- **Skin Health Restoration:**

  improves skin quality, appearance, and tolerance and slow down the signs of aging

  prevents or delays the need for a procedure

  long-term approach: daily program, variable strength to maintain skin health indefinitely

SHORT- AND LONG-TERM PHYSIOLOGICAL OBJECTIVES

The physiological objectives of skin health restoration and skin conditioning are to 1) improve the quality of the epidermis, 2) improve the quality of the dermis, 3) increase skin tolerance, and 4) improve skin circulation. These objectives are achieved by regulating the function of key cells—keratinocytes, melanocytes, and fibroblasts and angioblasts, increasing collagen production, increasing growth factors release, decreasing the inflammatory response, promoting angiogenesis (improving circulation), improving dermal or epidermal hydration, and up-regulating immunological function. These lead to the clinical improvements of increased skin firmness and elasticity, a rosy skin glow, increased skin hydration, increased tolerance to external irritants, and shortened postprocedure recovery time.

The specific agents selected to achieve the clinical and physiological objectives of the Obagi program and their mechanisms of action are discussed in the next chapter.

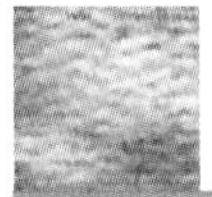

REFERENCES

1. Lever L, Marks R. Current views on the etiology, pathogenesis, and treatment of acne vulgaris. *Drugs.* 1990;39:681–692.
2. Sanchez NP, Pathak MA, Sato S, et al. Melasma: A clinical, light microscopic, ultrastructural and immunofluorescent study. *J Am Acad Dermatol.* 1980;2:295–302.
3. Grimes P. Melasma: Etiologic and therapeutic considerations. *Arch Dermatol.* 1995;131:1453–1457.
4. Kligman L. Skin changes in photoaging: Characteristics, prevention, and repair. In: Kligman AM, Balin AK, eds. *Aging and the Skin.* New York, NY: Raven Press; 1993:331–346.
5. Kligman AM. Perspectives and problems in cutaneous gerontology. *J Invest Dermatol.* 1979;73:39–46.
6. Sams WM Jr. Sun-induced aging: clinical and laboratory observations in man. *Dermatol Clin.* 1986;4:509–516.
7. Kligman LH, Kligman AM. The nature of photoaging: its prevention and repair. *Photodermatology.* 1986;3:215–227.
8. West MD. The cellular and molecular biology of skin aging. *Arch Dermatol.* 1994;130:87–95.
9. Lavker RA. Cutaneous aging: chronological versus photoaging. In: Gilchrest BA, ed. *Photodamage.* Cambridge, England: Blackwell Scientific; 1995:123–135.
10. Yaar M, Gilchrest BA. Biochemical and molecular changes in photoaged skin. In: Gilchrest BA, ed. *Photodamage.* Cambridge, England: Blackwell Scientific; 1995:168–184.
11. Kligman AM, Kligman LH. Photoaging. In: Fitzpatrick TB, Eisen AZ, Wolff K, et al, eds. *Dermatology in General Medicine.* New York, NY: McGraw-Hill; 1993;2972–2979.
12. Montagna W, Kirchner S, Carlisle K. Histology of sun-damaged skin. *J Am Acad Dermatol.* 1989;21:907–918.
13. Calderone DC, Fenske NA. The clinical spectrum of actinic elastosis. *J Am Acad Dermatol.* 1995;32:1016–1024.

14. Taylor CR, Stern RS, Leyden JJ, Gilchrest BA. Photoaging, photodamage, and photoprotection. *J Am Acad Dermatol.* 1990;22:1–5.

15. Kligman AM. Early destructive effects of sunlight on human skin. *JAMA.* 1969;210:2377–2380.

16. NIH Health Consensus Development Conference. Sunlight, Ultraviolet Radiation, and the Skin [conference statement]. Bethesda, Md: National Institutes of Health; 1989;7:1–9.

17. Kochevar IE. Molecular and cellular effects of uv radiation relevant to chronic photodamage. In: Gilchrest BA, ed. *Photodamage.* Cambridge, England: Blackwell Scientific; 1995:51–67.

18. Draelos, ZD. Skin cleansers. In: Draelos ZD, ed. *Cosmetics in Dermatology.* 2nd ed. New York, NY: Churchill Livingstone; 1995:207–214.

19. Draelos, ZD. Facial foundations. In: Draelos ZD, ed. *Cosmetics in Dermatology.* 2nd ed. New York, NY: Churchill Livingstone; 1995:1–14.

20. Kligman AM, Grove GL, Hirose R, Leyden JJ. Topical tretinoin for photoaged skin. *J Am Acad Dermatol.* 1986;15:836–859.

21. Hevia O, Nemeth AJ, Taylor R. Tretinoin accelerates healing after trichloroacetic acid chemical peel. *Arch Dermatol.* 1991;127:678–682.

22. Kim IH, Kim HK, Kye YC. Effects of tretinoin pretreatment on TCA chemical peel in guinea pig skin. *J Korean Med Sci.* 1996;11:335–341.

23. Kligman AM, Grove GL, Hirose R, Leyeden JJ. Topical tretinoin for photoaged skin. *J Am Acad Dermatol.* 1986;15:836–859.

CHAPTER

3

SKIN HEALTH RESTORATION AND SKIN CONDITIONING: AGENTS USED

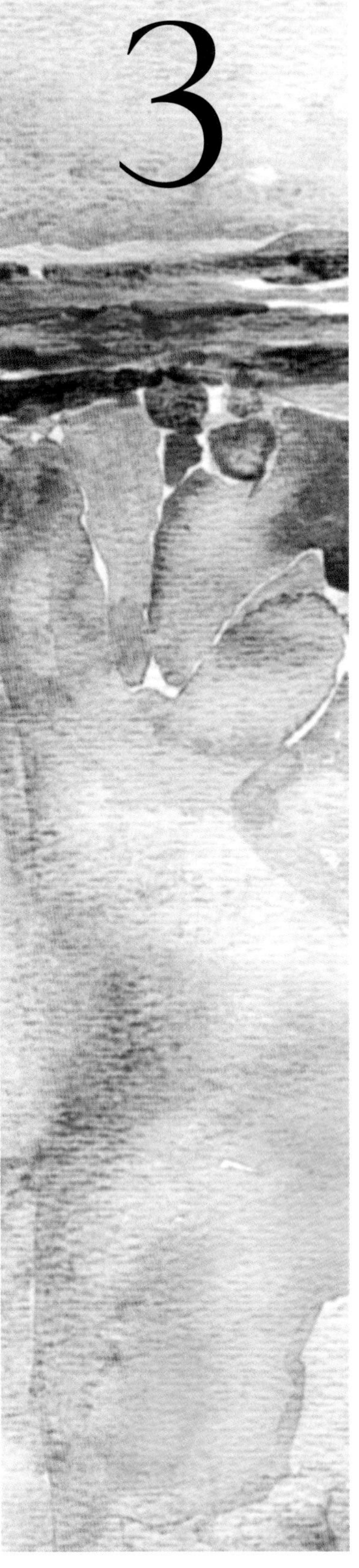

AGENTS USED IN SKIN HEALTH RESTORATION AND THEIR MECHANISM OF ACTION

In a survey of people age 50 and over, it was recorded that virtually all had photodamage and 65% had significant skin disorders.[1] Furthermore, individuals of all ages have shown little understanding of their skin problems by accepting blindly the many misleading claims of various cosmetics manufacturers and aestheticians. Consumers have been persuaded to believe, for example, that light fruit acid will significantly rejuvenate facial skin, that sun damage can be remedied by moisturizing make-up, and that "active" agents applied at the outer layer of the skin can influence and repair underlying dermal damage.

Unlike the agents with questionable efficacy in many skin care programs, the agents recommended for use in the Obagi Skin Health Restoration and Skin Conditioning programs have been selected based on their solid scientific evidence and safety. Relatively few agents are to be used, and they are easy to apply.

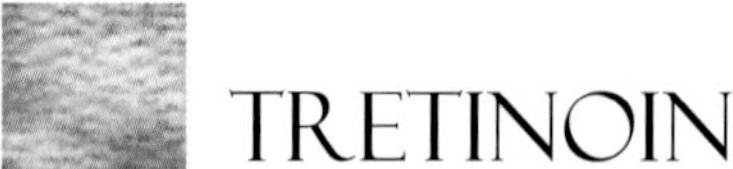

TRETINOIN

CLINICAL EVIDENCE OF ACTIVITY

The beneficial effects of topically applied tretinoin (vitamin A derivative) on signs of photoaging were first observed on women treated for persistent acne who demonstrated the incidental finding following treatment of smoother, less wrinkled skin.[2] In subsequent studies, tretinoin was shown to affect the visible signs of skin damage due to sun exposure,[3–10] to treat actinic keratosis, prevent skin cancer,[11–14] and to improve recent stretch marks.[15] Specifically in the photodamage studies, investigators' objective evaluations and the patients' self-assessments showed the most consistent improvement in fine wrinkling, mottled hyperpigmentation, and facial skin roughness. In self-assessments, 83% of the patients rated their skin as improved after 6 months of treatment with 0.05% tretinoin cream.[7,8]

Statistically significant improvement in fine line, coarse wrinkles, and skin texture was sustained after treatment with tretinoin was extended for up to 22 months, despite a decrease in dose or frequency of application.[6] Lentigines decreased by 71%. Histological findings included a statistically significant thickening of the epidermis.

Tretinoin in a 0.1% concentration was shown to lighten hyperpigmented lesions in photoaged Chinese and Japanese skin,[9] as previously demonstrated on white skin.[16] In the Asian skin study stratum corneum compaction, increased granular cell layer, and epithelial thickening were also observed. Because actinic lentigines cleared through use of topical tretinoin neither relapse nor repigment after cessation of treatment, the mechanism for lightening is believed to be a result of melanin reduction.

HISTOLOGICAL RESULTS

The histological effects of varying concentrations of topical tretinoin on photodamaged skin have been investigated in a randomized study.[17] At the end of 6 months of daily application of 0.05% tretinoin, significant differences from the control group were seen in stratum corneum compaction, increased epidermal thickness, increased granular layer thickness, and decreased melanin content. The permanence and clinical significance of the changes have not yet been determined. For that reason the author recommends that tretinoin be used indefinitely.

Biopsy specimens taken from patients treated with tretinoin for up to 4 years showed a 34% reduction in the dermal area occupied by elastosis and an increase in papillary dermal thickness between 1 and 4 years.[18] This study also showed specimens to have a normal epidermis with no atypical keratinocytes or melanocytes, demonstrating long-term safety of use.

Another biopsy study[19] showed that average synthesis of collagen type I was reduced by more than half in photodamaged skin, and the reduction was correlated with the severity of the photodamage. Treatment with tretinoin increased collagen I formation an average of 80%. This study suggested that wrinkle effacement following tretinoin therapy may be due to the restoration of collagen synthesis. Thus the ability of topical tretinoin to clinically reduce the effects of photodamage is not simply cosmetic and temporary, but rather is based on the active repair of dermal collagen.[8]

MECHANISM OF ACTION

Although collagen formation with tretinoin treatment has been demonstrated, its exact mechanism of action is not well known. Retinoids in general are liposoluble materials, and they will pass easily through cell membranes. They then work at the molecular level by binding to proteins in the cytoplasm and receptors in the nucleus. Tretinoin actions mediated through the receptors in the nucleus may involve regulation of gene transcriptions.[19] Effects of tretinoin action include increased cell division and turnover, altered cell differentiation, and formation of new collagen.[20] Tretinoin may temporarily increase proliferation of normal keratinocytes and fibroblasts but decrease proliferation in certain hyperproliferative diseases.[2] Melano-cyte activity has decreased, while anchoring filament and fibril formation and new collagen at the dermal/epidermal junction have both increased with 0.1% tretinoin.[22]

The extent of clinical improvement with tretinoin has been called modest by some, but cytological and histological studies have revealed extensive changes in the epidermis and dermis.[23] Kligman has stressed that the naked eye "greatly underestimates the corrective effects of this drug" and believes that the most important changes are evident at the histological and not the clinical level.[24]

According to Kligman, tretinoin substantially improves not only the structure of the skin but also its physiological functions. The formation of new blood vessels (angiogenesis) improves blood flow to allow rapid clearance of potentially toxic substances. Clinically this translates to a desirable rosy glow. The stimulation of the immune function restores the density of antigen-presenting Langerhans cells, for increased protection against viral and fungal infections and the inhibition of neoplastic growths. The deposition of collagen increases skin firmness. Increased elasticity, demonstrated by rapid recovery after the skin has been deformed by suction, has also been shown[24]; also, the dermal matrix is strengthened to reduce the occurrence of solar purpura. Tretinoin has also been shown to accelerate healing after TCA peeling.[25,26]

ENHANCING THE MECHANISM OF ACTION OF TRETINOIN

Several steps can be taken to enhance the beneficial effect of tretinoin. Bringing the skin to an appropriate pH prior to application can enhance penetration, as does the removal of skin sebum with proper cleansing. The skin should saturated by applying an adequate amount of tretinoin cream at each application, and it should be rubbed in until completely absorbed. When tretinoin is used in combination with other active agents, the mixture should be freshly prepared because compounded tretinoin products are less effective after a few weeks.[27]

The physician should attempt to obtain the maximum skin reaction that can be tolerated by the patient. In the early stages, when tolerance is low, the patient whose reactions become troublesome, can be advised to stop the tretinoin treatment and use moisturizers for a few days. The patient should resume treatment after comfort has been reestablished and continue treatment until natural tolerance has been attained. This usually occurs in an average of 6 weeks (Fig. 3-1).

Box 3-1

ACTINIC KERATOSES

Actinic keratoses are the most common premalignant skin lesions. They are found in areas of increased sun exposure and are characterized by macular erythema with an overlying tan-colored scale. These lesions are significant because of their disfigurement and potential for malignancy. Because actinic keratoses are confined to the epidermis, treatment modalities are targeted at superficial destruction or modification of the differentiation of abnormal keratinocytes. Cryosurgery, electrodessication, curettage, and topical application of 5-fluorouracil or Masoprocol have been effective therapies. More recently, systemic and topically applied retinoids, through their activity on cellular differentiation, have also been successful in treating those lesions.

Box 3-2

TRETINOIN PERSONAL OBSERVATIONS

The author has applied tretinoin on his own face for more than 15 years and has followed patients using it for more than 10 years. The benefits of using 0.05% to 0.1% tretinoin as part of the Obagi process of correction, stimulation and blending are

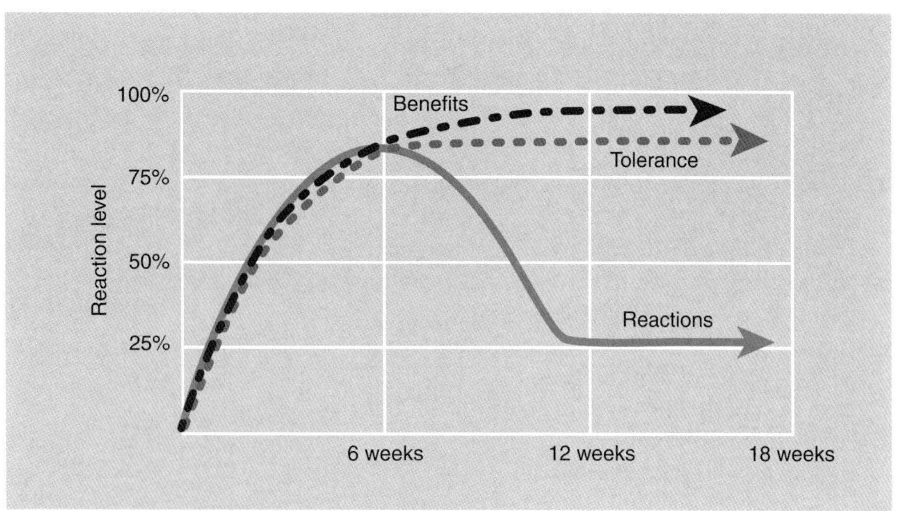

FIGURE 3-1. *Relationship between benefits, reaction and tolerance while using tretinoin over time.*

shown in Table 3-1. The response was generally better when tretinoin was applied twice daily, but good result can be obtained with once-daily application.

SIDE EFFECTS

In clinical trials, the most frequently reported side effects from tretinoin treatment were initial skin irritation consisting of exfoliation, burning, stinging, redness, and itching.[6,7] These reactions were generally mild to moderate in severity and often diminished after temporary reduction in application frequency. Signs and symptoms of irritation peaked at the second week of tretinoin use and usually decreased thereafter. Only 4% of the patients dropped out of the clinical trials because of adverse skin reactions. Existing telangiectasias may appear worse after treatment with tretinoin, but this is not a reason to discontinue treatment, since these can be easily treated with a vascular laser.

Treatment failures with tretinoin are generally the result of a patient's stopping the treatment prematurely, insufficient explanation by the physician of the objectives and their importance to the patient, or lack of motivation on the part of the patient. The physician should take the time to properly motivate the patient, telling her or him the expected side effects and explaining that these are a desirable sign of response to the treatment. The term "Retin-A dermatitis" should be avoided, for it has a negative connotation and suggests that the treatment should be terminated to stop the side effect. Since there is no substitute for tretinoin activity in the dermatological arsenal, the anticipated reaction should be presented in a positive light.

Table 3.1

BENEFITS FROM LONG-TERM USE OF TOPICAL TRETINOIN

General

- An increase in skin tolerance to external factors
- An increase in skin thickness and firmness with minimal aging signs
- Good response in certain types of dermal pigmentation
- Restoration of even color tone and resistance to development of uneven pigmentation and PIH
- Resolution of dark circles around the eyes
- More hydrated skin that does not need moisturizers
- Less irritation from shaving in men and less pseudofolliculitis barberi in Afro-American men
- Response of minor skin laxity
- Reversal of stretch marks in the early stages (pink) and improvement of older stretch marks

Medical

- Ideal treatment for acne vulgaris, acne rosacea, seborrheic dermatitis, and many other inflammatory conditions
- Improvement in patients with vitiligo (no progression) by stimulating melanocyte regeneration in areas with sufficient adnexal structures
- Improved quality of life in patients with atopic dermatitis of the face when used gradually and with increasing strength and frequency of application (tolerance is built up and hydration is increased)
- Effective treatment of keratosis pilaris seen in upper arms and thighs
- Ideal for smoothing, relaxing, and softening skin grafts in burn patients. Improvement in skin texture, color, and mobility
- Localized morphea (burned out and not progressing) brought back to normal texture and color in 8 months
- Skin damage from radiation or steroid atrophy restored nearly to normal
- Response of advanced actinic keratoses (except hypertrophic form) with long-term treatment
- Disappearance of dermal hemosidrine deposits which cause long-term discoloration after sclerotherapy
- Good response of chronic, superficial, pigmented scars on legs, i.e., insect bites
- Good response in some patients suffering from alopecia areata on face and scalp
- Some cases of early male-pattern baldness reversed while on treatment for facial conditions. Increased growth of facial hair has also been seen.

Procedure-Related

- Faster and better wound healing and less chance of scarring after rejuvenation procedures or trauma
- Shortening of the erythema phase after CO_2 laser resurfacing
- Scars from acne, burns, and trauma made softer and less noticeable; better response than to chemical peels or CO_2 laser resurfacing
- Softening of keloids and hypertrophic scars and acceleration of their response to laser treatment or corticosteroid injections

Box 3-3

"I prefer aggressive usage [of tretinoin] in patients with photoaging, since the beneficial effects can be realized earlier and to a greater degree." (Albert M. Kligman. *Cutis.* 1996;57:142–144)

Box 3-4

The patient should be told to expect a reaction to tretinoin and that a reaction is a desirable sign of response to the treatment. Since no substitute exists for tretinoin, the anticipated reaction should be presented in a positive light.

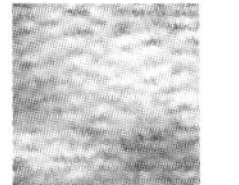

ALPHA HYDROXY ACIDS

CHEMICAL PROPERTIES AND TOPICAL USE

Alpha hydroxy acids (AHAs) are a group of weak hydroscopic acids that contain an alcohol (hydroxy) function in the alpha position relative to the carbon atom bearing the carboxyl function. These fruit acids are very popular in cosmetics such as facial moisturizers, cleansers, and toners and are also used in superficial chemical peels. While these acids are now produced synthetically for cosmetic use, glycolic acid can be derived from sugar cane, lactic acid from fermented milk, citric acid from fruits, and malic acid from apples.[19,28–30]

Glycolic and lactic acids are the AHAs most commonly used in skin care products. Glycolic acid is hydroscopic, binding to water in the skin, and also decreases corneocyte bonds. In higher concentrations, it detaches the epidermis from the dermis (epidermolysis) through lysis of desmosomes. It can be used alone or in combination with other chemicals in some facial peels.[31–35] The AHAs have different molecular sizes. Glycolic acid is the smallest and thus has the better penetrating activity.

The acidic pH of these acids is buffered for facial application to approximately 2.8 to 3.5.[36] Cosmetic products currently on the market claim to be "neutralized" or "buffered" for less irritation. However, neutralized products would have little cutaneous efficacy.[37]

AHAs are classified by the U.S. Food and Drug Administration as a cosmetic and, consistent with this, over-the-counter cosmetic products containing AHAs have virtually flooded the market in the past decade. The recent trend has been to increase the concentration and thereby decrease the pH to obtain a "stronger" product. Acidity alone, however, does not predict acantholytic effect, since electrostatic, inductive, and steric effects, as well as hydrogen bonding, are also involved.[36]

AHAs: MECHANISM OF ACTION AND BENEFITS

The effectiveness of AHAs at different concentrations and pH values has been examined.[34] For example, decreasing the pH of glycolic acid increases efficacy but increases irritation and untoward effects. The relationship of glycolic acid concentration to its pH value is shown in Table 3-2.

Cutaneous surface pH changes induced by AHAs should be taken seriously, since the changes can remain up to 4 hours following application. Low concentrations can change the pH of the outer three layers of the stratum corneum, while a 10% concentration can affect 10 to 20 layers.

Moderate concentrations of glycolic acid, i.e., at 30% or below, have been used for "refresher" or "lunch-time" peels performed by medical personnel as well as aestheticians. This procedure removes epidermal corneocytes to produce exfoliation at the lower levels of the stratum corneum.[38,39] It is not a true peel. It can produce a short-lived smoother skin and improve comedogenic acne, but it has no effect on wrinkles or scars and cannot tighten skin.

Concentrated solutions of glycolic acid tend to penetrate more deeply, producing epidermolysis and, possibly, stimulation of dermal macrophages and fibroblasts. In vitro studies with fibroblast cultures have shown that, depending on exposure time, glycolic acid in higher concentrations may induce dermal effects such as collagen synthesis.[29,39] There has been no evidence from human studies, however. There is no stimulation of angiogenesis with AHAs. One of the studies[40] shows increases of the production of glycosaminoglycans following use of ammonium lactate. There are also reports that glycolic acid has anti-inflammatory activity and antioxidant properties.[41]

TABLE 3.2

pH VALUES OF DIFFERENT CONCENTRATIONS OF GLYCOLIC ACID

Concentration (%)	*pH*
5	1.7
10	1.6
20	1.5
30	1.4
40	1.3
50	1.2
60	1.0
70	0.6

The exact mechanism of action of AHAs is not totally elucidated, but the dermatological effects are believed to be mostly epidermal. Much remains to be learned about optimal formulations and use of AHAs, and more studies need to be performed to fully explain their mechanism of action. However many claims made by manufacturers of AHA products are exaggerated and unsubstantiated by scientific data.

AHAs: SAFETY ISSUES

AHAs are chemicals capable of producing safety concerns even though they are available without prescription. Attempts to use AHAs in concentrations high enough to produce a true chemical peel (wounding of the dermal layer) can produce focal dermal necrosis and possible scar formation. In a few cases surface scarring, hypertrophic reactions, and pigmentary changes have been observed, especially in thin-skinned persons and those with severe photodamage. However these effects are rare in thick-skinned persons, because the acid cannot penetrate deep enough to be damaging. The true therapeutic value of AHAs and their role in treating photoaged skin, as well as the associated risks, are not known at this time.

MISINFORMATION ON GLYCOLIC PEELS

Misleading and inaccurate information about glycolic acid peels has led to inappropriate use. Patients are now being given such peels for the correction of wrinkles and scars, problems that often do not respond to glycolic acid peels. Procedures with deeper penetration are needed for these conditions, such as medium-depth TCA peel, CO_2 laser resurfacing, or dermabrasion.

The cosmetic industry has inaccurately attributed the beneficial effects of glycolic acid in a peel concentration to creams, lotions, foundations, and other cosmetic products that contain 2% to 10% glycolic acid or other AHAs. This misinformation has been widely transmitted through cleverly worded advertising.

AHAs are extracellular agents that have no regulatory or intracellular effects (Figure 3-2). Products containing AHAs in concentrations less than 10% can produce short-lived smoothness and help remove comedones with continued use. They cannot repair damaged DNA or suppress tyrosinase to reduce melanin production. Superficial improvement in pigmentation, for example, is a result of exfoliation, and not from a regulatory effect on melanocytes. Actinic keratoses do not respond to AHAs, and skin cancer is not prevented by them. The principal reason that AHAs have had significant impact on skin treatment is due to their ability to reduce corneocyte adhesion and accelerated cell proliferation within the basal layer. AHAs should be properly positioned among skin care products as only exfoliants that help to remove the stratum corneum or upper layers of the epidermis.

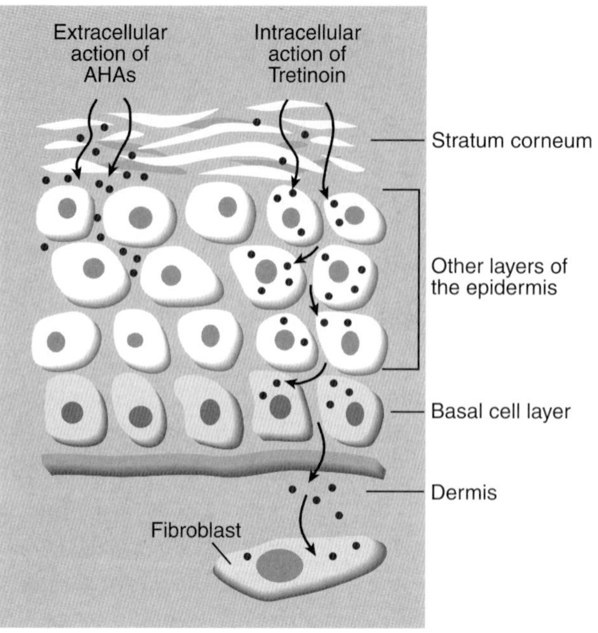

FIGURE 3-2. *Extracellular action of AHAs vs intracellular action of tretinoin.*

Box 3-5

"A 70% concentration, such as used in a glycolic acid peel, can rejuvenate skin. Concentrations of 4% to 15%, however, do not remove wrinkles—they do not rejuvenate skin—they can only exfoliate."

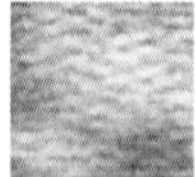

OTHER EXFOLIATOR: PHYTIC ACID

Phytic acid (hexaphosphate inositol) is a natural component of plant seed. The hexaphosphate structure suggests strong acid properties; however, the internal resonance system between the hydrogen atoms makes the product less acidic and thus more suitable for alpha hydroxy type effects. Concentrations of 3% to 10% have valuable exfoliating properties. The advantage of phytic acid over currently used AHAs is its ability to act at low pH without causing stinging or irritation.

Phytic acid has shown efficacy superior to that of AHAs in a cell turnover study, as well as increased mildness in a 48-hour patch test (3% phytic acid formulation, pH 1.0, compared with 10% AHAs, pH 3.0). Phytic acid can be beneficial in black or dark Hispanic skin and also sensitive skin that reacts to AHAs.

HYDROQUINONE AND OTHER DEPIGMENTING AGENTS

HYDROQUINONE: AN OVERVIEW

Hydroquinone is a topical depigmenting agent that specifically targets the melanocyte system to interfere with the formation of new melanin. Pigmentary disorders such as melasma, postinflammatory hyperpigmentation (PIH), and freckling have been treated successfully with topical hydroquinone. The agent works by causing structural changes in organelles of melanocytes, thereby decreasing the formation of and increasing the degradation of melanosomes. It also inhibits the activity of tyrosinase.[42] Skin lightening is not immediate, because hydroquinone only prevents the formation of new melanin and production resumes when its use is discontinued. Side effects, which are rare, include burning, stinging, rash, irritation, and allergic reactions.

CONCENTRATION AND FORMULATION

Topical preparation of hydroquinone are available in 2% (nonprescription strength) and 4% (prescription strength) concentrations of cream, lotion, gel, or liquid that is applied to the area to be lightened once or twice daily. These concentrations are capable of suppressing skin melanin production. Higher concentrations (6% and 8%) have not been shown to be more effective and carry the risk of inducing idiosyncratic reactions during or after discontinuation of treatment (similar to ochronosis). The mechanism of this reaction is unknown, and further investigation is needed. Liquid or gel forms result in uneven application and are not suitable for delivering hydroquinone to the skin. Cream or lotion preparations are preferable.

Hydroquinone preparations that have oxidized (turned brown) have weaker activity.

APPLICATION REGIMEN

For best results, the epidermis should be saturated with hydroquinone during the application. A dosage of 1.5 g of the hydroquinone preparation (similar to the amount in an inch of toothpaste) should be applied and massaged in until totally absorbed. The entire area should be covered, not just the spots. Because contact of the product with skin will shift the skin's pH toward neutral and also facilitate oxidation, the activity of hydroquinone is short-lived. Thus, skin should be saturated with the product twice daily. Once an even color tone has been obtained, the frequency of application can be reduced gradually. Application should not be discontinued abruptly.

EFFICACY

Hydroquinone is a very effective depigmenting agent, but its efficacy can change when it is used together with other products. Hydroquinone penetration, and therefore its activity, is increased when it is used together with AHAs and tretinoin. Furthermore, the presence of AHAs in hydroquinone-containing products prevents its oxidation and thus preserves its activity. Hydroquinone is unstable, however, when compounded with tretinoin, and the two products should be combined just before application.

Hydroquinone penetration can also be increased by using it with certain penetrating agents and adjusting the pH of the skin before treatment. That is the approach taken by the Skin Health Restoration program for correcting pigmentation problems such as melasma. This combination, when used for several weeks before a procedure such as the Blue Peel, decreases the skin's ability to create melanin, thereby reducing the occurrence of PIH. If it does occur, postpeel hydroquinone use reduces its intensity.

SKIN TYPE AND THE EFFECTIVENESS OF HYDROQUINONE

Failure to correct epidermal pigmentation problems with hydroquinone should not be attributed to a lack of agent efficacy. It is more likely due to a lack of knowledge of the proper delivery of active hydroquinone to target areas. For optimal efficacy, skin type must be taken into consideration and the regimen adjusted for skin thickness, oiliness of the stratum corneum, and whether skin color is original or deviated. To saturate thicker skin, more than 1.5 g of a 4% hydroquinone preparation should be used for each application. Oily skin requires proper washing to remove sebum and the use of topical or systemic agents that reduce oiliness and increase penetration of hydroquinone.

Most hyperpigmentation problems arise from the increased activity of melanocytes and the overproduction of melanin, which can be suppressed by hydroquinone to give a bleaching effect. However, when hydroquinone is mixed with tretinoin and AHAs in proper proportions and concentrations, the bleaching effect becomes less important and another effect in diminishing hyperpigmentation becomes evident. The author uses the term "blending" to describe the more even distribution of melanin to surround-

Box 3-6

Failure to correct pigmentation problems with hydroquinone can be due to improper use of the agent.

Box 3-7

- **Bleaching—suppression of the overproduction of melanin**
- **Blending—attaining a more even distribution of melanin to surrounding keratinocytes**

Box 3-8

Hydrocortisone suppresses the bleaching and blending effects of hydroquinone.

ing keratinocytes. The more even skin tone that can be obtained through blending supports its use for all hyperpigmentation problems. For faster and more effective results in treating hyperpigmentation, the bleaching step should be performed first, followed by blending. Hydrocortisone preparations should be avoided as much as possible, for they suppress both the "bleaching" and "blending" effects.

In very light skin with no pigmentation problems, the bleaching step in the Obagi Skin Restoration or Skin Conditioning programs can be omitted and only blending performed. However, when very light skin has the potential for PIH, as indicated by the presence of melasma, lentigo, or freckles, bleaching is helpful in addition to blending. Bleaching and blending are indicated for deviated (racially or ethnically mixed) white skin. Asian and Afro-American skin in the original color group (not racially mixed) needs a special approach to bleaching and blending that includes gradual discontinuation of bleaching when an even color tone has been obtained but a continuation of the blending step. However, for the same type of skin in the deviated (racially mixed) color group, including light and medium yellow and light and medium black, the bleaching step should be continued on a maintenance schedule (twice weekly for many months), after even skin color has been attained, while the blending step is continued daily, as before. The bleaching and blending should be continued longer in deviated skin than for other skin types, both before and after a procedure, such as the Blue Peel.

SAFETY OF HYDROQUINONE

Hydroquinone is the most effective and safest depigmenting agent available. Adverse effects usually do not occur, even after many years of use, and the incidence of allergic reactions is low when a 2% to 4% concentration is used. Patients about to start extended treatment should undergo a patch test with hydroquinone. Systemic absorption or toxicity from prolonged exposure to 2% to 4% topical concentrations has not been reported, and even if ingested accidentally, hydroquinone seldom produces systemic toxicity. This contrasts with depigmenting agents used in the past, such as mercurial compounds, which caused kidney damage, and monobenzone, which caused permanent melanocyte destruction.

Skin cancer has not been reported from the use of hydroquinone. It does not induce photosensitivity, but the lack of skin pigmentation will cause the skin to absorb more ultraviolet rays, and that leads to sun damage in the long term. Sun protection and sunscreens, preferably physical blockers, are recommended while hydroquinone is being used. Rarely, a high concentration of hydroquinone used for long periods can produce ochronosis, a blue-black hyperpigmentation reaction occurring in black-skinned people of certain tribal origins. The author has treated a few such cases with hydroquinone for bleaching and blending, along with a papillary dermis peel and Nd:YAG laser treatment, with excellent results.

OTHER DEPIGMENTING AGENTS

Inconsistent results or treatment failures in melasma and other forms of hyperpigmentation have led to efforts to find a substitute for hydroquinone. Kojic acid (and its ester kojic dipalmitate) and azelaic acid were introduced as new-generation alternatives to hydroquinone. The enthusiasm was short lived, however, and my personal experience with these agents has been disappointing. Overall, I have seen less than a 20% improvement in epidermal pigmentation with kojic acid, similar to what can be achieved with lactic acid, glycolic acid, or sunscreen alone. Improvement of melasma with azaleic acid is even less impressive. Because of their limited efficacy, kojic and azaleic acids cannot be considered as substitutes for hydroquinone.

Hydroquinone is the agent recommended for bleaching and blending in the Obagi Skin Health Restoration and Skin Conditioning programs. The best length of use of hydroquinone and its effectiveness when combined with other skin health products are discussed in Chapter 5.

Among various ways to enhance penetration of active materials such as hydroquinone, lipsomal encapsulation presents interesting immediate applications and the advantages of greater permeation, significant reduction or elimination of irritation, dosage optimization, sustained release at the epidermal level, and reduction of systemic absorption. Such formulations using low levels of hydroquinone can achieve activity equivalent to higher levels of hydroquinone response.

Kojic Acid

Kojic acid is related chemically to hydroquinone; it has a weaker tyrosinase inhibition property. Currently it is used as an alternative to hydroquinone to treat pigmentation disorders in individuals who are sensitive to hydroquinone. In a study comparing the efficacy of both combinations, hydroquinone/glycolic acid and kojic acid/glycolic acid proved to be effective in treating melasma; however, the latter combination proved to cause more irritation.[43]

Azeleic Acid

A naturally occurring saturated dicarboxylic acid, azeleic acid inhibits tyrosinase and hyperactive melanocytes. It is used in concentrations of 15% to 20% to treat hyperpigmentation and acne. It is well tolerated in the treatment of melasma, but it is not highly effective.[44]

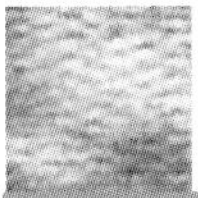

HYDROCORTISONE

Topical hydrocortisone 0.5% is the standard low-potency corticosteroid used to suppress inflammation during the Obagi Skin Health Restoration and Skin Conditioning program. Penetration of hydrocortisone can be affected by its vehicle. In general, occlusive petrolatum-based ointments are the most penetrating; creams, cosmetically more acceptable, are less efficient; alcohol-containing liquid solutions and gels are more irritating and less penetrating.[45] Skin thickness also affects hydrocortisone absorption; a thin skin absorbs a greater quantity of the agent in a shorter time.

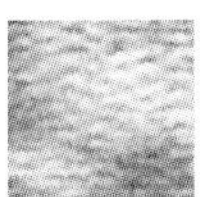

REFERENCES

1. Beauregard S, Gilchrest BA. A survey of skin problems and skin care regimens in the elderly. *Arch Dermatol.* 1987;123:1638–1643.
2. Kligman AM, Grove GL, Hirose R, Leyden JJ. Topical tretinoin for photoaged skin. *J Am Acad Dermatol.* 1986;15:836–859.
3. Weiss JS, Ellis CN, Headington JT, Voorhees JJ. Topical tretinoin in the treatment of aging skin. *J Am Acad Dermatol.* 1988;19:169–175.
4. Weiss JS, Ellis CN, Headington JT, et al. Topical tretinoin improves photoaged skin: a double-blind vehicle-controlled study. *JAMA.* 1988;259: 527–532.
5. Ellis CN, Weiss JS, Hamilton TA, et al. Sustained improvement with prolonged topical tretinoin (retinoic acid) for photoaged skin. *J Am Acad Dermatol.* 1990;23:629–637.
6. Weinstein GD, Nigra TP, Pochi PE, et al. Topical tretinoin for treatment of photodamaged skin: a multicenter study. *Arch Dermatol.* 1991;127: 659–665.

7. Olsen EA, Katz HI, Levine N, et al. Tretinoin emollient cream: a new therapy for photodamaged skin. *J Am Acad Dermatol.* 1992;26:215–224.

8. Griffiths CE, Russman AN, Majmudar G, et al. Restoration of collagen formation in photodamaged human skin by tretinoin (retinoic acid). *N Engl J Med* 1993;329:530–535.

9. Griffiths CE, Goldfarb MT, Finkel LJ, et al. Topical tretinoin (retinoic acid) treatment of hyperpigmented lesions associated with photoaging in Chinese and Japanese patients: a vehicle-controlled study. *J Am Acad Dermatol.* 1994;30:76–84.

10. Bhawan J, Gonzales-Serva A, Nehal K, et al. Effects of tretinoin on photodamaged skin. *Arch Dermatol.* 1991;127:666–672.

11. Moon TE, Levine N, Cartmel B, et al. Retinoids in the prevention of skin cancer. *Cancer Lett.* 1997;114:203–205.

12. Sankaranarayanan R, Matthew B. Retinoids as cancer-preventive agents. *IARC Sci Publ.* 1996;139:47–59.

13. Drake LA, Ceilley RI, Cornelison RL, et al. Guidelines of care for actinic keratoses. *J Am Acad Dermatol.* 1995;332:95–98.

14. Noble S, Wagstaff AJ. Tretinoin: a review of its pharmacological properties and clinical efficacy in the topical treatment of photodamaged skin. *Drugs Aging.* 1995;6:479–496.

15. Kang S, Kim KJ, Griffiths CE, et al. Topical tretinoin (retinoic acid) improves early stretch marks. *Arch Dermatol.* 1996;132:519–526.

16. Rafal ES, Griffiths CEM, Ditre CM, et al. Topical tretinoin (retinoic acid) treatment for liver spots associated with photodamage. *N Engl J Med.* 1992;326:368–374.

17. Bhawan J, Palko MJ, Lee J, et al. Reversible histologic effects of tretinoin on photodamaged skin. *J Geriatr Dermatol.* 1995;3:62–67.

18. Bhawan J, Olsen E, Lufrano L. Histologic evaluation of the long-term effects of tretinoin on photodamaged skin. *J Dermatol Sci.* 1996;11:177–182.

19. Draelos ZD. Photoaging, sunscreens, and cosmeceuticals. In: Draelos ZD, ed. *Cosmetics in Dermatology.* 2nd ed. New York, NY: Churchill Livingstone; 1995:233–244.

20. Mangelsdorf DJ, Umesono K, Evans RM. The retinoid receptors. In: Sporn MB, Roberts AB, Goodman DS, eds. *The Retinoids, Biology, Chemistry, and Medicine.* 2nd ed. New York, NY: Raven Press; 1994:319–349.

21. Goldfarb MT, Ellis CN, Weuss JS, Voorhees JJ. Topical tretinoin therapy and photoaged skin. *Cutis.* 1989;43:476–482.

22. Eichner R. Epidermal effects of retinoids: in vitro studies. *J Am Acad Dermatol.* 1986;15(suppl):789–797.

23. Zelickson AS, Mottaz JH, Weiss JS, et al. Topical tretinoin in photoaging: an ultrastructural study. *J Cutan Aging Cosmet Dermatol.* 1988;1:41–47.

24. Kligman AM. Topical retinoic acid (tretinoin) for photoaging: conceptions and misconceptions. *Cutis.* 1996;57:142–144.

25. Hevia O, Nemeth AJ, Taylor R. Tretinoin accelerates healing after trichloroacetic acid chemical peel. *Arch Dermatol.* 1991;127:678–682.

26. Kim IH, Kim HK, Kye YC. Effects of tretinoin pretreatment on TCA chemical peel in guinea pig skin. *J Korean Med Sci.* 1996;11:335–341.

27. Leyden JJ. Retin-A for wrinkles inactivated by aldehydes. *Skin and Allergy News.* 1988;19:3.

28. Van Scott EJ, Yu RJ. Hyperkeratinization, corneocyte collusion, and alpha hydroxy acids. *J Am Acad Dermatol.* 1984;5:867–879.

29. Van Scott EJ, Yu RJ. Alpha hydroxy acids: procedures for use in clinical practice. *Cutis.* 1989;43:222–229.

30. Van Scott EJ, Yu RJ. Alpha hydroxy acids: therapeutic potentials. *Can J Dermatol.* 1989;1:108–112.

31. Murad H, Shamban AT, Premo PS. The use of glycolic acid as a peeling agent. *Dermatol Clin.* 1995;13:285–307.

32. Moy LS, Murad H, Moy RL. Glycolic acid peels for the treatment of wrinkles and photoaging. *J Dermatol Surg Oncol.* 1993;19:243–246.

33. Piacquadio D, Dobry M, Hunt S, et al. Short contact glycolic acid peels as a treatment for photodamaged skin: a pilot study. *Dermatol Surg.* 1996;22:449–452.

34. DiNardo JC, Grove GL, Moy LS. Clinical and histological effects of glycolic acid at different concentrations and pH levels. *Dermatol Surg.* 1996;22:421–424.

35. Coleman WP, Futrell JM. The glycolic acid trichloroacetic acid peel. *J Dermatol Surg Oncol.* 1994;20:76–80.

36. Draelos ZD. Dermatologic considerations of AHAs. *Cosmet Dermatol.* 1997;10:14–18.

37. Daniello NJ. Glycolic acid controversies. *Int J Aesthetic Restor Surg.* 1996;4:113–116.

38. Newman NN, Newman A, Moy LS, et al. Clinical improvement of photoaged skin with 50% glycolic acid. *Dermatol Surg.* 1996;22:455–460.

39. Moy LS, Howe K, Moy RL. Glycolic acid modulation of collagen production in human skin fibroblast culture in vitro. *Dermatol Surg.* 1996;22:439–441.

40. Lavker RM, Kaidbey K, Leyden JJ. Effects of topical ammonium lactate on cutaneous atrophy resulting from a potent topical corticosteroid. *J Am Acad Dermatol.* 1992;26:535–544.

41. Perricone NV, DiNardo JC. Photoprotective and anti-inflammatory effects of topical glycolic acid. *Dermatol Surg.* 1996;22:435–437.

42. Gilman AG, Goodman LS, Gilman A. *The Pharmacologic Basis of Therapeutics.* 6th ed. New York, NY: Macmillan; 1980:959.

43. Garcia A, Fulton JE Jr. The combination of glycolic acid and hydroquinone or kojic acid for the treatment of melasma and related conditions. *Dermatol Surg.* 1996;22:443–447.

44. Grimes PE. Melasma: etiologic and therapeutic considerations. *Arch Dermatol.* 1995;131:1453–1457.

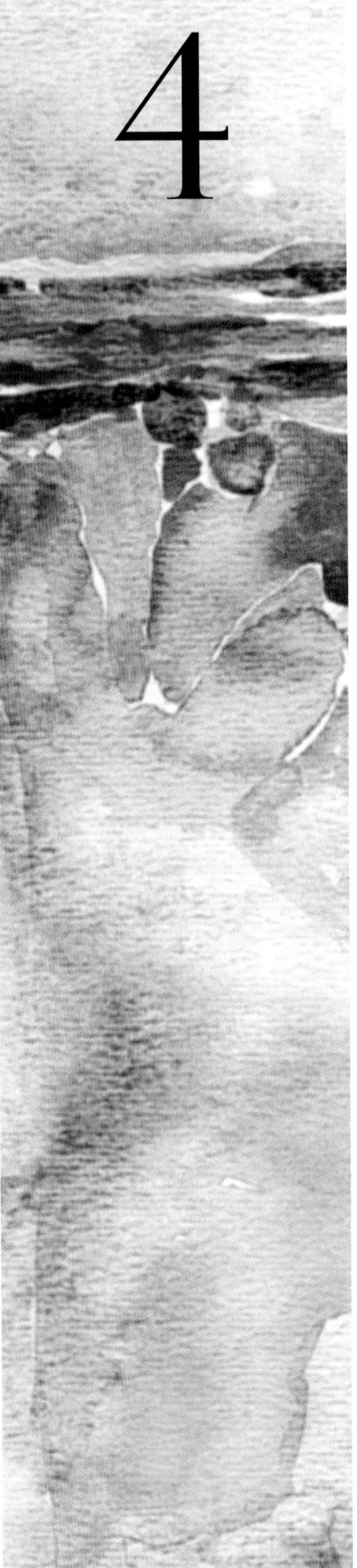

SKIN CLASSIFICATION

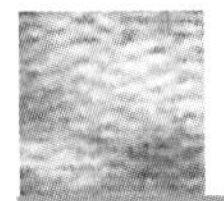

SKIN CLASSIFICATION SYSTEMS

EXISTING SYSTEMS

Clinical appearance and skin color are the bases for classifying skin in existing classification systems. While these systems have been helpful in providing a common language for treatment, teaching, and the reporting of study results, they have not contributed valuable practical information toward the selection of an appropriate rejuvenation procedure for a particular patient. They do not take into account factors relevant to skin rejuvenation procedures, such as: 1) the appropriate procedure for a specific skin type, 2) the depth of procedure that will give the most improvement while maintaining natural appearance, 3) the kind of conditioning needed for different skin types before and after a procedure, and 4) the reactions to anticipate postoperatively and their treatment.

The Fitzpatrick skin classification system (Table 4-1)[1] links skin color to a response to ultraviolet light, a connection which is beneficial since it is known that skin color determines a patient's suitability for skin rejuvenation procedures. Fitzpatrick skin types I to III have been considered the ideal skin types for these procedures, while types IV through VI have been considered the more difficult types because of the high incidence of postinflammatory hyperpigmentation (PIH), and the possibility that a procedure will permanently change skin color.

Another skin classification system, developed by Glogau,[2] groups skin into four possible types from the standpoint of the presence of sun damage, wrinkling, and acne scarring. This system is useful in classifying patients according to their degree of photodamage, wrinkling, and scarring, but it does not help in selecting the procedure or treatment needed for each group or help in the prediction of a patient's response to different levels of depth of chemical peeling or other procedures.

A photonumeric scale has been developed for assessing the improvement of photodamaged skin following treatment compared with its condition at baseline.[3] This scale was developed in response to the difficulty of obtaining standardized photographs of patients pre- and posttreatment. It enables even subtle changes to be appreciated and graded similarly by more than one observer. The system uses a 9-point scale in which 0 equals no photodamage and 8 equals severe photodamage. For standardization purposes, photographs were selected to illustrate grades 0, 2, 4, 6, and 8. The standards were developed based on their ability to demonstrate the easily photographable (nontactile) factors of photodamage, such as coarse and fine wrinkles, dyspigmentation, elastosis, etc. The authors of the study believe the main role of this system will be to help increase interobserver agreement in categorizing groups of patients prior to and after treatment for skin repair in multicenter studies.

TABLE 4.1

FITZPATRICK CLASSIFICATION OF SUN-REACTIVE SKIN TYPES

Skin Type	*Color*	*Reaction to First Sun Exposure*
I	White	Always burns, never tans
II	White	Usually burns, tans with difficulty
III	White	Sometimes mild burn, tan average
IV	Moderate brown	Rarely burns, tans with ease
V	Dark brown	Very rarely burns, tans very easily
VI	Black	No burns, tans very easily

THE EVOLUTION OF THE OBAGI SYSTEM

The Obagi Skin Classification System is an integral part of the Skin Conditioning and Skin Health Restoration programs. This system arose from the realization in 1981 that guidelines were needed to control for various factors so that TCA peels could be performed more accurately. The resulting current Obagi Skin Classification System takes into consideration a number of variables and their relevance to 1) pre- and postoperative skin conditioning, 2) reaction to procedures, and 3) postprocedure management (Table 4-2).

TABLE 4.2

RELEVANCE OF VARIABLES IN OBAGI SKIN CLASSIFICATION SYSTEM

Skin Variable	*Pre- and Postprocedure Skin Conditioning*	*Suitable Procedures and Potential Reactions to Procedure (TCA peel, dermabrasion, CO_2 laser)*	*Postprocedure Management*
Color	Darker skin: Aggressive conditioning before procedure and after healing to minimize PIH	Hypopigmentation: • Light procedures: rare • Medium-depth procedures: possible Hyperpigmentation: common • More likely	Dark skin: Condition aggressively to minimize PIH
Oiliness	Interferes with effectiveness of preprocedure conditioning.	Topical treatment needed to reduce surface oil prior to procedure	Intereferes with effectiveness of postprocedure conditioning. Topical treatment needed to reduce surface oil
Thickness	Thick skin needs correction and stimulation; thin skin needs more stimulation (further details in Chapter 5)	Thick skin: best for chemical peels, dermabrasion Medium-thick skin: best for TCA peels, dermabrasion, CO_2 laser Thin skin: lighter procedures such as Blue Peel: erbium resurfacing	Correction and stimulation, as needed
Laxity	Long-term stimulation to prevent further laxity	Skin laxity: medium-depth peel or several Blue Peels are ideal Muscle laxity: face-lift, alone or combined with a Blue Peel to correct associated skin laxity, may be needed	Correction and stimulation, as needed
Fragility	Aggressive stimulation to strengthen the skin	Correlates with postsurgical scarring. In fragile skin, procedure depth should be limited to papillary dermis	More cycles of correction and stimulation, as tolerated

PIH = postinflammatory hyperpigmentation

TABLE 4.3	
OBAGI SKIN COLOR TYPES	
Skin Color Category	***Stability during Procedures and Treatments***
Original (not racially or ethnically mixed)	Stable
Deviated (racially or ethnically mixed)	Moderately stable
Complex (e.g., South Asian, Latino-Indian)	Extremely unstable

For example, a given variable may have a high degree of relevance to preoperative skin conditioning but less relevance to postoperative management.

SKIN TYPE ACCORDING TO COLOR

The Fitzpatrick system proved to be inadequate after various new skin treatments and rejuvenation procedures were developed because patients in the same Fitzpatrick group may react differently to a given procedure and because ethnic background, not discussed in the Fitzpatrick system, can profoundly affect the outcome of treatments. For example, Asian and African-American patients, who are both classified in the Fitzpatrick type V category, do not react in the same fashion to the same treatments and procedures. Similarly, White type III and light Asian type III skin types respond differently to procedures, and PIH (postinflammatory hyperpigmentation) is more likely to occur in the Asian patients. The Obagi Skin Classification system divides skin color into Original, Deviated, and Complex categories that relate to their stability during treatments and procedures, thus providing for a more detailed and useful skin classification system (Table 4-3).

Original Skin Color Category

The Original skin color type is found in persons who are not racially or ethnically mixed (Table 4-4, Figures 4-1–4-3), and is stable after most rejuvenation procedures. Melanocytes reappear and resume their normal function after healing has been completed, and skin returns to its original color. There may be short-lived PIH, but this responds rapidly to treatment. Light White, dark Black, and dark Asian (yellow) are original skin colors.

The exception to this is when Original skin color undergoes deep procedures (below the immediate reticular dermis [IRD]), such as phenol peels, medium-depth TCA peels, CO_2 laser resurfacing, and dermabrasion, that produce variable degrees of melanocyte destruction and subsequent textural changes, resulting in lighter color tone. This occurs quite commonly after such deep procedures.

When the Obagi Skin Classification System is compared with the Fitzpatrick system, a given skin type may overlap (have characteristics of) the

TABLE 4.4

OBAGI CLASSIFICATION: ORIGINAL SKIN COLOR TYPES

Original Color Type	*Corresponding Fitzpatrick Type*	*Description*
Very Light and Light White	I, II	Very light in color; does not tan; possibly light freckles; unprotected areas chronically exposed to sun commonly show telangiectasia, redness, actinic keratoses, and other forms of photodamage
Normal White	III, IV, V	White; tans well; pigmentary skin problems common; photodamage changes commonly seen
Dark (jet) Black	VI	Very dark, sun-exposed and nonexposed areas are mostly similar in color
Dark Asian	V	"Brownish" color. Mildly darker in areas exposed to the sun

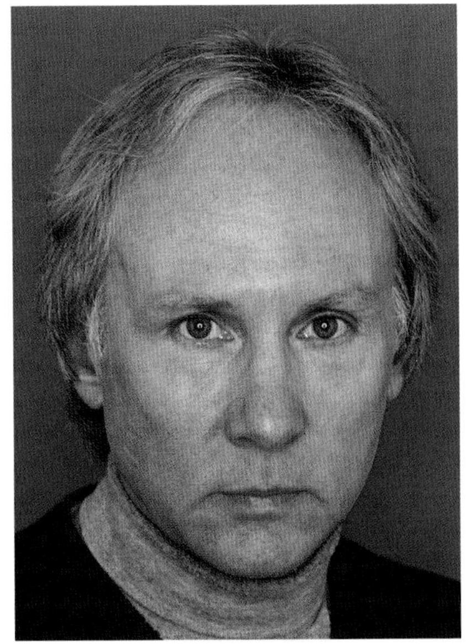

FIGURE 4-1. *Original White skin type (Light).*

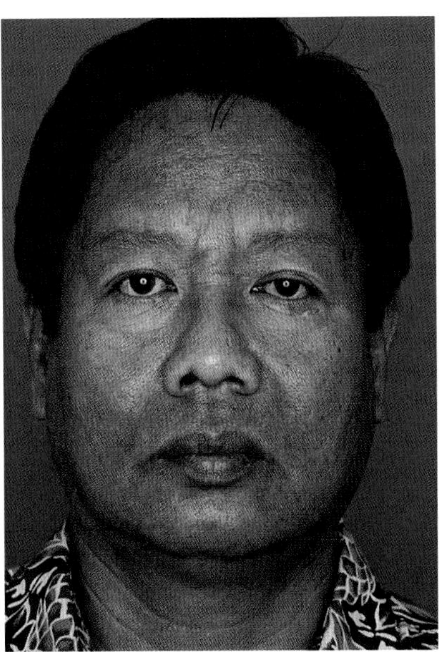

FIGURE 4-2. *Original Asian skin type (Dark).*

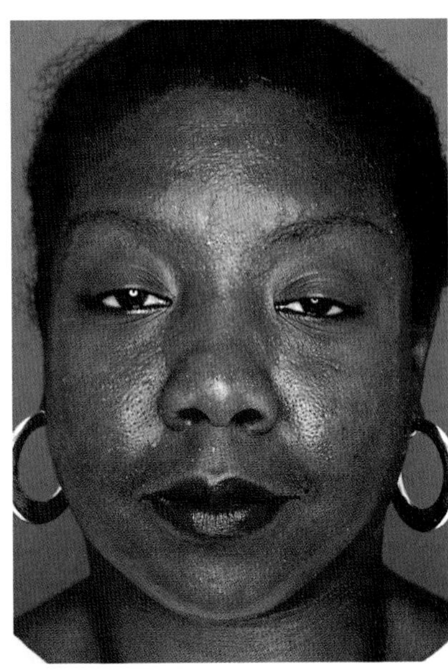

FIGURE 4-3. *Original African-American skin type (Dark).*

type preceding or immediately following it. In certain circumstances, this may be beneficial to the outcome of the procedure. For example, if a patient with deviated Fitzpatrick type I skin has some Fitzpatrick type II skin characteristics, he or she may respond to a procedure like a patient who has skin in the Original category, i.e., more favorably because Original type skin usually responds better to procedures than the deviated type. This explains why it is wrong to assume that persons in the Fitzpatrick darker skin groups will be more difficult to treat than lighter-skinned individuals.

Skin conditioning before and after a procedure must be performed in a specific way for each Obagi color group. The Light White group needs 1 skin cycle of conditioning, while the dark-skinned groups may need 2 to 3 cycles. After the procedure, all color groups need at least 1 cycle to stabilize skin color, and the darker-skin groups may need 2 to 3 cycles.

Deviated Skin Color Category

The Deviated skin type is found in persons who are racially or ethnically mixed. Their skin color is unstable and more sensitive to the effects of procedures, and this skin takes longer than skin in the Original category to return to its natural color after a procedure. Furthermore, while procedures that reach below the IRD, such as phenol peels, deep TCA peels, deep CO_2 laser resurfacing, and dermabrasion, produce variable degrees of melanocyte reduction or destruction and a lighter color tone in all skin types, they are even more likely to lighten skin color in the Deviated category. Skin darkening in the form of PIH is also more likely, and it may persist longer and require more aggressive bleaching and blending.

As can be seen in Figure 4-4 and Tables 4-5 and 4-6, Asian, Black, and White Fitzpatrick skin types fall along a spectrum of Original to Deviated

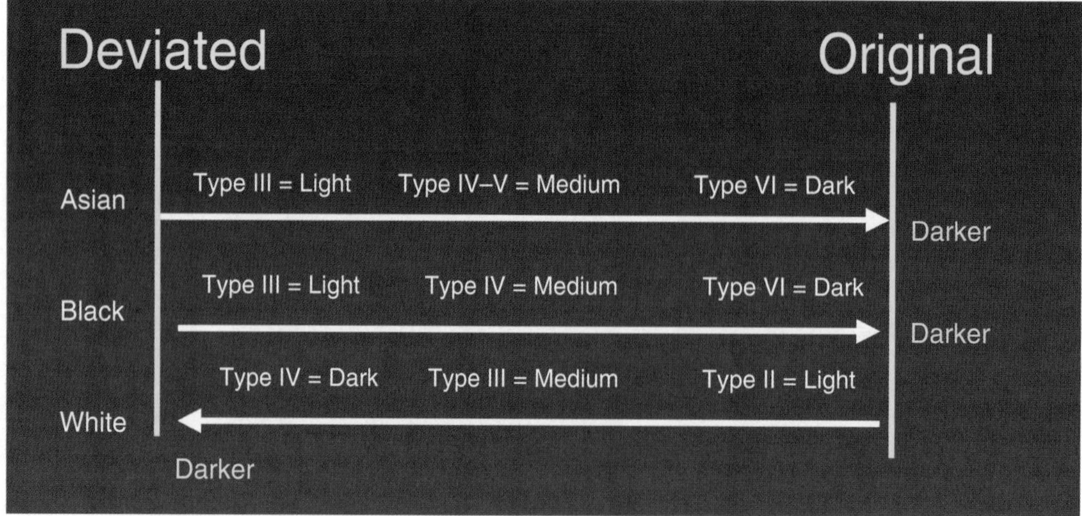

FIGURE 4-4. *Spectrum of Original to Deviated Fitzpatrick skin types in Asian, Black, and White Skin. In Asian skin, dark yellow is the original type and the skin becomes more deviated as it gets lighter. In Black skin, dark black is the original type and the skin becomes more deviated as it gets lighter. In White skin, the original is light and the skin becomes more deviated as it gets darker.*

TABLE 4.5

RELATIONSHIP OF OBAGI SKIN COLOR TYPES AND FITZPATRICK COLOR TYPES IN DEVIATED SKIN

Obagi Deviated Color Type	*Fitzpatrick Type*					
	Type I	*Type II*	*Type III*	*Type IV*	*Type V*	*Type VI*
Dark White[1]	5%	—	90%	5%	—	—
Brunette	—	—	5%	90%	5%	—
Light and Medium Asian	—	10%	40%	40%	10%	—
Light and Medium Black (AA)	—	—	25%	50%	25%	—

[1]For example, in the Fitzpatrick system, the Obagi Dark White Color Type would be classified as type III in 90% of the cases, and either type I or IV in the rest of the cases.

types. The original types of Asian and Black skin are dark—dark yellow for Asian and dark black for African-American (AA)—and the lighter the skin, the more deviated it is within these categories. The more highly deviated the Asian or Black skin, the greater the tendency for postprocedure pigmentary changes such as PIH. With White skin, the original type is light, and the darker the skin, the more deviated it is within the White category. Examples of White, Asian, and Black Deviated skin types are shown in Figures 4-5 to 4-10. In persons with the Deviated Black skin type, considerable variation in color tone can be seen on the face and hands (Figure 4-11).

Patients with skin in the Deviated color categories need more aggressive conditioning before undergoing a procedure and should have a procedure only after color has been controlled and tolerance has been achieved, which is usually after 1 to 3 skin conditioning cycles. The physician should not wait for PIH to appear before starting postprocedure treatment. Bleaching and blending in the most aggressive form warranted (aggressive to moderately aggressive, as needed) should begin immediately after healing. The patient should be informed in advance that 1 to 2 cycles will probably be needed after the procedure to stabilize skin color.

TABLE 4.6

RELATIONSHIP OF OBAGI SKIN COLOR TYPES AND FITZPATRICK COLOR TYPES IN COMPLEX SKIN

	Fitzpatrick Type					
	Type I	*Type II*	*Type III*	*Type IV*	*Type V*	*Type VI*
Obagi Complex Type	—	—	—	35%	50%	15%

In the Fitzpatrick system, the Obagi Complex Type would be classified as type IV (35% of cases), type V (50% of cases), or type VI (15% of cases).

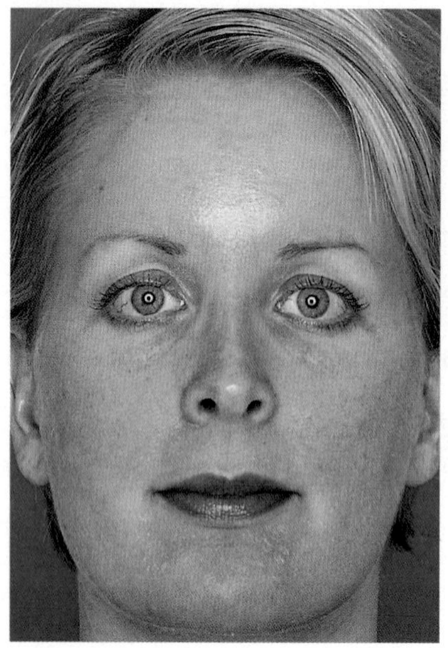

Figure 4-5. *Deviated White skin type: Light White.*

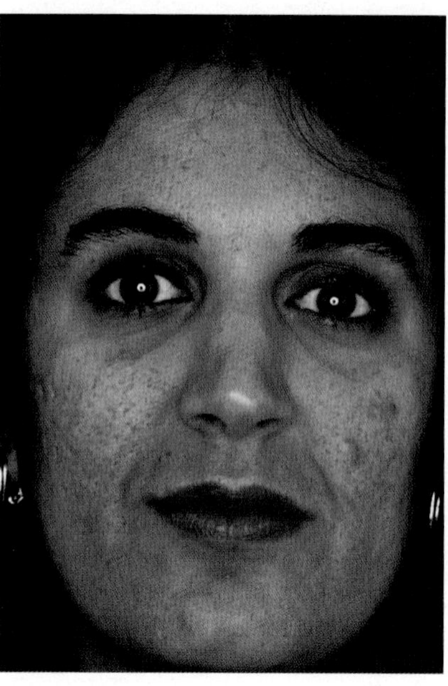

Figure 4-6. *Deviated White skin type: Dark White (Brunette).*

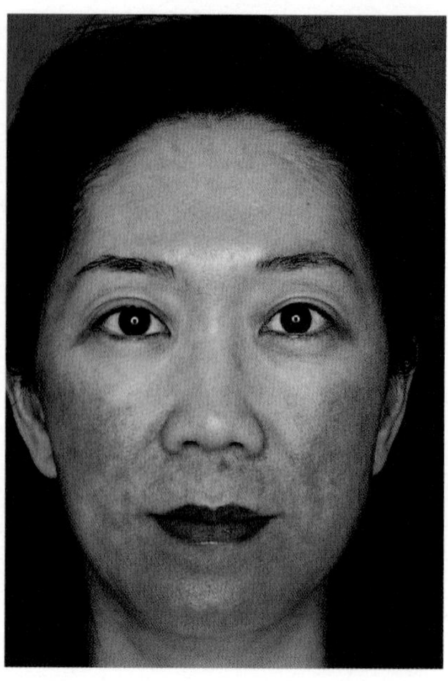

Figure 4-7. *Deviated Asian skin type: Light Asian.*

Complex Skin Color Category

Skin in the Complex color category is variable, dark in some areas and lighter in others, and is extremely unstable and photosensitive (Figure 4-12). This kind of skin naturally has an uneven, variable skin color tone that is accentuated by sun exposure and tanning. Examples include per-

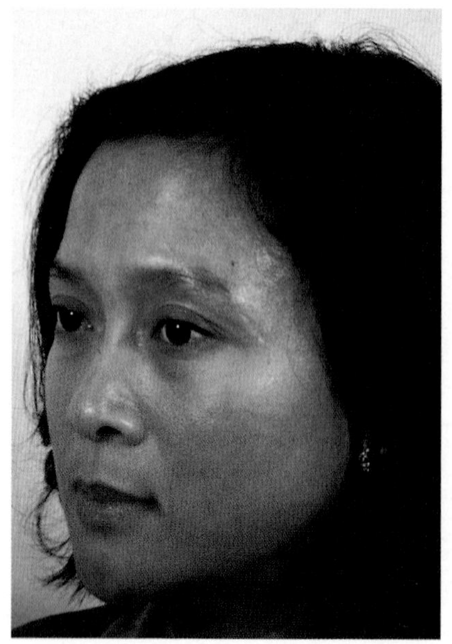

Figure 4-8. *Deviated Asian skin type: Medium Asian.*

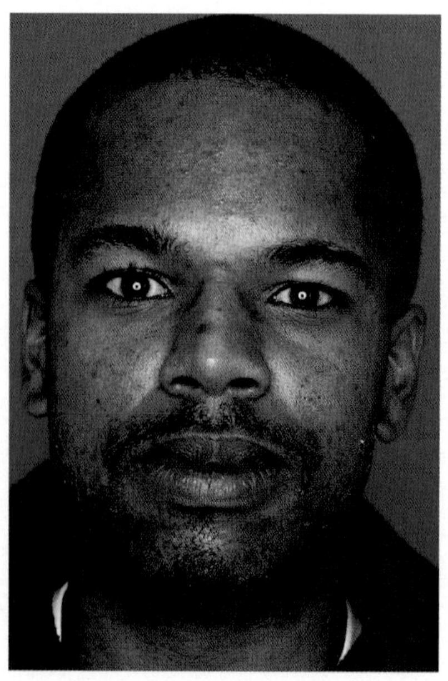

Figure 4-9. *Deviated Black skin type: Medium Black (AA).*

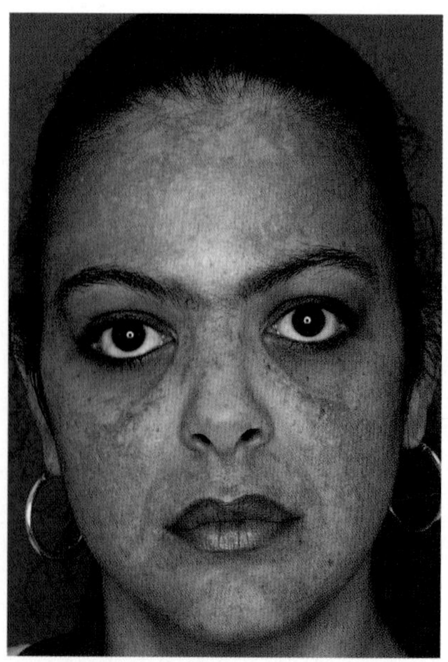

Figure 4-10. *Deviated Black skin type: Light Black (AA).*

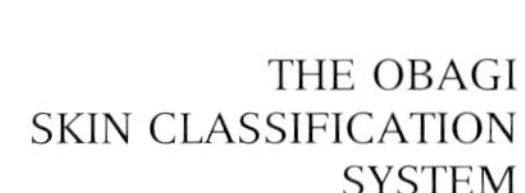

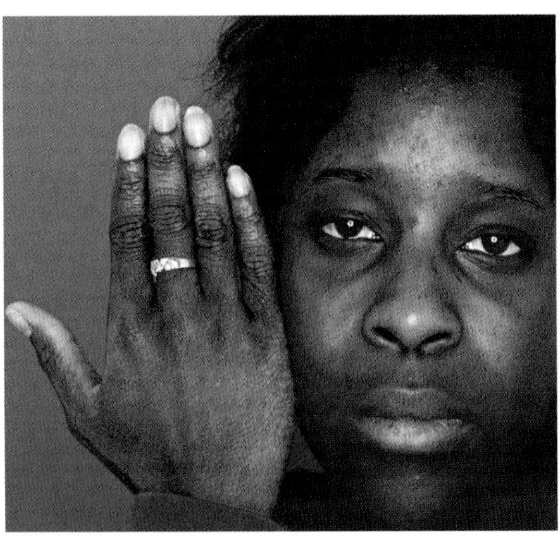

FIGURE 4-11. *Deviated Black skin type showing variation in color depth on face and hands.*

sons of South Asian and Amerindian ethnic origin and some persons of mixed racial origin. Most people in the Complex category fall into Fitzpatrick type V, but some are type IV or VI (Table 4-6). Certain patients have a combination of all 3 Fitzpatrick types.

Patients with skin in the Complex category need 2 to 3 cycles of aggressive skin conditioning to stabilize color before a procedure. They usually have severe and long-lasting PIH following a procedure despite adherence to a postprocedure conditioning program. Hypopigmentation can also occur, and therefore, procedures in these patients should not reach deeper than the IRD. Skin must be feathered during a procedure to prevent demarcation lines. These patients should be told in advance that it will take some time for their skin to return to normal after a procedure.

Table 4-7 outlines the different types of reactions to skin conditioning and rejuvenation procedures that occur in the various skin color types.

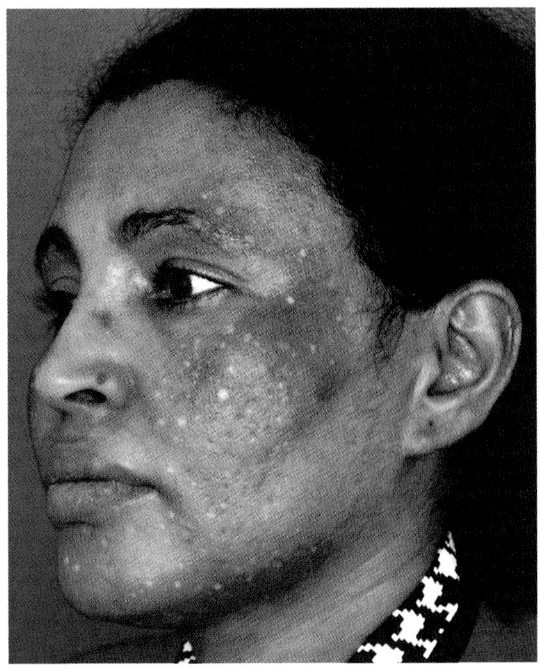

FIGURE 4-12. *Complex skin type: South American Indian.*

TABLE 4.7

VARIABILITY OF REACTIONS TO SKIN CONDITIONING AND PROCEDURES IN DIFFERENT SKIN COLOR TYPES

Skin Color	*Reaction to Skin Conditioning of 4–6 Weeks*	*Reaction 2–6 Weeks Postprocedure*	*Recommended Care following Procedures*	*Reactions with Increasing Depth*	*Long-Term Effects/ General Comments*
White: 1. Very Light White, 2. Light White, 3. Normal White	1. very red 2–3. red	1–2. Redness lasts longer 3. Often back to normal	1. Very Light and 2. Light White: sunscreen and moisturizer; 3. Normal White: conditioning regimen with the standard approach of bleaching and blending	More depth = more redness	All White Categories: redness may last 6 months or more in Very Light skin, esp. after CO_2 laser
Brunette: 1. Light; 2. Dark	All Brunette categories: variable redness	1. Light Brunette: mild PIH 2. Darker Brunette: moderate PIH	All Brunette categories: sun-screen essential; aggressive bleaching and blending	1–2. More depth = more PIH 1–2. More depth = possible hypopigmentation	Dark Brunette: Lighter procedures are recommended. With deeper procedures hypopigmentation possible
Asian (yellow): 1. Light Yellow, 2. Medium Yellow, 3. Dark Yellow	All Asian categories: Variable redness;	Light & medium: strong PIH, common, dark, Mild to strong PIH	All Asian categories: sunscreen essential; aggressive bleaching and blending	1–2. More depth = more PIH 3. More depth = more hypopigmentation	All Asian categories: spot peels to correct Persistent PIH may be needed & longer time & more aggressive reconditioning
Black (AA): 1. Light Black, 2. Medium Black 3. Dark Black	Loss of tan: some red-ness Loss of tan; not red	1–2. Deviated Black: strong PIH 3. Dark Black: mild to strong PIH	All Black categories: Bleaching Bleaching Reduce bleaching when skin color is even (to twice a week) continue with blending for 1–2 cycles (daily)	More depth = more PIH More depth = possible hypopigmentation	All Black categories lighter color tone can persist for 6–12 months; spot peels to correct persistent PIH may be needed Less bleaching (short period) More blending (stronger & longer period)

PIH = postinflammatory hyperpigmentation

Box 4-1

Conditioning of dark skin needs to be stronger and to be continued longer than conditioning of light skin.

SKIN TYPE ACCORDING TO THICKNESS

Skin thickness is determined genetically and can be categorized into 1) thin, 2) medium-thick, 3) thick, and 4) hamartomatous (Figures 4-13, 4-14). Distinctions between each type are not clear-cut and must be made by clinical examination of firmness, tightness, bulkiness, and the ease with which the skin can be folded by the action of underlying muscles.

An individual's skin thickness varies with anatomical location. For example, the epidermis and papillary dermis are of approximately the same thickness in all anatomical locations, the stratum corneum is thickest in the palms and soles, and the dermis is thickest on the back and thin on the eyelids. As expected, the skin of the face varies in thickness, depending on the location: In each skin thickness category in general, cheeks are thicker

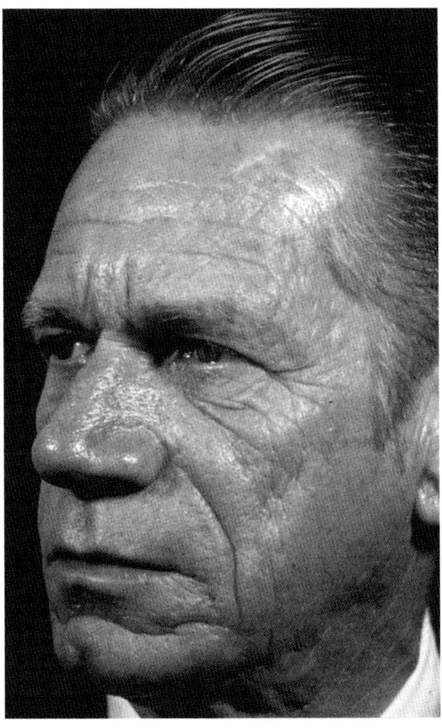

FIGURE **4-13.** *Patient with very thick skin (kamartomatous). Notice enlarged pores; dominant dynamic lines.*

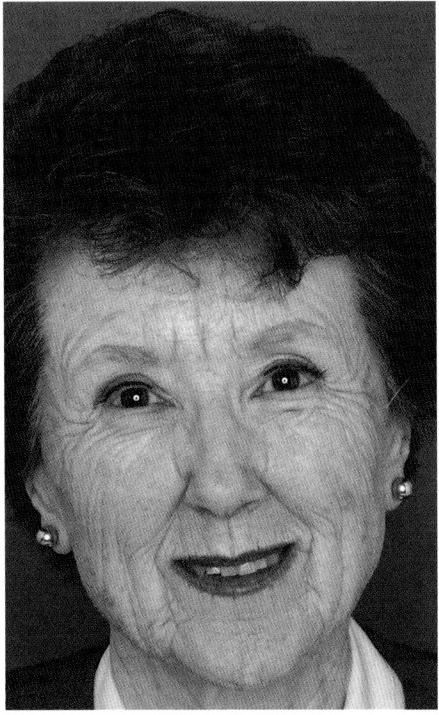

FIGURE **4-14.** *Patient with thin skin. Skin appears thick due to solar elastosis. Notice skin is poor with adnexal structures (pores hardly visible); exaggerated dynamic lines.*

Box 4-2

Skin thickness has an influence on:

- **strength and duration of skin conditioning**
- **selection of a procedure and procedure depth**
- **predictability of procedure results**
- **suitability of skin for a certain depth or repeated procedure**
- **the chance of complications (permanent color changes and scarring)**

relative to the rest of the face, the forehead varies, and the jawline is thinner than the cheeks. Eyelid skin in every patient is thin. Skin thickness is not related to the fullness of appearance, which is due to the thickness of the underlying subcutaneous layer and the amount of fat deposits. Efforts have been made to standardize the measurement of skin thickness through biopsies, ultrasound, and other methods, but results have been inconclusive.

There are racial differences in skin thickness. In my observation, Blacks have predominantly thick or medium-thick skin, while Asians are more likely to have medium-thick skin. The skin of Whites can vary widely in thickness, with some having fairly thick skin and others such as very fair, or many red-haired persons having very thin skin with visible blood vessels. Men have thicker skin than women in all racial groups.

Determination of Skin Thickness

Expression Lines: Expression lines (dynamic lines) are folds in the skin seen when the underlying muscles contract during expression (Figure 4-15), lifting of the eyebrows (Figure 4-16), smiling (Figure 4-17), or pursing the lips (Figure 4-18). They are more prominent in persons with thin skin and in thin skin areas of a particular individual, such as the periorbital and perioral areas, the forehead, and the cheeks. Skin thickness can be determined by evaluating the extent of the folds made with facial expression. Ask the patient to contract a muscle or muscle group to the extreme by frowning, smiling, lifting the eyebrows, pursing the lips as if whistling, etc. Observe for the following: 1) the width of the "mountains" and depth of the "valleys," 2) the degree of extension of fold length, and 3) the appearance when the muscle is relaxed.

Expression folds (the "mountains") are a result of underlying muscle contraction. In thin skin, the folds are thin, 2 to 4 mm wide, and numerous, 6 to 10 in each location. The valleys are shallow: 2 to 3 mm deep. The folds extend beyond the anatomical location of the muscle to the surrounding skin. They

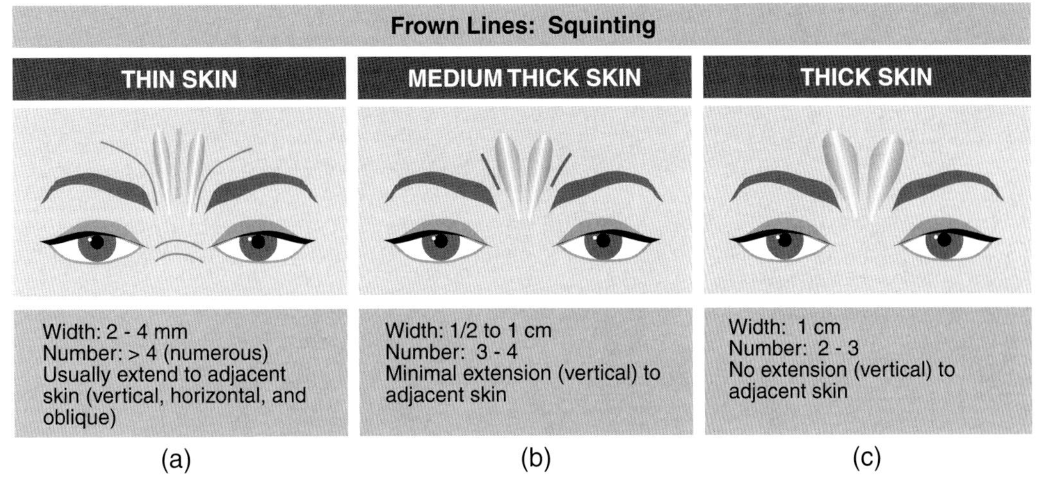

FIGURE 4-15 a, b, c. *Effect of skin thickness on expression lines of patients while frowning (squinting lines).*

can be made to appear without extreme muscle contraction (i.e., with only mild expression) and are present at a trace level when the muscles are relaxed.

In skin of medium thickness, the folds are 5 to 10 mm wide, with deeper valleys (5 to 10 mm). There are 2 to 4 folds in each anatomical location that extend just slightly beyond the muscle location to the surrounding skin. Some expression effort is required to make the folds appear, and they are not apparent when the muscles are relaxed.

Thick skin has fewer folds (1 to 3) which are 1 to 2 cm wide and do not extend to the surrounding skin beyond the anatomical location of the muscle. The valleys are 4 to 6 mm deep. Effort is required to make folds

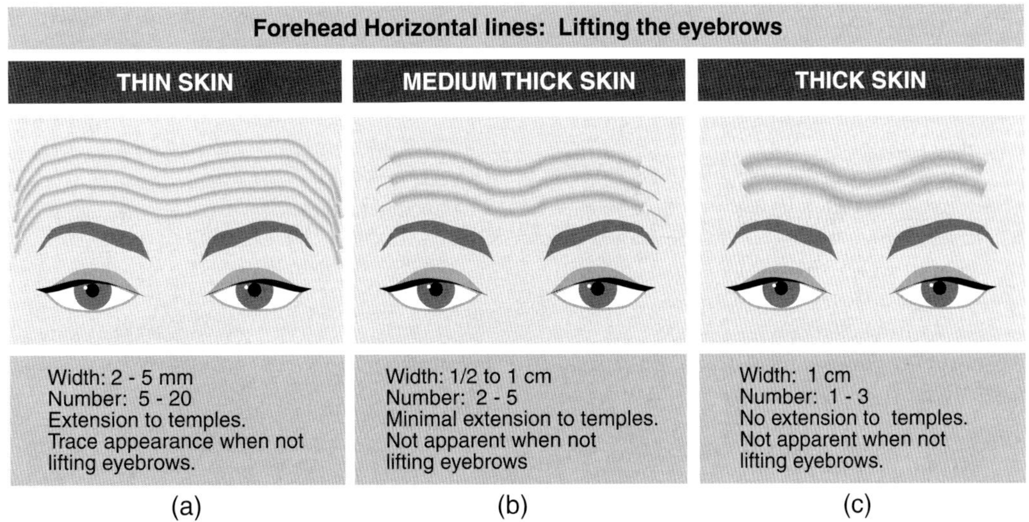

FIGURE 4-16 a, b, c. *Effect of skin thickness on expression lines of patients while lifting eyebrows (horizontal forehead lines).*

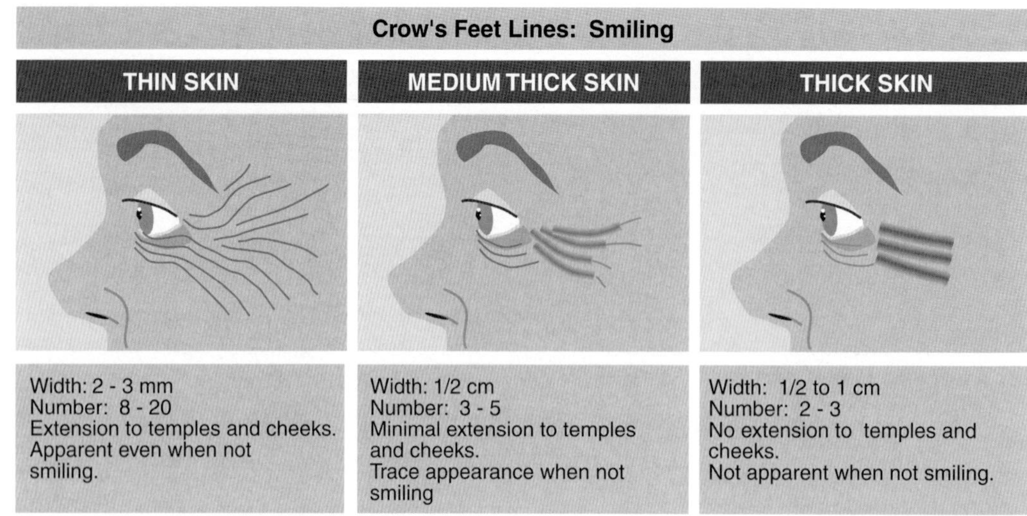

FIGURE 4-17 a, b, c. *Effect of skin thickness on expression lines of patients while smiling (crow's-feet).*

in thick skin appear, and the folds are not apparent when the muscles are relaxed. Longstanding dynamic lines may be present even without facial expression, as the skin texture is changed by the prolonged underlying muscle action (ironing effects). In summary, skin is considered thin if a clip reveals a fold thinner or less than 1 cm thick; medium if a clip reveals a fold 1 to $1^1/_2$ cm thick; and thick if a clip reveals a fold more than $1^1/_2$ cm thick.

Skin Pinching: Thickness of skin can also be determined by pinching the skin instead of using a clip to determine the thickness of the folds. Grasp the skin with the thumb and index finger and pull it away slightly. The pinched fold will be less than 1 cm in thin skin, 1–$1^1/_2$ cm in medium-thick skin, and more than $1^1/_2$ cm in thick skin.

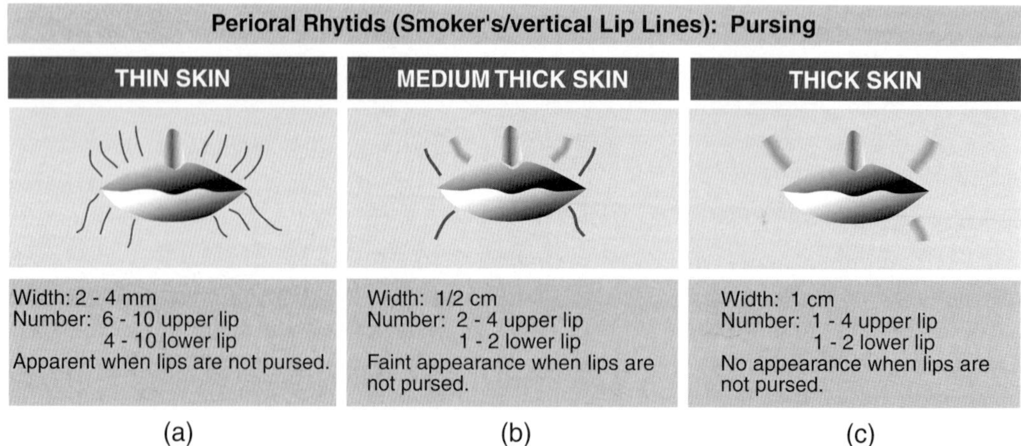

FIGURE 4-18 a, b, c. *Effect of skin thickness on perioral rhytids of cigarette smokers.*

Box 4-3

Quick Identification of Skin Thickness: Skin thickness is a range, not one specific measurement. The ranges are very thin to thin, thin to medium, medium to thick, and thick to very thick. Measured by skin pinching or using a clip to grasp a skin fold, the scale is as follows:

- **Very thin skin = Fold less than $1/2$ cm in thickness**
- **Thin skin = Fold less than 1 cm in thickness**
- **Medium thin skin = Fold between 1 and $1\,1/2$ cm in thickness**
- **Thick skin = Fold more than $1\,1/2$ cm in thickness**

These measurements are an approximation.

Box 4-4

During the aging process:

- **thick skin sags more than it wrinkles; wrinkles appear late**
- **thin skin wrinkles more than it sags; wrinkles appear early**

Clinical Evaluation: Thin skin is only weakly firm, usually translucent with some visible blood vessels (including telangiectasia), and is poor in adnexal structures. In thin skin, jowling is minimal, while wrinkling is common at an early age. The face has extreme expression lines that appear easily when the person expresses him- or herself. Pushing the skin gently with your hand in one direction can create many folds.

Skin of medium thickness is firmer, does not usually show underlying blood vessels, and is moderate or rich in adnexal structures. With aging, both jowling and wrinkling are common. Expression lines do not extend markedly to adjacent skin and folds are not easily created by pushing.

Thick skin is the most firm, has no visible underlying blood vessels and is moderate or rich in adnexal structures. Jowling is usually the first sign of aging and wrinkles usually follow but to a lesser degree than in medium-thick skin. Expression lines do not extend to adjacent skin, and the skin does not fold when pushed. Instead, it will bulge and form a pouch.

Hamartomatous skin is abnormally very thick, glabrous, and hyperplastic. Hyperplasia or adenomas of the sebaceous glands are common, as are rough texture, large pores, and density of adnexal structures. All of the features of thick skin are exaggerated in hamartomatous skin. Hamartomatous skin may occur together with thick skin, as in the case of a person with rhinophyma of the nose. In these patients, with aging skin sagginess is predominant, while wrinkles are minimal.

Relevance of Skin Thickness

Effect of Skin Thickness on Skin Conditioning: Skin thickness influences many aspects of a skin conditioning and skin health restoration programs. With thin skin, the goal is to increase skin thickness and to build up the dermis for firmness, tightness, and longer postprocedure effect. Long-term skin stimulation (action on the dermis and basal epidermis) is required to accomplish this. Medium-thick and thick skin needs a moderately aggressive approach with emphasis on stimulation to help to smooth the skin surface, tighten large pores, and maintain firmness. Long-term stimulation of thick skin to keep pores small and maintain skin firmness can be delivered by alternating 1 cycle of an aggressive approach using enhanced retinoic acid with 3 to 4 cycles of a slow, twice weekly maintenance approach.

Effect of Skin Thickness on Skin Rejuvenation Procedures: As discussed in Chapter 7, the goal of rejuvenation procedures can vary: 1) to produce leveling (CO_2 laser, dermabrasion, medium deep peels), 2) tightening (Blue Peel) and exfoliation (Blue Peel, AHA peel), 3) dermal matrix build-up (from stimulation with topical creams), 4) filling (fat injection), or 5) immobilization (Botox) effects. Thin skin is ideal for a tightening effect. Leveling procedures, on the other hand, are risky in thin skin for they may make it even thinner and accelerate aging in the long term.

Thin Skin: Procedures in thin skin should not exceed the IRD in depth. This depth will provide sufficient tightening and mild leveling and will not make the skin thinner or most likely change its color. The procedure can be repeated at intervals of 6–8 weeks or longer for gradual improvement. If a thin-skinned patient needs leveling for deep wrinkles or scars, CO_2 laser resurfacing is safer than a medium-depth peel or dermabrasion for the inexperienced physician. The treatment should be restricted to the affected areas and reach to the upper reticular dermis only. The rest of the face should be blended with a tightening procedure, such as the Blue Peel. Aggressive leveling should be avoided because it is safer to perform a second procedure later, if necessary. Thin skin is not suitable for leveling procedures or facelift combined procedures producing both. Tightening and mild leveling are preferred. Combined procedures are discussed in greater depth in Chapter 9.

Medium and Thick Skin: Skin of medium thickness is the ideal type for leveling and tightening and for all procedures. Guidelines for skin color should be followed in selecting a procedure and its depth. The safest type for any procedure is thick skin, and good results at any desired depth can be achieved. However, CO_2 laser resurfacing for deep wrinkles or scars in thick skin has variable results in this skin type, as thick skin requires more passes, that can create permanent changes due to the excessive heat generated by the laser that will adversely affect skin texture. A medium-depth peel or dermabrasion are more effective for nonstretchable scars and deep wrinkles in thick skin.

Box 4-5

Skin thickness is the most important factor in determining the depth of a procedure.

Effect of Skin Thickness on the Predictability of Procedure Results

Thin Skin: In thin skin, tightening effects (papillary dermis or IRD level procedures) are more remarkable and are seen sooner than in thick skin, and the effects of dermal matrix build-up using tretinoin are excellent. Tightening procedures will reduce but not eliminate the appearance of expression lines. Compared with thick skin, the results from mechanical tightening (face-lift) in thin skin do not last as long, nonstretchable scars from acne or trauma do not improve as much because the dermis has less regenerative ability in deeper procedures which carry a high degree of risk as erythema and skin sensitivity may be more severe and longer lasting than in thick skin.

Medium-thick Skin: In skin of medium thickness, both leveling and tightening effects can be achieved with satisfaction. Expression lines can be significantly minimized, and some can be eliminated entirely for a long period of time. Dermal matrix build-up is not clinically as dramatic as is seen in thin skin. In this skin type, topical treatment effects can be appreciated only years later by maintaining skin firmness and tightness. Mechanical tightening (face-lift) results last longer than in thin skin, and the chances of improving scars are better because this skin type can tolerate deeper leveling procedures.

Thick Skin: In thick skin, leveling procedures can produce the most prominent effects, and it is not unusual for expression lines to be eliminated for years before returning. However, because of jowling and sagging, thick skin is likely to benefit more from a surgical face-lift procedure. In all other respects, thick skin is similar to medium-thick skin, described above.

Effect of Skin Thickness on Repeated Procedures

Thin Skin: Procedures in thin skin that penetrate to the papillary dermis can be repeated in 4 to 6 weeks and those that penetrate to the IRD, in 6 to 8 weeks. Procedures in thin skin that reach the upper reticular dermis should be repeated in no less than 4 to 6 months or not at all, and the repeated procedure should reach to the level of the papillary dermis and only rarely to the IRD. This is necessary because the initial deep procedure will have eliminated many adnexal structures and have made the skin thinner and no longer suitable for deeper procedures.

Medium-thick and Thick Skin: Like procedures in thin skin, procedures in medium-thick and thick skin that penetrate to the papillary dermis can be repeated in 4 to 6 weeks and those that penetrate to the IRD, in 6 to 8 weeks. Procedures that penetrate to the upper reticular dermis or mid dermis can be repeated in in 4 to 6 months and are generally well tolerated.

Effect of Skin Thickness on the Rate of Complications
Scarring (keloids) and permanent hypopigmentation are more common following deeper procedures. These complications are especially seen in patients with thin skin who have undergone deeper procedures that reach below the IRD. Thin skin has a narrow safety margin for deep procedures.

SKIN TYPE ACCORDING TO SKIN OILINESS

Skin can be classified as

1. oily, secreting excess sebum,
2. normal, secreting an average amount of sebum, or
3. dry, with below average sebum secretion.

People with oily skin tend to have medium-thick or thick skin. Oily skin does not age more slowly than dry skin, as is commonly believed, since aging is related to the amount of collagen, elastin, textural changes, and other factors. A reduction in sebum production is not the only mechanism for dryness; hydration levels due to epidermal and dermal glycosaminoglycan content are also important, and high levels of glycosaminoglycans are desirable to reduce the true skin dryness.[4,5,6]

Excessive skin oiliness impedes the penetration of active ingredients used in topical therapy and thus has a profound effect on the success of skin conditioning before and after a procedure and on skin health restoration in general. Excessive skin oiliness is the most common cause for topical treatment failure in acne, melasma, actinic keratoses, and other conditions.

Before a procedure, excessive skin oiliness must be brought to a normal level by means of special topical agents or a short course of systemic treatment with Accutane (isotretinoin) for 1 to 4 weeks, when necessary. Be sure to take the necessary precautions when using Accutane (avoid pregnancy, undergo liver function tests, etc.). The author does not believe that use of Accutane contraindicates a procedure to the level of the papillary dermis or the IRD. However, procedures deeper than the IRD should be avoided as Accutane therapy for 3 to 5 months will increase skin fragility for a period of 6 months or more.

Dryness or oiliness of skin is not a factor in the choice of procedure depth; skin thickness is the only determinant. However, it is more difficult to achieve an even peel or an even vaporization with CO_2 laser resurfacing in an oily yet poorly hydrated and prepared skin.

Proper skin conditioning to overcome excessive oiliness must be performed before a procedure; the objective is to normalize skin so that it is not oily or excessively dry. The goal is to restore a properly hydrated skin that has normal tolerance and is not excessively oily. Patients with improperly conditioned dry skin, on the other hand, tend to have a longer postprocedure recovery time with prolonged erythema and increased skin sensitivity. Conditioning of dry-skinned patients may need to be more gentle at the beginning and carried out for a longer time to build tolerance. Moisturizers that can be used more often in dry skin should be avoided in patients with oily skin.

SKIN TYPE ACCORDING TO LAXITY

Skin laxity is manifested clinically by wrinkles, dropping of the eyebrows, redundancy of upper and lower eyelid skin, deepened nasolabial folds, redundant skin on the cheeks, and jowling at the jawline with formation of platysmal cords. These changes begin at approximately the age of 30 with the appearance of fine lines and the loss of skin tightness and are accelerated by the degenerative effects of photodamage on elastic tissue. Histologically, lax skin has a thinner epidermis and dermis with reduced and possibly damaged collagen and elastic fibers and loss of anchoring fibrils in the papillary dermis.

Although they are often seen together in advanced cases of skin laxity, muscle laxity is distinguished from skin laxity for treatment purposes. Muscle laxity is evident when certain muscles such as the platyrma become redundant, leading to jowling, the orbicularis and frontalis muscles' laxity and weakness cause eyebrow dropping, and the overall picture is severe skin and muscle sagginess.

Box 4-6

In thin skin, laxity is revealed by wrinkling, while in thick skin it starts with jowling and sagging, to be followed later by wrinkling.

Box 4-7

Sensitive skin is a phenomenon, but not a skin type, and, with the exception of atopic dermatitis and certain other medical conditions, no one is born with sensitive skin. Sensitive skin is actually an informal term commonly used to describe skin with certain characteristics. These include the inability to tolerate cosmetics or other products on the skin, frequent irritation, "addiction" to moisturizers, and a high rate of discomfort when tretinoin and AHAs are used, which lead to frequent interruption of skin conditioning treatment and use of moisturizers and topical steroids for relief. This type of skin is not suitable for procedures until sufficient skin tolerance is restored.

Table 4.8	
RECOMMENDED PROCEDURES FOR SKIN LAXITY CORRECTION	
Laxity	***Correcting Procedures***
Level 1	(1–2) Standard Blue Peels + • dermal stimulation (3–6 cycles).
Level 2	(1–3) Standard or designed Blue Peels
Level 3	(1–2) Designed Blue Peel ± CO_2 laser resurfacing (localized)
Level 4	CO_2 laser resurfacing (for unstretchable wrinkles) & designed Blue Peel OR Medium depth TCA peel & designed Blue Peel.
Level 4	Face lift ± Blue Peel ± CO_2 laser resurfacing, etc.

Skin Laxity Classification

Facial skin laxity should be determined without facial expressions. The classifications are as follows:

Level 1: Fine lines, skin pinching elicits fine wrinkling (positive accordion sign).

Level 2: General fine wrinkles, exaggerated expression lines, expression lines present without facial expressions; all disappear with gentle skin stretching.

Level 3: Changes seen in levels 1 and 2 and general skin laxity as evidenced by deeper wrinkles and lines, deeper nasolabial folds, redundancy of eyelid skin, and falling eyebrows; all can be improved by gentle stretching and lifting.

Level 4: All of the above plus deeper wrinkles and general skin laxity that do not improve with gentle lifting.

Level 5: All of the above plus excessive facial and neck muscle laxity that do not improve with gentle lifting and skin stretching.

For skin laxity alone the ideal treatment is usually nonsurgical, but for muscle laxity the ideal treatments are surgical facelift, neck tightening, etc. (Table 4-8).

SKIN TYPE ACCORDING TO FRAGILITY

Skin fragility, a term used by the author to indicate the unsuitability of certain skins for deeper procedures, should be studied at the molecular level, as histological studies are not expected to be helpful, since fragile skin appears the same histologically and clinically as its opposite, tough skin. Thin, medium-thick, and thick skin can be fragile. The author has observed that fragile skin is more common in Asian skin and, to a lesser degree, in Black (AA) skin, but it can occur in all skin colors and types.

Fragile skin can be appreciated and somewhat identified clinically in 2 ways. The first is evaluation of the resistance to penetration of the skin by a needle or comedone extractor. Fragile skin offers no or minimal resistance, while tough skin resists penetration. The second is to pinch a skin fold with a firm squeeze. Fragile skin can be squeezed without resistance and feels like butter, while tough skin is firmer, resists squeezing, and feels like leather. In addition, patients with keloids or a history of scarring after minor trauma or bruising should be considered as having fragile skin.

Fragile skin is to be approached with care regarding conditioning and procedures. It reacts more strongly to procedures and tends to heal more slowly afterwards. Prolonged erythema and skin surface roughness, especially in areas where penetration was deeper than the IRD, occur frequently after procedures in fragile skin, and the incidence of textural changes and scarring is higher. Use of Accutane (isotretinoin) or oral corticosteroids for more than 3 to 4 months can induce skin fragility that may last up to 8 months. The mechanism for this drug-induced fragility is not currently known.

Procedures in fragile skin should not penetrate deeper than the papillary dermis and should never go below the IRD. These patients should be advised of the higher incidence of scarring from deeper procedures needed to correct deep wrinkles or scars. Conditioning of fragile skin needs to be much longer, 2 to 3 cycles longer than conditioning of normal skin, as skin conditioning tends to increase skin toughness and tolerance.

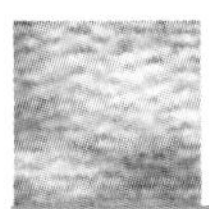

REFERENCES

1. Fitzpatrick TB. The validity and practicality of sun-reactive skin types I through VI. *Arch Dermatol.* 1988;124:869–871.
2. Glogau RG. Chemical peeling and aging skin. *J Geriatr Dermatol.* 1994;2: 30–35.
3. Griffiths CEM, Wang TS, Hamilton A, et al. A photonumeric scale for the assessment of cutaneous photodamage. *Arch Dermatol.* 1992;128:347–351.
4. Reiger MM, Skin, water, and moisturization. *Cosmet Toilet.* 1989;104: 41–43.
5. Pierard GE. What does 'dry skin' mean? *Int J Dermatol.* 1987;26:167–169.
6. Draelos Z. Moisturizers. In: Draelos Z, ed. *Cosmetic Dermatology.* 2nd ed. New York, NY: Churchill Livingstone; 1995:83–95.

CHAPTER

5

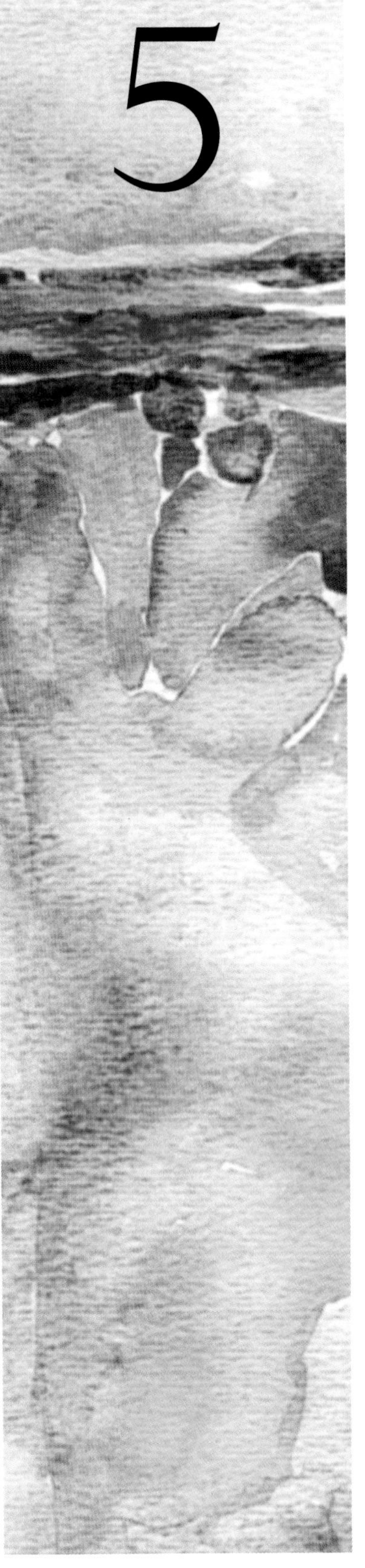

SKIN HEALTH RESTORATION AND SKIN CONDITIONING: CORRECTION AND STIMULATION

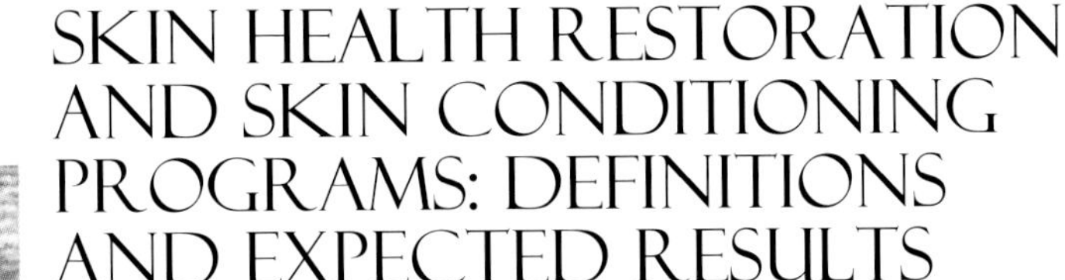

SKIN HEALTH RESTORATION AND SKIN CONDITIONING PROGRAMS: DEFINITIONS AND EXPECTED RESULTS

SKIN HEALTH RESTORATION

Skin Health Restoration is the process of restoring skin to a healthy state, free of disease and deterioration (Table 5-1). Experience with thousands of patients taught me that it was fruitless to treat any skin condition in isolation —the patient's underlying skin type and any other medical conditions that might be present must be taken into account. It became clear that many common skin disorders could be eliminated more effectively by a program designed to restore overall skin health than by a treatment aimed solely at the elimination of a single skin disorder. Such a program

TABLE 5.1

SKIN CONDITIONING AND SKIN HEALTH RESTORATION PROGRAMS: DEFINITIONS AND EXPECTED RESULTS

Skin at Baseline	*Program*	*Expected Results*
Minimal deterioration	Obagi Topical Skin Health Restoration program	Healthy skin
Advanced deterioration	Obagi Skin Conditioning program followed by a procedure	Healthy skin

includes topical application of specialty products to regulate skin cell functions and improve circulation and gives skin the opportunity to constantly renew itself, repair any damage, and act as an effective barrier with good tolerance. Skin Health Restoration can be accomplished utilizing two principles devised by the author, correction and stimulation, to restore or regulate skin functions. The steps are usually not related to procedures, and they can be utilized indefinitely as a program for life, unlike the same steps when utilized for one or more skin cycles to prepare the skin for a procedure and one or more cycles after the procedure to help in restoring the skin to normalcy. The limited approach is called Skin Conditioning. This process is utilized when a skin rejuvenation procedure is needed to correct deterioration that cannot be improved through topical treatment alone.

Box 5-1

Skin Health Restoration—Restores skin health with or without use of a procedure.
Skin Conditioning—Improves skin tolerance and skin quality before and after a procedure.

SKIN CONDITIONING

Skin Conditioning is intended to bring the skin to a tolerant state so that it responds better to a procedure and has a lessened chance of exhibiting an undesirable postprocedure response. It involves use of a topical skin care system for a number of skin renewal cycles before the procedure is performed, but it can also be continued for postprocedure maintenance and prevention. The steps to follow before initiating Skin Health Restoration and Skin Conditioning are presented in Table 5-2.

Both Skin Health Restoration and Skin Conditioning use the same components, but the emphasis can differ according to a particular patient's needs: Correction may be emphasized to manage younger patients with acne, Bleaching and Blending for patients with pigmentation problems, Stimulation to improve photoaged or thin skin, Prevention to prevent further damage, and Maintenance to prevent loss of improvement.

Table 5.2	
BEFORE PROCEEDING WITH SKIN CONDITIONING OR SKIN HEALTH RESTORATION	
Step	***Action***
Step 1	Identify the skin type
Step 2	Define the emphasis of the treatment • Correction • Stimulation
Step 3	Determine the type of procedure needed • Chemical peeling • Resurfacing • Surgery
Step 4	Inform the patient of • The purpose of conditioning before the procedure and how to perform it properly • The role conditioning plays in the successful outcome of a procedure • The importance of skin conditioning after the procedure • Prevention and treatment of expected reactions

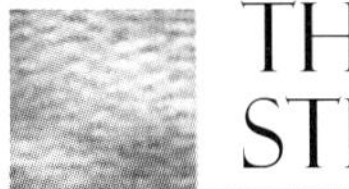

THE CORRECTION AND STIMULATION PROCESSES

SKIN CORRECTION

Skin correction works on the epidermal layer. After correction has been completed, the epidermis is healthier and shows the following features: The stratum corneum is compact and has less basket weaving; the stratum granulosum is thicker, with coarser granules; the stratum Malpighi has more uniform keratinocytes and no atypia; and the stratum basalis (basal layer) shows increased mitosis. Melanocytes are also functioning properly with even distribution of melanosomes. Clinically, this translates into an epidermis that is soft, resilient, evenly colored, moist, less sensitive to external factors, and free of medical problems (Table 5-3).

Table 5.3	
CHARACTERISTICS OF AN EPIDERMIS RESTORED TO HEALTH	
Histological Characteristics	***Clinical Characteristics***
Epidermis overall—thicker, has more mucinous material, healthy population of keratinocytes, more efficient renewability of cells, more stable and efficient melanocytes Stratum corneum—compact with less basket weaving Stratum granulosum—thicker with coarser granules Stratum Malpighi—more uniform keratinocytes, no atypia Stratum basalis (basal layer)—increased mitosis Melanocytes—decreased in number with fewer melanosomes	Soft, resilient, evenly colored, moist, less sensitive to external factors, free of medical problems

SKIN STIMULATION

Skin stimulation indicates topical agents effect on the papillary dermis and the basal layer of the epidermis. The papillary dermis shows improved circulation, which improves all skin functions, and an inhibition of collagenase activity, which reduces collagen degradation in the papillary dermis. Fibro-blasts in the papillary dermis are also stimulated, leading to the creation of new anchoring fibrils and the strengthening of the basement membrane. The tensile strength of the skin is improved, and skin fragility is reduced.

In the basal layer of the epidermis, mitosis is increased, leading to the enhanced production of keratinocytes and a thickening of the epidermis.

TABLE 5.4

CLINICAL EFFECTS OF AGENTS USED FOR SKIN CORRECTION AND STIMULATION

Agent	*Skin Conditioning Action*	*Clinical Response*
Tretinoin	• Enhances basal cell mitosis to produce new keratinocytes	Compact, smooth, soft, translucent keratinous layer
	• Compacts the stratum corneum	Improvement of acne, comedones, large pores, actinic keratoses
	• Increases epidermal thickness	Reduced bacterial flora
	• Normalizes atypical epidermal cells	Increased skin hydration
	• Controls pigmentary system	Increased skin firmness
	• Promotes angiogenesis	Even pigmentation, restored normal coloration
	• Induces fibroblast activity to increase collagen formation	Increased elasticity
	• Restores the population of antigen-presenting Langerhans cells	Increased protection against infections
	• Strengthens dermal matrix	Inhibition of neoplastic growths
	• Increases the production of glycosaminoglycans	Sallowness replaced with healthy, rosy glow
	• Increases skin tolerance	Reduced occurrence of solar damage
		Shortened postprocedure recovery time
AHAs	• Loosens epidermal corneocytes to produce exfoliation with low concentrations, epidermolysis with high concentrations.	Nonviable epidermal cells removed to expose smooth keratinous layer
	• Lightens skin by exfoliation; no direct effect on melanocytes	Improvement of acne, comedones
	• In low concentrations may improve skin tolerance, potentiate the action of other agents	Improvement of hyperpigmentation
	• No stimulation of angiogenesis	Increased skin hydration
Hydroquinone	• Decreases the formation and increases the degradation of melanosomes	Skin lightening
	• Changes the structure of membranous organelles of the melanocyte	Improvement of hyperpigmentation
	• Inhibits tyrosinase	

The stimulation of the keratinocyte maturation process leads to the gradual shedding of atypical, sun-damaged keratinocytes and can reduce the risk of skin cancer. The barrier function of the skin is improved, and skin tolerance is enhanced. Clinically, the skin becomes firmer and more elastic and has fewer fine wrinkles. Dermal stimulation should be a continuous process since the benefits are needed all life long, especially after age 30 when skin functions start to deteriorate. Benefits to the dermis can be appreciated by both patient and physician after three skin cycles, and they become quite evident after 1 year.

The following types of skin benefit most from the stimulation process:

1. thin skin, since stimulation actually thickens and firms the skin;
2. thick, rough-textured skin, since the process leads to smoother and softer skin;
3. large pores, since the process tends to tighten, shrink, and efface the large pores;
4. burn scars and skin grafts, which can become softer and more evenly pigmented;
5. acne scars, which can become softer and properly hydrated and respond better to peels and CO_2 laser resurfacing.

The clinical effects of agents used for skin correction and stimulation are shown in Table 5-4 and in Figures 5-1 to 5-11.

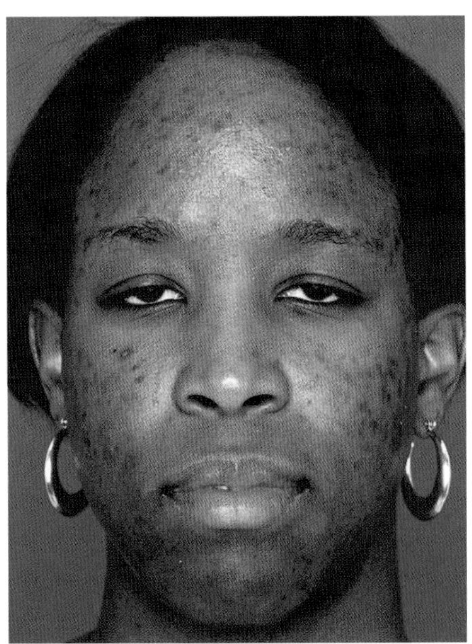

a

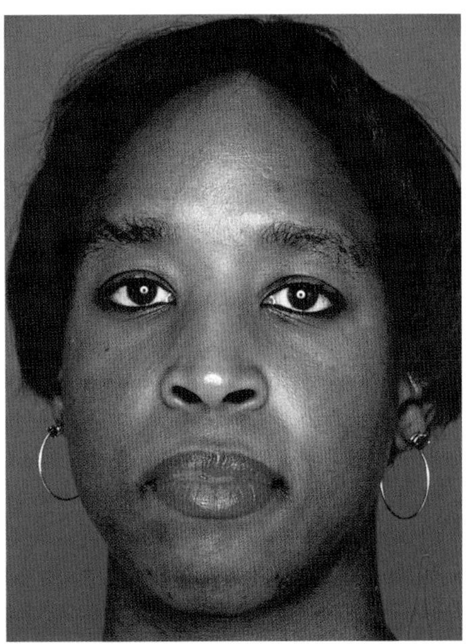

b

FIGURE 5-1. *(a) Before—Patient with cystic acne, scars, and PIH. (b) After—Treatment consisted of correction and stimulation, with emphasis on bleaching and blending. Bleaching was performed for 3 months and blending for 5 months. Isotretinoin (Accutane) 20 mg/day for 5 months was administered by another dermatologist prior to treatment.*

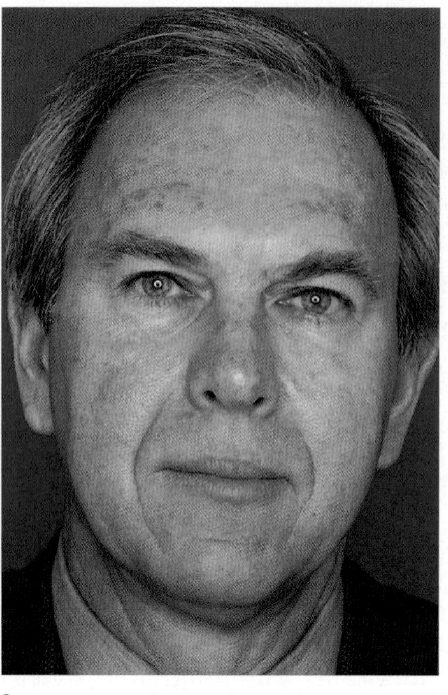
a

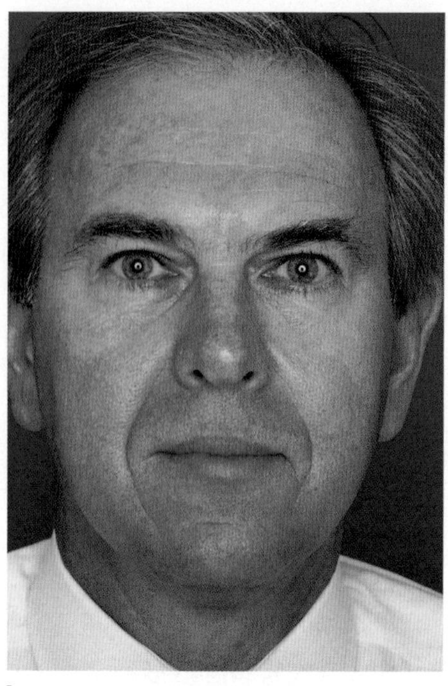
b

FIGURE 5-2. *(a) Before—Patient with actinic keratoses, early photodamage. (b) After—Treatment consisted of correction and stimulation for 5 months.*

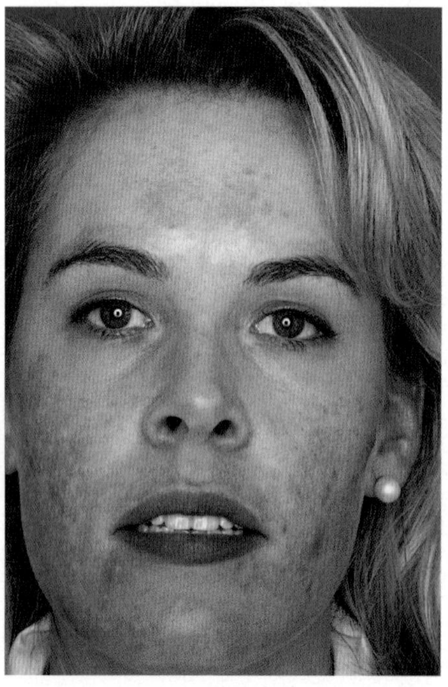
a

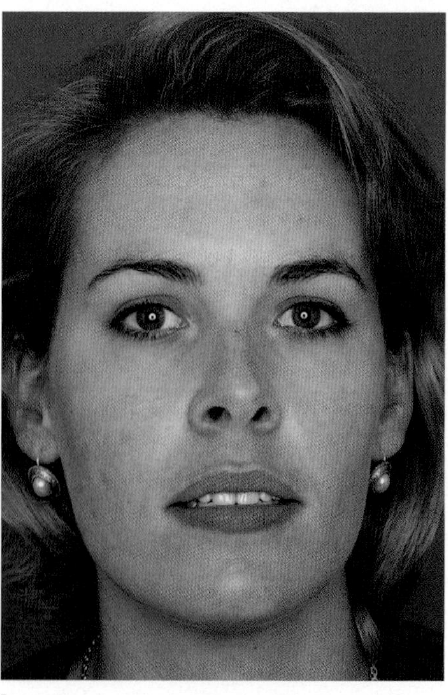
b

FIGURE 5-3. *(a) Before—Patient with acne vulgaris, large pores, PIH. (b) After—Treatment consisted of correction and stimulation for 5 months followed by maintenance program.*

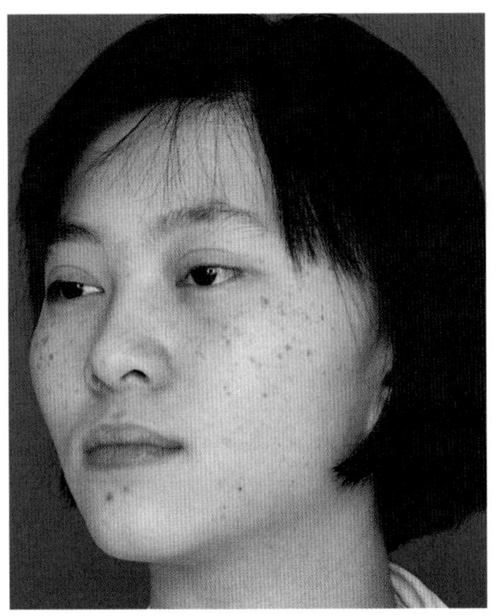
a

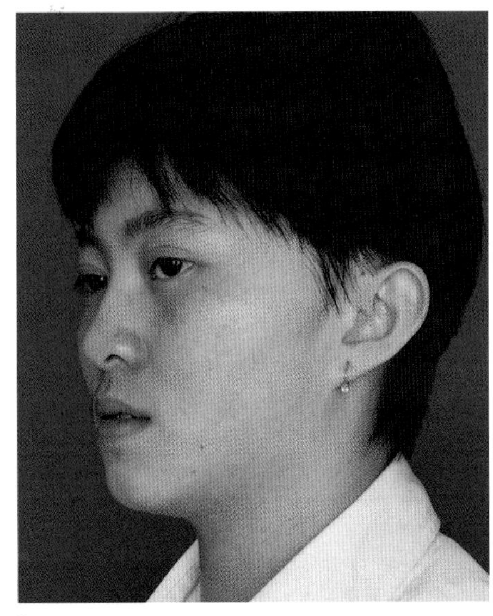
b

FIGURE 5-4. *(a) Before—Patient with lentigo and freckles. (b) After—Treatment consisted of correction and stimulation for 5 months with emphasis on blending. Maintenance is recommended in such cases to prevent recurrence.*

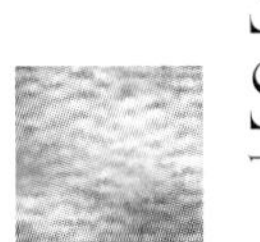

SKIN CORRECTION AND STIMULATION AGENTS AND THEIR ROLES

The agents used in the system for correction and stimulation are: tretinoin (0.05% or 0.1 %), AHAs (7 %), phytic acid (3%), hydroquinone (2% or 4%), and possibly antibiotic solutions. All those agents, except phytic acid, are well known in the dermatological field for treating acne, bleaching spots, reducing wrinkles, and use before and after a peel or laser treatment[1–5] to speed the healing process[6] and reduce the risk of postoperative hyperpigmentation[7–9].

In my system I use all those agents in cream form with variations of concentration (for correction or stimulation), type of skin, age of patient, and other factors that customize the treatment for each particular case. The number of skin cycles is very important, as is the level of aggressiveness. In an aggressive program, maximum skin correction requires at least 3 cycles, and maximum skin stimulation, at least 5 or 6 cycles. Less aggressive programs take longer to reach the maximum effects.

TRETINOIN

Tretinoin is the best agent for correction and stimulation and building skin tolerance. Tolerance is achieved when skin reactions start to diminish, usu-

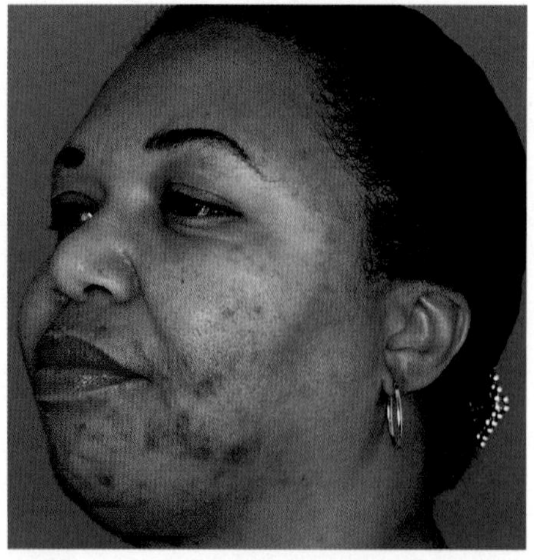

a

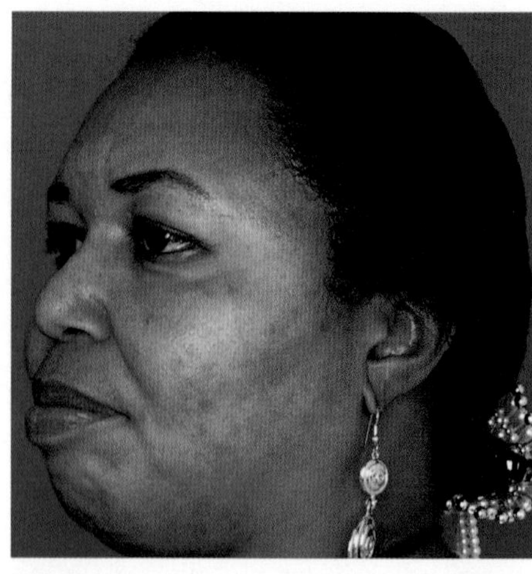

b

FIGURE 5-5. *(a) Before—Patient with pseudofolliculitis and excoriations with surface scarring and PIH. (b) After—Treatment consisted of correction and stimulation and aggressive blending.*

ally 4 to 6 weeks after initiation of therapy (Figure 5-12 and Table 5-5). The 0.05% and 0.1% concentrations of tretinoin are the best to achieve correction and stimulation.

The 0.025% concentration of tretinoin can produce proper correction (epidermal action) but is weak for stimulation. Thus, a lower concentration can be used for young individuals with a mild skin problem, but for severe photodamaged skin and for certain deteriorative changes affecting the dermis, dermal stimulation is needed along with epidermal correction. However, only a small, insufficent amount of the applied tretinoin is actually

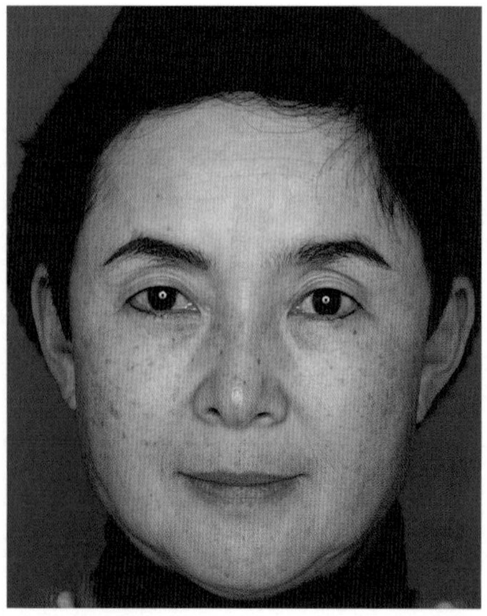

a

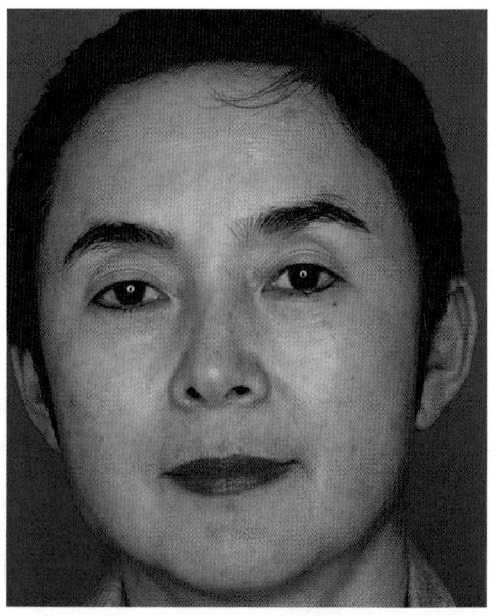

b

FIGURE 5-6. *(a) Before—Patient with lentigo, freckles, and laxity. (b) After—Treatment consisted of correction and stimulation for 1 year. The resulting skin tightening and clarity can be seen.*

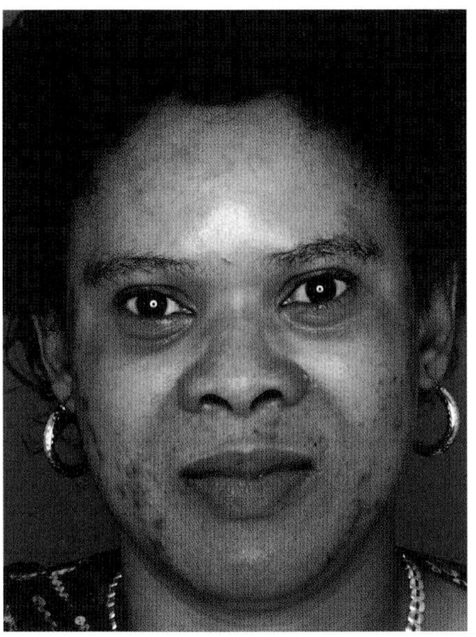
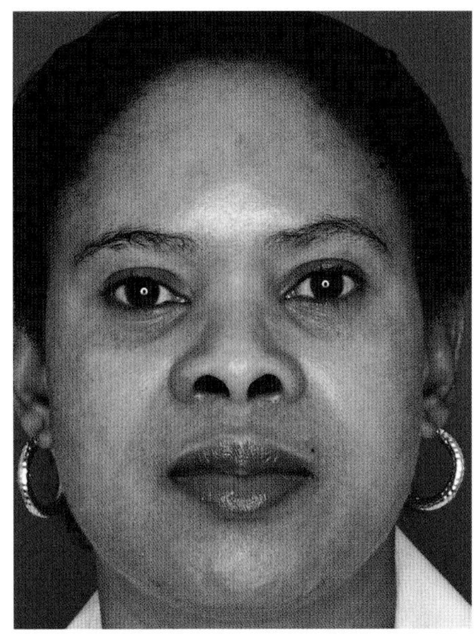

a b

FIGURE 5-7. *(a) Before—Patient with cystic acne and periorbital laxity. (b) After—Treatment consisted of correction and stimulation with emphasis on bleaching and blending. Bleaching was performed for 3 months and blending for 5 months, followed by maintenance. Isotretinoin (Accutane) 20 mg/daily was administered for 5 months.*

delivered to the basal layer or papillary dermis, and most remains in the epidermis. To enhance delivery of tretinoin to the dermis and thus hasten restoration of tolerance, I use creams with AHAs and phytic acid applied either before the application of retinoic acid or at the same time. This will in-

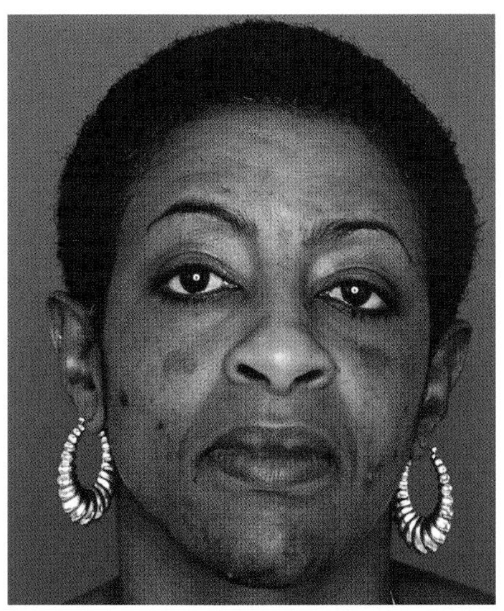
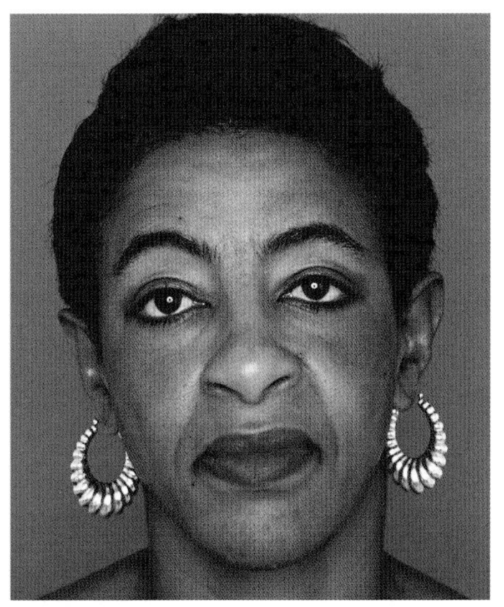

a b

FIGURE 5-8. *(a) Before—Patient who had CO_2 laser treatment by another physician for lentigo, with worsening of the condition. Postinflammatory hyperpigmentation, acne rosacea, and excoriations were also present. (b) After—Treatment consisted of correction and stimulation for 5 months; no procedure was necessary.*

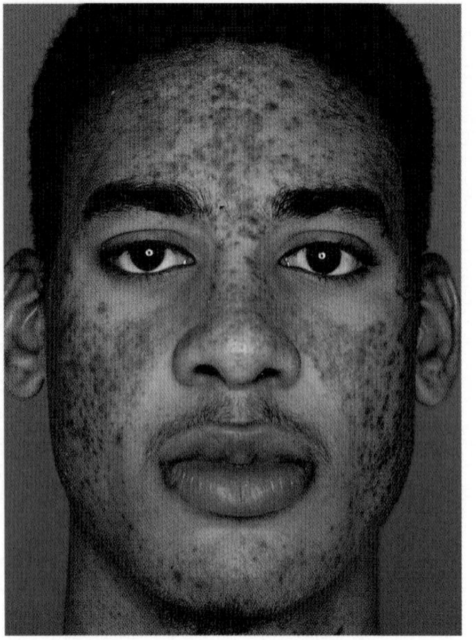

a

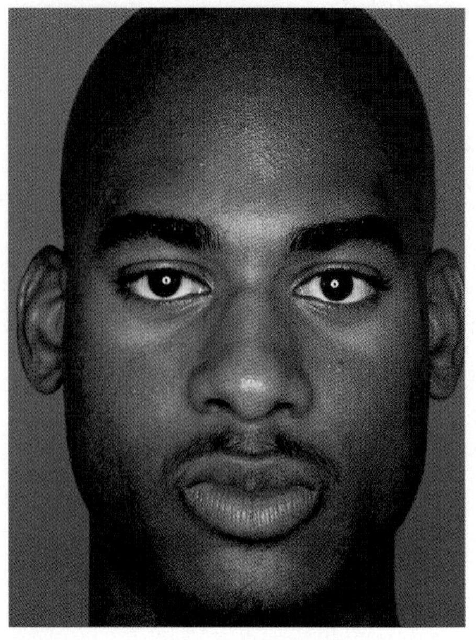

b

FIGURE 5-9. *(a) Before—Patient with acne vulgaris, PIH, and superficial scarring. (b) After—Treatment consisted of correction and stimulation with emphasis on bleaching and blending. Bleaching was performed for 3 months and blending for 5 months. Isotretinoin (Accutane) 20 mg/daily was also administered at the same time.*

crease the effectiveness and the penetration of tretinoin and hydroquinone. By exfoliating the outermost layers of stratum corneum while keeping the barrier function of the skin intact and by enhancing the penetration as I do in my system of topical skin treatment, the maximum desired effects of bleaching, blending, correction, and stimulation will be achieved, as both

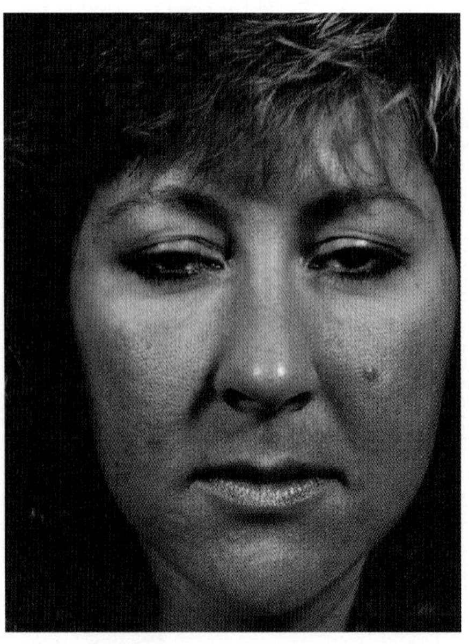

a

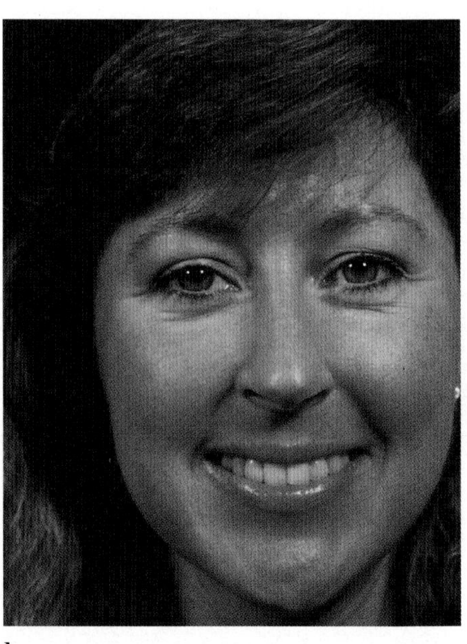

b

FIGURE 5-10. *(a) Before—Patient with acne vulgaris, large pores. (b) After—Treatment consisted of correction and stimulation with emphasis on stimulation and blending.*

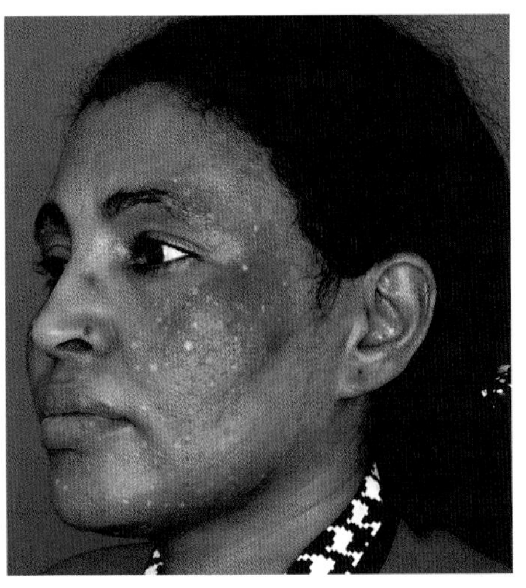

a

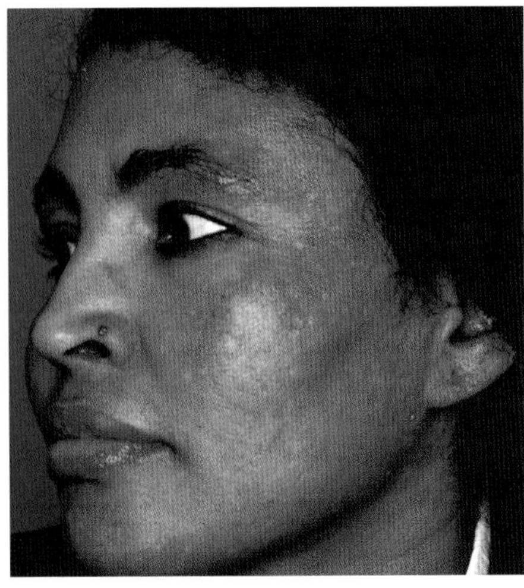

b

FIGURE 5-11. *(a) Before—Patient with PIH and round islands of depigmentation from shotgun blast. Previously treated by another physician with bleachers and AHA peels, with no improvement. (b) After—Treatment consisted of aggressive correction and stimulation and blending to even out skin color and regenerate melanocytes. Response occurred in 8 weeks.*

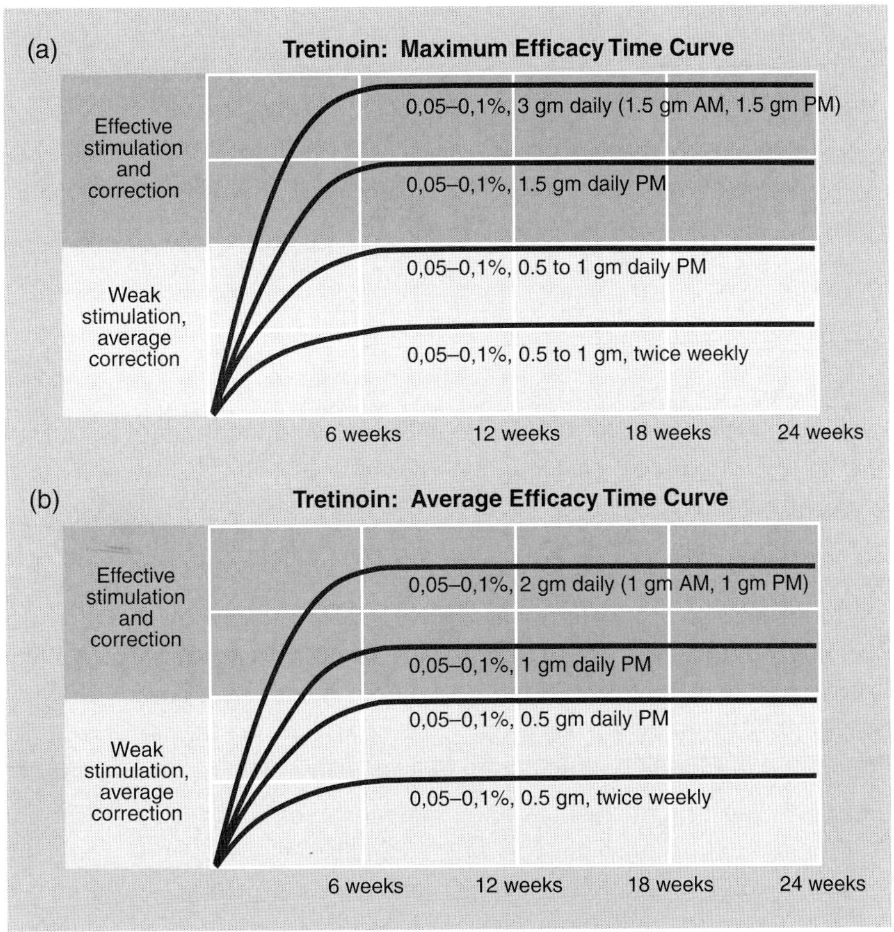

FIGURE 5-12. *(a) Relationship of tretinoin dosage with time to achieve maximum efficacy. (b) Relationship of tretinoin dosage with time to achieve average efficacy.*

TABLE 5.5	
EFFECTS OF SKIN CORRECTION AND STIMULATION	
Correction (affects the epidermis)	• Exfoliate to restore a soft, compact stratum corneum • Increase mitotic activity of basal layer (aided by stimulation) • Control keratinocytes and melanocytes functions
Stimulation (affects the dermis)	• Regulate fibroblast activity • Stimulate production collagen, elastin, and GAGs and improve circulation.

retinoic acid and hydroquinone have strong intracellular effects to regulate the functions of both the keratinocytes and melanocytes.

Depending on AHAs alone, without the use of retinoic acid, will result in minor benefits, limited to the epidermis. As AHA alone will induce exfoliation that will temporarily improve surface skin problems such as superficial pigmentation and surface sun damage. However, these agents do not exert any regulatory control of melanocytes, and higher concentrations can irritate and themselves create hyperpigmentation. Exfoliation induced by AHA is continuous (skin is always shedding) as long as the product is in use, while exfoliation with tretinoin stops when the stratum corneum is soft and compact and skin tolerance has been established. AHA should not be used for 3 weeks after CO_2 laser resurfacing or for 1 week after papillary-dermal-level TCA peeling to allow the epidermis to mature and allow a stable stratum corneum to be formed. For Black (AA), dark Hispanic, or sensitive skin that reacts to AHAs, I use another exfoliator—phytic acid. This agent has good exfoliation activity, increases mitosis in the basal layer, and is gentle and nonirritating, even for very sensitive skin. It also helps tretinoin and hydroquinone to penetrate evenly.

HYDROQUINONE

Bleaching: Hydroquinone regulates melanin production and is thus integral to the correction process. It lightens ("bleaches") the skin by inhibiting the enzyme tyrosinase, which converts tyrosine to L-dopa, thus decreasing the skin's ability to create melanin. This effect only lasts for the duration of treatment, and tyrosinase and normal enzyme levels are restored within 2 to 3 days after discontinuation of hydroquinone. In rare cases, hydroquinone can cause a paradoxical overproduction of tyrosinase (ochronosis), leading to an overproduction of melanin in spite of the continuous application of hydroquinone. This can occur in some native African patients, but is relatively unusual in African-Americans.

Blending: Regulating the dispersion of melanosomes is important in the control of pigmentation problems, as is the regulation of melanin production. Uses of hydroquinone and tretinoin in combination produces a unique effect I call "blending" that produces a more even dispersion of melanosomes throughout the epidermis and dampens the strong bleaching action of hydroquinone. Skin blending can be performed with or without bleaching to create a more even skin tone in patients with either hyper- or hypopigmentation. It is also useful for controlling the pigmentary system prior to any

Box 5-2

- **Hydroquinone used alone produces bleaching.**
- **Hydroquinone + tretinoin + (AHA) produces blending.**

or

(phytic acid)

surgical procedure, thereby reducing the risk of postoperative pigmentary changes. By varying the ratio of bleaching and blending, two apparently contradictory effects can be achieved: 1) melanocyte activation, which leads to a more even skin tone through both enhanced melanin production and melanosome dispersion (excellent for the treatment of facial vitiligo); or 2) melanocyte suppression through both decreased melanin production and melanosome dispersion that leads to a more even skin tone. The bleaching effects will usually be achieved within 2 to 3 months, but the process should not be ended abruptly; rather, it ought to be slowed down to a level of control, such as once daily, then twice a week, etc.

Blending effects are usually achieved in 1 to 2 months, but the process should be continued for 5 to 6 months, daily or less, for best control and prevention of recurrences. If hyperpigmentation starts to appear after treatment has been slowed down, daily treatment should be resumed for no less than 1 year. Several procedures (Blue Peels) to the level of the papillary dermis should be performed during that time and repeated every time the dermal dyspigmentation starts to reappear. These peels will gradually reduce the number of hyperactive melanocytes.

Thus, bleaching and blending and one or more Blue Peels to the level of the papillary dermis, repeated at intervals of 4 to 6 weeks or when dark pigmentation starts to reappear, will lead to a total cure at the end of the treatment program. CO_2 or erbium lasers are less effective in treating melasma and PIH and might even worsen the condition. Qs Nd YAG laser and other pigment-treating lasers should be reserved for congenital dermal pigmentation (dermal melanosis, nevus of ota) and tattoos.

AGGRESSIVENESS AND TREATMENT EFFICACY

Skin correction and stimulation can be achieved at variable strengths by varying the concentration of tretinoin used and the frequency of application. Four different approaches can be used: aggressive, moderately aggressive, standard, and maintenance (Table 5-6). The daily regimen for facial skin in different levels of treatment aggressiveness is shown in Table 5-7, and for nonfacial skin in Table 5-8. The three phases of skin restoration are shown in Table 5-9.

Efficacy of the programs is related to treatment aggressiveness. Aggressiveness can be controlled as needed for different skin types and sensitivities by varying the concentration, amount, and frequency of

TABLE 5.6

SKIN HEALTH RESTORATION REGIMEN ACCORDING TO TREATMENT AGGRESSIVENESS

Aggressiveness of Approach	*Correction*	*Bleaching**	*Stimulation/Blending**
Aggressive	1 to 1.5 g 6–10% AHA (AM) or 2–10% phytic acid	1 to 1.5 g hydroquinone (AM and PM)	1 to 1.5 g of 0.1% or 0.05% tretinoin (AM and PM) mixed with 0.5 g hydroquinone in in a **penetrating base
Moderately Aggressive	1 g 6–10% AHA (AM) or 2–10% phytic acid	1 to 1.5 g hydroquinone (AM and PM)	1 to 1.5 g of 0.1% or 0.05% tretinoin mixed with 0.5 g hydroquinone in a penetrating base (PM)
Standard	0.5 to 1 g 6–10% AHA (AM) or 2–10% phytic acid	1 g hydroquinone (AM and PM)	0.5 to 1 g of 0.1% or 0.05% tretinoin mixed with 0.5 g hydroquinone in a penetrating base (PM)
Maintenance	0.5 to 1 g 6–10% AHA (AM) or 2–10% phytic acid	0.5 g hydroquinone (twice weekly)	0.5 to 1 g of 0.1% or 0.05% tretinoin mixed with 0.5 g hydroquinone in a penetrating base (twice weekly)

1 g = amount in approximately 3/4 in of toothpaste. This provides average efficacy.

1.5 g = amount in approximately 1 in of toothpaste. This provides maximum efficacy.

AHA = alphahydroxy acid

*Stimulation and blending are combined into one step. Some patients may not need the bleaching step.

****The penetrating base:** contain saponins and pH balancing agents.

application of each preparation. The more damaged the skin, the more aggressive the program should be. In the aggressive approach, skin correction is fast and skin stimulation is strong, while in the mild approach, skin correction is slow and skin stimulation is minimal (Figure 5-13).

The amount of the agents applied to the skin is critical and can be described through an analogy with the amount of toothpaste usually used for brushing teeth. One g (which is equal to 1.5 cm of toothpaste) of any product in the programs, when applied equally on 5% of the skin surface, will provide average efficacy. One and one-half g (equal to 2.5 cm of toothpaste), applied similarly, will provide maximum efficacy (Figure 5-14).

EXPECTED REACTIONS

A keratinocyte requires approximately 6 weeks to mature, reach the stratum corneum, and exfoliate (1 skin cycle). During this first cycle, tretinoin produces redness, dryness, exfoliation, and occasionally itching or burning. Concomitant use of AHA or phytic acid and hydroquinone intensifies the reactions. The severity of reaction is correlated with the skin type, degree of skin damage, and level of aggressiveness.

TABLE 5.7

SKIN HEALTH RESTORATION: DAILY REGIMEN FOR FACIAL SKIN

Obagi Specialty Products and Ingredients

Steps	*Products and Active Ingredients*	*Type of Skin*	*Time*	
			AM	*PM*
Preparation	Cleanser	All	Yes	Yes
	Toner	All	Yes	Yes
	Topical antibiotic	All	If indicated	If indicated
Correction (repairing and balancing skin color)	Clear® (2% to 4% HQ)[1]	All	0.5 to 1 g	Yes except for patients with dark skin
	Exfoderm® (3% phytic acid)[1]	Hispanic/dark	0.5 to 1 g	Yes
	Exfoderm Forte® (7% AHA)[1]	White	0.5 to 1 g	Yes
Stimulation (development of new skin)	Tretinoin			
	0.1%	All	No	Yes
	0.05%	All	No	Yes
	Obagi Blender			
	2% HQ[1]*	All	No	2% HQ
	4% HQ[1]	All	No	2% HQ
	Exfoderm® (3% phytic acid)[1]	Hispanic/dark	Yes	With 0.1% tretinoin + 4% HQ
	Exfoderm Forte® (7% AHA)[1]	White	Yes	With 0.1% tretinoin and 4% HQ
Protection	Sunfader® Rx	All	Yes	No
	Sunblock	All	Yes	No
Moisturizing	Action™	All	As needed	As needed
	Eye Cream	All	As needed	As needed
Control	Tolereen®™** (0.5% hydrocortisone)[1]	All	As needed to relieve surface tightness, itching, and dryness	Both as needed to relieve surface tightness, itching, and dryness
	Moisturizer (Action™ and Eye Cream)	All		

HQ = hydroquinone

[1]Active chemical ingredient in parentheses

*2% lipomized

**Also available with HC

APPLICATION INSTRUCTIONS

Correction: Apply Clear evenly on entire face, including eyelids, extending to the hairline, over the ears, and ending with a feathering motion. Wait until the cream is absorbed, removing any excess around the eyes with a tissue. Wait 2 minutes and apply a second coat over the dark spots. *Note*: If you have dark skin, apply Clear on the entire face only once daily and apply at night only on the darkest areas. Once a desirable color tone has been reached, use Clear only as needed. Apply Exfoderm evenly over the entire face, but avoid the eyelid area. For the Maintenance program, apply Clear and Exfoderm only twice weekly.
Stimulation: Mix 1/2 gram of Blender with the prescribed amount of tretinoin on the palm of your hand. Apply evenly on the entire face, including the eyelids, entending to the hairline, over the ears, and ending with a feathering motion.
Protection: Apply Sunfader or Sunblock in the morning under makeup. Reapply often while in the sun. Avoid prolonged exposure to the sun for the first month.
Control: Use moisturizers sparingly and only if skin is uncomfortably dry. Can be used to cut strength of Exfoderm. Eye Cream can be used daily on top of other creams. Apply Tolereen when needed for itching, burning, or redness. Use only temporarily as hydrocortisone slows down the skin restoration process.

Table 5.8

SKIN HEALTH RESTORATION DAILY REGIMEN FOR NONFACIAL SKIN (NECK, BACK, ARMS)[1]

Step	*Agents*	*Morning*	*Evening*	*Special Instructions*
Correction and bleaching	Clear™ + Exfoderm™ (2% to 4% HQ + 4% AHA)[2] or 3% phytic acid	Yes	Yes	Concentrate application on lesions and feather out
Stimulation and blending	Tretinoin + Blender™ + Exfoderm™ (tretinoin + hydroquinone + 4% AHA)[2] or 3% phytic acid	No	Yes[3]	If redness, dryness, exfoliation are extreme, stop for 1 to 2 days and use moisturizer and control agents

[1]Treatment of nonfacial skin should continue for 3 cycles.

[2]Active chemical ingredient in parentheses

[3]On neck and chest, start with twice weekly and increase gradually, as tolerated. On arms, hands, legs, and back, start once daily and increase amount and frequency to induce a reaction

Table 5.9

THE THREE PHASES OF RESTORATION

Phase of Restoration	*What the Patient Can Expect*	*Duration*
1. ***Reaction Phase: "Out with the Old"*** Initial correction and stimulation phase	In about 6 weeks, the damaged top layers of skin are replaced by new layers of healthier cells. One or more of these symptoms can be expected: • Dryness • Itching • Peeling • Burning • Redness • Wrinkles may look worse • Sensitive skin • Acne may look worse Reactions are a sign that skin restoration is in process.	6 weeks or 1 skin cycle (for most skin conditions)
2. ***Tolerance Phase: "In with the New"*** Correction and stimulation continue	Skin has built tolerance to the treatment, and skin improvement becomes visible. Even more important, the regimen is increasing the production of collagen and elastin, helping to diminish wrinkles and pore size. Expected: • Reactions subside • Good skin (color even and clear, skin smooth, supple, translucent, and naturally hydrated)	***Aggressive*** 6 weeks (1 skin cycle) ***Moderately Aggressive*** 12 weeks (2 skin cycles) ***Standard*** 24 weeks (4 skin cycles)
3. ***Corrected Phase: "Healthy Glow"*** Correction and stimulation have peaked.	Skin tolerance is now complete. Surface problems have been corrected, and skin is healthy. This level can be maintained with the Maintenance program. Expect: • Reactions to almost disappear • Best skin (healthy, younger-looking)	6 weeks (1 skin cycle)

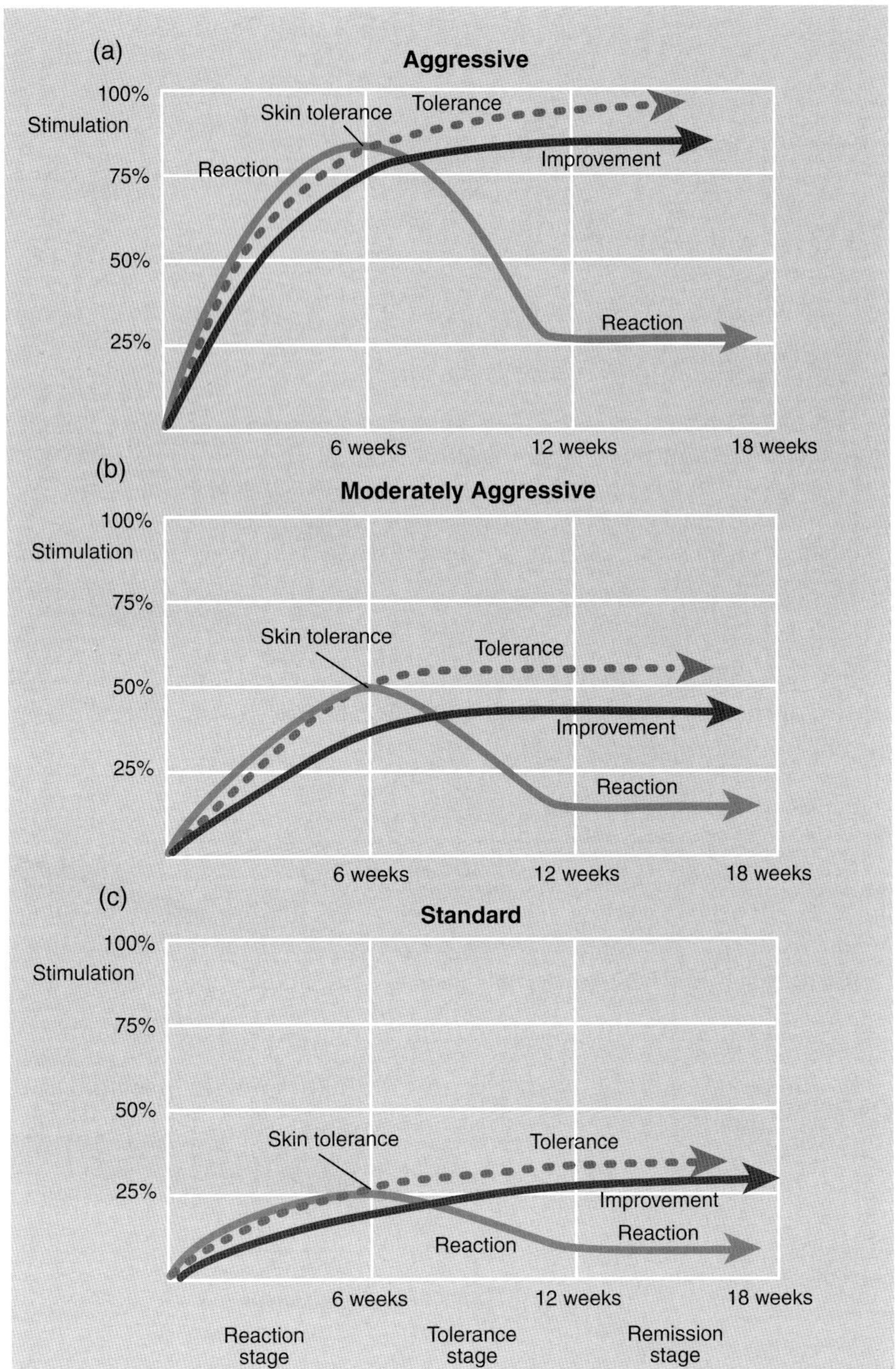

FIGURE 5-13. *Time for reaction, tolerance, and improvement stages with an aggressive, moderately aggressive, or standard program.*

Such reactions are to be expected and usually indicate that the treatment is being used effectively and that the skin is responding. The reactions also indicate the initial lack of skin tolerance, which the programs are meant to build up. The physician must support and encourage the patient during the reaction stage. Frequently restating that the worsening of the skin appearance is expected, beneficial, and temporary does much to en-

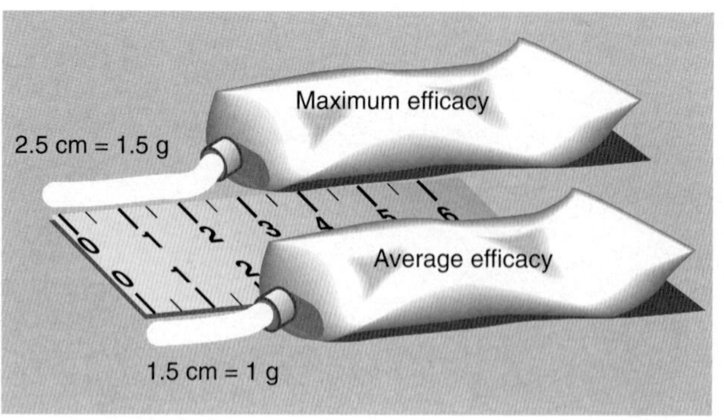

FIGURE 5-14. *Toothpaste drawing. The amount and frequency of agents used in Skin Conditioning are important for maximal efficacy. One g (which is equal to 1.5 cm of toothpaste) of any product in the programs, applied equally on 5% of the skin surface, such as the face, will have average efficacy. One and one-half g (equal to 1 in or 2.5 cm of toothpaste), applied similarly, will give maximum efficacy.*

courage compliance. Upon completion of 1 skin cycle, the intensity of the reaction diminishes, the skin begins to tolerate the treatment, and the patient become more comfortable.

Box 5-3

The patient undergoing Skin Health Restoration or Skin Conditioning should be told:

- **to anticipate skin reactions while tolerance is being built**
- **that reactions are desirable and indicate effectiveness of the treatment**
- **that reactions can be controlled and tailored, if desired.**

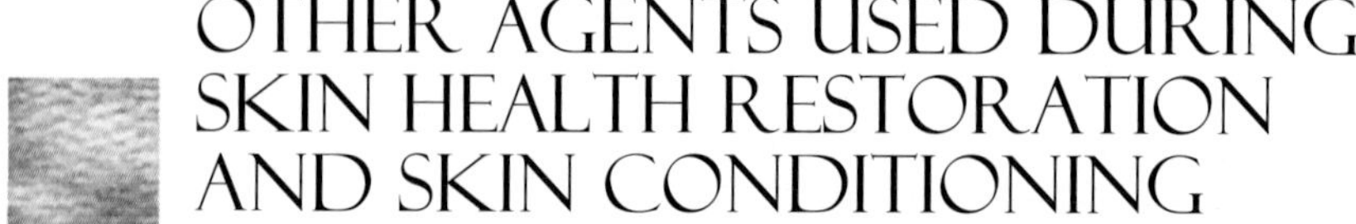

OTHER AGENTS USED DURING SKIN HEALTH RESTORATION AND SKIN CONDITIONING

TAMING REACTIONS WITH TOPICAL CORTICOSTEROIDS

A short course of topical corticosteroids is indicated for 1) decreasing skin sensitivity and providing some comfort while building skin tolerance for a rejuvenation procedure; 2) reducing sensitivity just after a skin rejuvena-

Box 5-4

Patients are advised to minimize use of hydrocortisone and moisturizers while building skin tolerance and while recovering from a procedure.

tion procedure; and 3) treating keloids and hypertrophic reactions. Potency of topical corticosteroids ranges from the very potent (clobitasol) through midpotency (triamcinolone) to the very weak (plain hydrocortisone). The weaker agents (which penetrate to the papillary dermis) can be used after superficial procedures or in the program for building skin tolerance in patients with highly irritable skin. Weak topical corticosteroids can reduce erythema after a procedure, suppress melanocyte hyperactivity, and prevent or minimize postinflammatory hyperpigmentation through their specific anti-inflammatory properties.

The high-potency agents (which penetrate to upper and mid reticular dermis) can be useful for suppressing or preventing the development of hypertrophic reactions and early keloids. However, they should be used only after deep procedures (medium-depth peel or CO_2 laser resurfacing and infrequently after superficial procedures, such as a Blue Peel) for 5 to 7 days. Longer use is discouraged because potent corticosteroids have profound suppressive effects on skin functions as well as the potential for side effects, such as skin atrophy and telangiectasias, and they can increase skin sensitivity to external agents.

The desired bleaching and blending effects that arise from using tretinoin in combination with hydroquinone can be significantly suppressed by concomitant use of topical corticosteroids. Also, after prolonged use patients can develop a strong addiction, since discontinuation of corticosteroids makes the skin feel dry and irritable. If needed, I use 0.5% of hydrocortisone in a cream base during the first 6 weeks of the Skin Health Restoration or Skin Conditioning programs while building tolerance as well as after the procedure, but not for more than 1 week at a time.

SKIN PREPARATION AGENTS

Cleanser: As part of the daily regimen, facial skin should cleaned in the morning and evening to remove sebum, makeup, environmental dirt, bacteria, and dead skin cells. The cleanser should be mild, respect the physiological pH of the skin (which is approximately 5.5), and not contain soapy material (fatty acids neutralized by strong base). It should also be readily removable and leave no residual. The presence of active plant extracts in the cleanser can be beneficial. The skin should not be rubbed during cleaning or drying. Only cold or warm water should be used for washing. Hot water can stimulate oil secretion in oily skin and exacerbate dryness and irritation in dry skin.

Toner: Toner, the second component of the system, enhances the cleaning of oily skin, makes it feel tight, and helps to prepare the surface for the next step of treatment.

Astringent/Topical Antibiotics: Astringents and topical antibiotics (2% erythromycin or 1% clindamycin) are used when indicated as part of the Skin Conditioning and Skin Health Restoration programs to restore skin to normalcy prior to any procedure so that infection and recurrence of acne are less likely during the healing stage. This also helps to reduce bacterial effects and inflammation in patients with acne, folliculitis, acne rosacea, or oily skin. Patients are to apply the antibiotic 2 times daily after application of the toner and leave it to dry on the skin. Patients with dry, noninflamed skin do not need astringents.

MOISTURIZERS

The Physiology of Dry Skin

For the epidermis to be normally hydrated, the water content of the stratum corneum must be above 10%, but the cosmetic companies believe between 20% and 35% is desirable.[10] Water that is lost from the skin through evaporation must be replaced by water from the lower epidermis and dermis, and the stratum corneum must have the ability to retain this moisture. However, it is known that dry skin is a result of more than low water content of the stratum corneum that produces abnormal desquamation of corneocytes,[11] since electron micrographs show dry skin with a thicker, fissured, and disorganized stratum corneum. Intracellular lipids are important in proper epidermal barrier function that prevents excessive water loss. For remoisturization to occur, barrier function must be restored and intracellular lipid synthesis brought to normal. This cannot be accomplished with the mere application of moisturizers.

Moisturizing Products

Moisturizers are commercially very successful, and cosmetics companies put much effort into creating and presenting new and elegant products. Most marketed dry skin moisturizers contain water, mineral oil, petrolatum or lanolin, propylene glycol, and a variety of so-called "special ingredients" with supposedly magical propereties. These creams and lotions do not and cannot live up to their claims because they do not penetrate into the dermis to have any measurable effect. Products sold as "lubricants," "moisturizers," and "anti-aging" or "skin repair" agents are all essentially emollients; that is, they temporarily make the skin feel smooth and soft by filling in the spaces between desquamating skin cells. This causes the skin to be smooth, but it does not correlate with decreased epidermal water loss, and the effect is temporary.[10–12] Moisturizers have no role in restoring normal skin functions, reversing or preventing skin aging, or producing other effects on the dermis. In actuality, moisturizers are suppressive of skin functions and,

Box 5-4

Moisturizers do not restore the barrier function of the skin or normalize lipid synthesis. They simply fill in the spaces between desquamating cells in the stratum corneum. Long-term use of moisturizers may actually increase skin sensitivity and decrease tolerance.

like topical steroids, may increase skin sensitivity and cause loss of normal tolerance. With long-term usage, this may lead to faster aging.

In the Obagi Skin Conditioning and Skin Health Restoration programs, moisturizers are to be used only when needed for a soothing effect while skin is undergoing the corrective and stimulative processes. This includes times when a patient may desire to reduce the normal skin reaction to tretinoin and AHAs for a short period of comfort or for social events.

It must be kept in mind that both correction and stimulation will eventually bring back hydration to normal levels in the epidermis, especially the stratum corneum, and in the dermis through GAG formation, which often eliminates the need for moisturizers. Only in the dry skin type (Obagi skin classification), which cannot become properly hydrated because of genetic influence, can moisturizers be used freely. For most patients, I recommend that moisturizers be used only occasionally when the weather can adversely affect the stratum corneum (e.g., cold, low humidity, extensive outdoor exposure, etc.).

UV LIGHT DAMAGE, SUNSCREENS, AND SUN-PROTECTIVE AGENTS

Ultraviolet (UV) light consists of UVA (320–400 nm) UVB (290–320 nm), UVC (100–290 nm), and vacuum UV (10–100 nm). UVC, vacuum UV, and the shortest UVB waves are trapped by the ozone layer. Longer-wave UVB and all UVA pass through the atmosphere and affect skin. I strongly believe that infrared rays (heat) also contribute to the formation of photodamage in general and solar elastosis in particular, and that protection from this wavelength is important (time of exposure).

Factors affecting radiation intensity and effects on the skin are time of day, season, elevation (5% UV increase with each 1,000 ft), reflection from snow, ice, water, or sand, and the use of moisturizers. The latter, by hydrating and thickening the stratum corneum, reduces reflectiveness to UVB and causes skin to absorb 4 times more UVB light than dry skin does.

UVB Properties: Only 10% to 20% of UVB penetrates to the dermis, while most of the effect is in the epidermis—photodamage, melanogenesis, and skin cancer. The minimal erythemal dose (MED) is the minimal amount of UVB that produces detectable erythema in the skin. It is used to create an

Box 5-5

- **UVA exposure increases melanin content only.**
- **UVB exposure increases both melanin content and the number of melanocytes.**

appropriate SPF (sun protection factor) in sunscreens. Exposure to UVA and UVB leads to melanogenesis from increased melanin oxidation and production as well as an increased number of active melanocyte-keratinocyte units, while the number of melanocytes remains the same. In Fitzpatrick type IV to VI individuals, tanning gives the same protection as an SPF of 5.

UVA Properties: All UVA that reaches the skin penetrates easily to the dermis. In the epidermis, UVA oxidizes existing melanin to cause immediate tanning. UVA is capable of producing erythema and melanogenesis, but it does not stimulate stratum corneum thickening or reduce the damage from further UVA exposure. UVA is responsible for elastosis changes in the skin and many of the allergic reactions to UV light. Furthermore, the infrared component of the sun's rays plays a major role in the development of solar elastosis, and proper protection from this wavelength is necessary as well.

One type of skin melanin, eumelanin, when oxidized, is a stable compound that protects skin from further exposure to UV light with an SPF of approximately 5. Oxidized pheomelanin, on the other hand, forms unstable compounds that break down upon subsequent UV exposure and release oxygen free radicals. These damage DNA, and, with chronic exposure, lead to precancerous lesions and skin cancer. Eumelanin is the dominant type of melanin in Fitzpatrick skin types III to VI. Pheomelanin is present in all skin colors in varying percentages; however, it is more dominant in light skin colors, and this accounts for the higher incidence of skin cancer in light-skinned persons.

Sunscreens

Sunscreen agents absorb specific waves of UV light, UVB, UVA, or both. An agent with both UVA and UVB protection is best. Recently there have been concerns that some UVC will start to reach the earth's surface because of erosion in the earth's ozone layer, and protection from UVC may soon be needed.

The SPF of sunscreens indicates the length of time that the product gives protection from the sun. The MED is the base, so that a product with an SPF of 4 protects for a shorter time than one with an SPF of 15, and so forth. Some sunscreens are waterproof, which is useful for prolonged outdoor activity with water exposure. Physical sunblocks (zinc oxide, titanium oxide) can scatter, reflect, and absorb all UV wavelengths. These offer better protection and are waterproof.

Patients undergoing Obagi Skin Conditioning or Skin Health Restoration programs should use sunscreens and sunblock routinely because the essential agents, tretinoin, AHAs, and hydroquinone, make skin more sun sensitive and susceptible to sun damage.

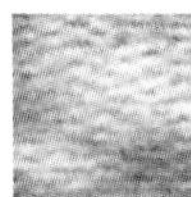

REFERENCES

1. Effendy I, Kwangsukstith C, Lee JY, Maibach HI. Functional changes in human stratum corneum induced by topical glycolic acid: comparison with all-trans retinoic acid. *Acta Derm Venereol.* 1995;75:455–458.
2. Jimbow K, Obatha H, Pathak MA, Fitzpatrick TB. Mechanism of depigmentation by hydroquinone. *J Invest Dermatol.* 1974;62:436–449.
3. Kligman AM. Compatibility of combinations of glycolic acid and tretinoin in acne and in photoaged facial skin. *J Geriatr Dermatol.* 1995;3 (Suppl A):25–28.
4. Dolezal J. Basic concepts in skin peeling: pharmaceutical considerations. In: Rubin MG, ed. *Manual of Chemical Peels.* Philadelphia, Pa: JB Lippincott, 1995:44–50.
5. Hevia O, Nemeth AJ, Taylor JR. Tretinoin accelerates healing after trichloroacetic acid chemical peel. *Arch Dermatol.* 1991;127:678–682.
6. Vagotis FL, Brundage SR. Histologic study of dermabrasion and chemical peel in an animal model after pretreatment with Retin-A. *Aesthetic Plast Surg.* 1995;19:243–246.
7. West TB, Alster TS. Effect of pretreatment on the incidence of hyperpigmentation following cutaneous CO_2 laser resurfacing. *Dermatol Surg.* 1999;25:15–17.
8. Nemeth AJ, Eaglstein WH, Falanga V. Methods to speed healing after skin biopsy or trichloroacetic acid chemical peel. *Prog Clin Biol Res.* 1991;365:267–277.
9. Kim IH, Kim HK, Kye JC. Effects of tretinoin pretreatment on TCA chemical peels in guinea pig skin. *J Korean Med Sci.* 1996;11:335–341.
10. Reiger MM. Skin, water, and moisturization. *Cosmet Toilet.* 1989;104:41–43.
11. Pierard GE. What does 'dry skin' mean? *Int J Dermatol.* 1987;26:167–169.
12. Draelos Z. Moisturizers. In: Draelos Z, ed. *Cosmetic Dermatology.* 2nd ed. New York: Churchill Livingstone; 1995:83–95.

CHAPTER

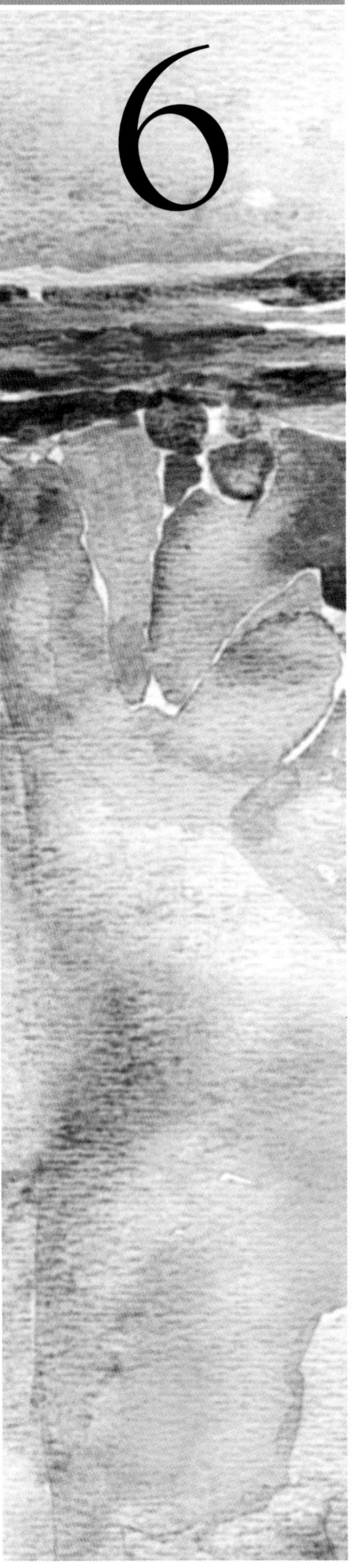

OVERVIEW OF TCA AND OTHER CHEMICAL PEELS

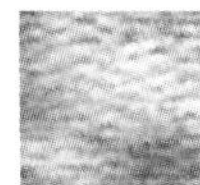

HISTORY AND DEVELOPMENT OF CHEMICAL PEELS

PHENOL PEELS

Although the ancient Egyptians used various herbs and chemical extracts as treatments to rejuvenate and beautify the skin,[1] peeling agents such as salicylic acid, resorcinol, phenol, and trichloroacetic acid (TCA) were not scientifically described until 1882 with the work of German dermatologist P. G. Unna.[2] Use of phenol to treat soldiers with gunpowder burns during World War I built up the knowledge base of this chemical peeling agent, which was used predominantly for the next 30 years.

BAKER-GORL
3 ml 88% USP phenol
8 drops liquid soap (Septisol,

MacKee used full strength phe early as 1903, and his biopsy findin ... wed compact collagen bundles and fibers a ... urface.[3] In 1960 Ayres[4] essentially confirmed MacK ... he reported on a subepidermal band of new collagen wi ... ibers arranged horizontally following application of phenol to a ... ically damaged skin of the neck. Litton, in 1962, described an increase in the number and thickness of collagen fibers following a phenol peel.[5]

While TCA chemical peels were described in reports in 1926,[6] 1945,[7] and the early 1960s,[8] and use of other chemical peeling agents, including sulfur and resorcinol pastes, salicylic acid, carbon dioxide snow, and β-naphthol, was described in the 1940s,[9] the introduction of the Baker-Gordon formula for the phenol peel in the 1960s[10–12] (Table 6-1) eclipsed the refinement of other phenol peel protocols. This formula penetrated deeper (to the midreticular dermis) than full-strength 88% phenol and eliminated severe photodamage and deep rhytids. Baker, Stuzin, and Baker[13] believe that phenol peeling produces the most predictable degree of dermal penetration followed by a predictable degree of neocollagen formation and dramatic, long-term, clinical improvement (Tables 6-1, 6-2).

However, the striking clinical results of phenol peels came at the price of potential for serious systemic toxicity (cardiac, renal, and hepatic), toxicity to melanocytes that caused permanent hypopigmentation and a "china-doll" skin color,[14–21] obvious lines of demarcation, and prolonged

TABLE 6.2

SUGGESTED TIMING AND SEQUENCE FOR FULL-FACE BAKER-GORDON PEEL

8:30 AM	Perioperative preparation: skin cleaning, analgesia, IV access, cardiac monitoring
9:00 AM	Solution applied to forehead
9:15 AM	Solution applied to first cheek
9:30 AM	Solution applied to contralateral cheek
9:45 AM	Solution applied to nose and glabella
10:00 AM	Solution applied to perioral and vermillion areas
10:15 AM	Solution applied to lower eyelids
10:30 AM	Solution applied to upper eyelids
11:00 AM	Patient monitored for 30 min before dressing of wound

recovery. Furthermore phenol peels were not suitable for peeling of darker skin types or the peeling of nonfacial skin. Despite its toxicity, phenol was considered the "gold standard" for facial skin peeling[22] and was widely used. In a 1981 survey, 74% of the plastic surgeons reported using phenol for facial peeling.[23]

To prevent systemic and hypopigmentation as complications, only fair-skinned patients should undergo phenol peels, and the treatment needs to be applied slowly and cautiously.[24] Brody recommended dividing the face into 5 to 8 segments with application of phenol to each of the segments at 10- to 20-minute intervals.[25] Heart rhythm had to be monitored during the procedure and intravenous fluids administered.[26]

A number of safer and equally effective alternatives to phenol peels are now available. Dermabrasion is very effective for treating coarse rhytids and scars in the perioral, cheek, and forehead regions and does not have the same bleaching effect. However, it is not recommended for all skin types, cannot be used to treat rhytids around the eyes, and is a difficult procedure to master. CO_2 laser resurfacing and deeper TCA peels such as the Obagi Controlled-Depth TCA peel can produce very effective results with full-face treatment and are replacing phenol peels for the treatment of deeper wrinkles and scars for most patients (Table 6-3). These modalities produce fewer changes in facial pigmentation when depth is controlled and thus can treat a wider spectrum of skin-color types. The sharing of knowledge from multiple disciplines such as dermatology, plastic surgery, and cosmetic surgery has resulted in the availability of many techniques and makes it possible for us to improve the appearance of all skin types and colors, in facial and nonfacial areas, with a quality of results and safety not imagined 20 years ago.

TCA PEELS

The feasibility of performing a chemical peel that was less deep than a phenol peel became apparent in the 1980s as trichloroacetic acid (TCA) peel techniques were refined to increase their efficacy and safety. Stagnone showed

TABLE 6.3

MECHANISM OF ACTION OF CHEMICAL PEEL AGENTS

Agent	*Mechanism*
TCA	Coagulation of dermal and epidermal proteins (keratolytic)
Phenol	Coagulation of dermal and epidermal proteins
Jessner's	Breaking of intracellular bridges to enhance effects of keratolytic agents
AHAs	Low concentrations decrease corneocyte adhesion; high concentrations cause epidermolysis

the absence of toxicity of 50% TCA.[11] Other investigators demonstrated the histological changes that correlated with peel penetration depth in humans and in animal models[27–29] and provided clinical descriptions of patient peels.[30–32] Following these and other reports, the clinical spectrum of TCA skin peeling came to be recognized, ranging from exfoliation to eradication of lines, wrinkles, elastotic deposits, and mottled pigmentation (now called skin rejuvenation) by penetration to the papillary dermis or below.

Today TCA peels are a widely practiced modality for depths ranging from exfoliation to mid-dermal penetration. These chemical peels are currently performed in a variety of ways including

1. used alone in concentrations ranging from 35% to 50%,
2. combined with augmenting agents for increased penetration,
3. combined with acid penetration–slowing modifying agents in concentrations of 25% to 40%, known as as the Obagi Controlled Depth Peel, and
4. combined with color and acid penetration–slowing modifying agents in concentrations of 15% or 20%, known as the Obagi Blue Peel.

This book will emphasize the latter 2 types of TCA peels mentioned above, which are the author's techniques.

Box 6-1

METHODS USED FOR MEDIUM TO DEEP FACIAL SKIN REJUVENATION

Chemical Methods

- **Phenol**
- **Conventional TCA, 35% to 50%**
- **35% TCA augmented with solid CO_2**
- **35% TCA augmented with Jessner's solution (resorcinol, salicylic acid, lactic acid, and ethanol)**
- **35% TCA augmented with 5% to 10% methylsalicylate, 1% polysorbate 20**
- **70% Alpha hydroxy acid (AHA) alone**
- **50%–70% AHA plus 20%–35% TCA**

Nonchemical Methods

- **Dermabrasion**
- **CO_2 laser resurfacing**
- **Erbium laser resurfacing**

TCA PEELS AS PERFORMED TODAY

35% TO 50% TCA USED ALONE

While conventional TCA peels have produced good results in the hands of certain peelers, many other physicians have experienced poor depth control and variable results. In concentrations over 40%, TCA penetrates the skin very fast and the therapeutic effects are hindered by the high risk of caustic effects (Figure 6-1). Postinflammatory hyperpigmentation (PIH) and potential scarring are continuing concerns with higher concentrations. Other problem areas are a generally poor understanding of the mechanism of a TCA peel and poor control of the many variables involved. Conventional, deeper TCA peels are difficult to perform and are not recommended for anyone but the most experienced physician.

IMPORTANCE OF DEPTH

The most important variable in the quality of outcome and safety of a TCA peel procedure is the depth of acid penetration. Light penetration (to basal layer) generally improves the epidermis and superficial coloration. If the upper papillary dermis is reached, improvement in texture, increased tightness, removal of fine lines, and correction of deeper pigmentation problems and some scars can be expected. Medium-depth wounding (reaching the upper reticular dermis to mid dermis) generally improves deeper wrinkles and scars, softens the texture, corrects deep discoloration, and increases skin firmness. Deep wounding (below the mid dermis to the lower reticular dermis) improves certain deep wrinkles and scars.

TCA peels in concentrations of 10%, 35% and 50% have been classified as superficial, medium, or deep with the erroneous assumption that a certain concentration penetrates to a certain depth.[33] As will be explained later, TCA concentration determines only the speed at which the acid penetrates the skin (higher concentrations penetrate faster), and any concentration can be made to penetrate to any depth.

As with other rejuvenation procedures, TCA complications are correlated with depth, and deeper TCA peels have a higher incidence of com-

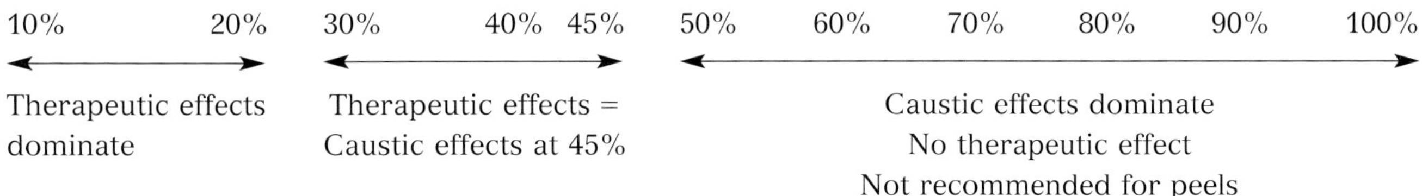

FIGURE 6-1. *Therapeutic and caustic effects of TCA are related to concentration.*

TABLE 6.4

GENERAL CHARACTERISTICS OF TRICHLOROACETIC ACID CHEMICAL PEELS

Characteristic	*Comment*
Histological Goal	■ To increase collagen and elastin in the dermis and maintain the 3-dimensional alignment of collagen
Mechanism of Action	■ Coagulation of skin proteins
Neutralization	■ Self-neutralizing; no need to apply external neutralizing agents
Penetration	■ Higher concentrations penetrate skin faster ■ Penetration with a given concentration can be increased with additional applications or an increase in volume applied ■ With continuous application, deep penetration can be achieved with any concentration
Quality of Results	■ Depth reached generally determines the postpeel quality of skin texture and color
Skin Conditioning	■ Conditioning before and after a TCA peel improves the quality of the skin after the peel and expedites healing
Complications	■ Related to depth; deeper procedures have a higher risk of complications, such as keloids and hypopigmentation

plications than lighter TCA peels. Two common misconceptions about TCA peels are that high concentrations cause scarring, that lower concentrations are thus safer, and that lower concentrations cannot penetrate deeply. Table 6-4 shows the general characteristics of the TCA peels known today, and Table 6-5 shows the the problem areas of conventional, nonstandardized TCA peels. The Obagi Controlled Medium-Depth TCA Peel and the Obagi Blue Peel were developed to address and prevent these problems. The Obagi peel modalities are discussed in depth in subsequent chapters.

Box 6-2

PREVAILING MISCONCEPTIONS ABOUT TCA PEELS

- **High concentrations cause scarring.**
- **Lower concentrations cannot penetrate deeply and are thus safer.**

TABLE 6.5	
PROBLEMS ASSOCIATED WITH CONVENTIONAL, NONSTANDARDIZED TCA PEELS	
Area	***Characteristic***
Definition of peel depth	Not consistent—a "superficial peel" can range from stratum corneum to papillary dermis penetration
Existing skin classification systems	Not complete for proper patient selection
Pre and post skin conditioning programs	Erratic and arbitrary
TCA concentration can vary from 20% to 50%	Numerous techniques with different concentrations
Depth monitoring signs	None
Use of augmenting agents to remove the stratum corneum prior to TCA application	Unpredictable depth

CONTROL OF TCA PEEL VARIABLES

The practitioner must keep in mind that a 100% safe chemical peel or procedure does not exist; however, the risk can be significantly lowered with procedures that give the physician more control of the variables associated with the peel (Table 6-6). Control of the variables can lead to more predictable acid penetration depth, thus increasing the likelihood of good results and avoidance of complications.

TABLE 6.6	
FACTORS INFLUENCING TCA PEEL OUTCOME	
Variable	***Comment***
Skin type	■ Original deviated colors ■ Skin thickness, laxity, fragility, and depth selection
Preoperative and postoperative skin conditioning	■ Skin tolerance ■ Even TCA penetration ■ Recovery time ■ Complications rate
TCA concentration, and method used for monitoring depth of peels	■ Peel depth ■ Require precise endpoints

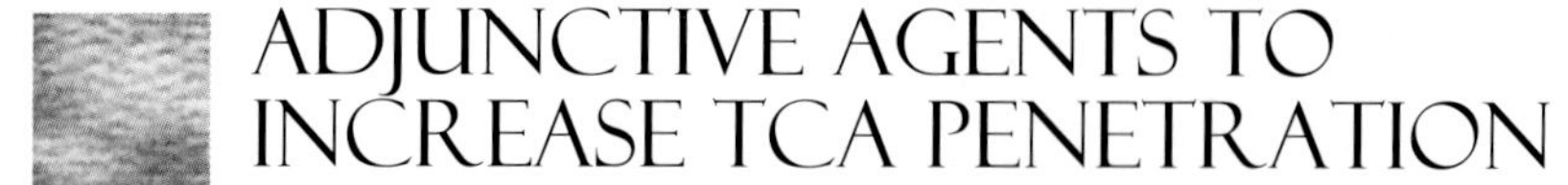

ADJUNCTIVE AGENTS TO INCREASE TCA PENETRATION

To increase the penetration of TCA into the skin, various agents can be applied to the skin prior to the application of TCA.

SOLID CARBON DIOXIDE PLUS TCA

Adjunctive agents are used with 35% TCA to increase the depth of penetration and to augment its action.[22,34] In 1986 Brody and Hailey reported satisfying clinical results from the application of solid carbon dioxide, followed by application of 35% TCA, to enhance the penetration of the TCA solution.[35] Actinic damage, edges of atrophic scars, light rhytids, and irregular hyperpigmentation were improved with this "medium-depth" peel. Histological specimens showed an expanded papillary Grenz zone (neocollagen formation in the subepidermal region of the dermis) and a midreticular dermal band consisting of elastic fibers and collagen. This technique was reported to penetrate to the upper reticular dermis, a wound depth that was similar to full-strength phenol, and to be more effective than Jessner's plus TCA in the treatment of scars.[36]

PEELS USING SOLID CARBON DIOXIDE PLUS TCA: THE AUTHOR'S VIEW

Solid carbon dioxide has not been scientifically demonstrated to add any benefit to a TCA peel. The clinical results are similar to those obtained with TCA alone, and histological studies show the same pattern seen after peels performed with TCA alone. In the author's opinion, solid carbon dioxide should not be used with TCA for several reasons:

1. it will produce edema with poorly defined boundaries at the site of application that can result in uncontrolled deeper penetration in certain areas;
2. it can destroy melanocytes, not only in the epidermis, but also in the adnexal structures, leading to hypopigmentation, especially in darker skin; and
3. there are no clear endpoints for using the agent along with TCA.

This form of TCA peel is poorly controlled and gives variable results. It should be considered a questionable variation of a TCA peel until clinical studies demonstrate its value.

PEELS USING JESSNER'S, METHYLSALICYLATE, OR GLYCOLIC ACID PLUS TCA

Jessner's Plus TCA

Monheit developed a medium-depth peel that incorporated Jessner's solution (resorcinol 14 g, salicylic acid 14 g, lactic acid 14 cc, and ethanol 100 cc), an agent that destroys the epidermal barrier function by breaking the intracellular bridges between keratinocytes.[37,38] His procedure involved vigorous degreasing with Septisol and acetone, then application of Jessner's solution to remove the stratum corneum and "open" the epidermis to TCA penetration, followed by application of 35% TCA. Formation of a white frost indicated protein coagulation. According to Monheit, the application of Jessner's solution allows TCA to penetrate to the papillary dermis and leads to the formation of new collagen that clinically decreases wrinkles and improves skin texture. Treatment with Jessner's solution plus TCA has been shown to reach the same depth and achieve similar results as solid carbon dioxide (CO_2) plus TCA, with the exception of the treatment of scars.

Methylsalicylate Plus TCA

Fulton[39] developed a "hot rod" TCA peel which contained 35% TCA with 5% to 10% methylsalicylate for augmentation and 1% polysorbate 20 as a surfactant. Dermabrasion was suggested 4 to 6 weeks after the peel to remove scars or remaining perioral and periorbital wrinkles.

Glycolic Acid Plus TCA Peels

Glycolic acid 70% has also been applied before the application of 35% TCA. This is believed to allow TCA to frost more evenly and to penetrate deeper.[40] After 2 minutes of contact with the skin, the glycolic acid is removed with water and the 35% TCA is applied. The skin sloughs between the fourth and sixth postoperative day, and after 7 days the patient can usually wear make-up. Postoperative histology specimens showed effects similar to those of other medium-depth peels. According to the investigators, this peeling method has the advantage of not requiring storage of solid CO_2, the precise mixing of components needed for Jessner's solution, or vigorous prepeel scrubbing with acetone.

JESSNER'S, METHYLSALICYLATE, OR GLYCOLIC ACID PLUS TCA: THE AUTHOR'S VIEW

Removing the stratum corneum prior to the application of 35% TCA to enhance TCA penetration appears to have no clear advantage, and histological studies have not shown results to be any different from those obtained

Box 6-3

Trichloroacetic acid (TCA) is a very versatile peeling agent that can be used for a peel depth ranging from the stratum corneum to the lower reticular dermis. The ability of TCA to correct skin conditions is controlled by 2 factors: 1) the depth of the problem, which is especially important in the case of scars, and 2) the depth of the peel that is performed. Augmenting agents simply add confusion to these controlling factors.

after a peel in which TCA alone was used. Subjecting the skin to 2 injurious agents is not necessary when TCA as a single agent can penetrate very well, and the second agent simply complicates the penetration issues. Acid penetration depth with peels that use augmenting agents is arbitrary, and the peels do not have clear endpoints that clarify when application of the peeling agent should stop. Furthermore, papillary dermis peels performed with augmenting agents have erroneously been labeled "medium-depth" peels. Peels to this depth are in reality superficial peels (See the author's recommended terminology, Chapter 7).

Augmentation of TCA by removing the stratum corneum with methylsalicylate (the Fulton "hot rod" peel) is similar to using Jessner's.

GLYCERIN AND POLYSORBATE PLUS TCA

In 1994, Dinner reported good cosmetic results with less irritation and easier and more even application when using a mixture of 40% TCA and glycerin that was emulsified with the surfactant polysorbate 20.[42] He believed that the concentration of TCA used for a peel was actually of limited importance and that factors such as volume of the acid, the force of application, and the susceptibility of the skin determined the depth of penetration and subsequent tissue destruction. He attributed the beneficial clinical effects and ease of application to the emollient action of glycerin. To this, Laub added that Complex 272, present in the Obagi TCA peel formula, not only emulsifies like polysorbate 20 but also increases acid penetration through the skin through an interaction with polar compounds.[43] Complex 272 is described in Chapter 8.

Collins[44] reviewed the variables that affect penetration of TCA, including concentration of the acid, technique of application, prior use of retinoic acid, prepeel skin degreasing, sebaceous gland density and activity, and application of prepeel keratolytic agents and solutions. He believed a 15% to 25% concentration would produce mild epithelial sloughing while a 45% concentration would produce necrosis of the epidermal proteins and a dermal, inflammatory infiltrate. With vigorous rubbing, however, a 35% solution could penetrate to the same depth as a 45% solution. Similarly, he stated that repetitive application of TCA would increase penetration, so that several TCA peels with a lower concentration, separated by intervals of weeks to months, could be as effective as a single, more concentrated peel.

GLYCERIN AND POLYSORBATE PLUS TCA: THE AUTHOR'S VIEW

Dr. Dinner's peel follows Obagi's principles and techniques to a certain extent, but his use of polysorbate 80, a well-known penetrating agent, makes it necessary to categorize this peel in the augmented TCA peel group. TCA penetrates skin very well, and agents that increase its penetration, such as polysorbate 20, lead to faster appearance of frost and give the physician less time to observe depth signs. Complex 272 in the Obagi preparations slows down the penetration of TCA so that depth signs can be observed and contains glycerin, which is less invasive and less irritating than polysorbate 20.

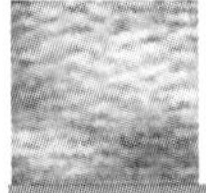

MODIFIED TCA PEELS (OBAGI PEELS)

The modified TCA peel category includes the Obagi Blue Peel and the Obagi Controlled Depth Peel. Both of these peels are unique in that most of the variables associated with TCA peels are better controlled through the use of standardized agents and protocols. By using the modified solutions and following the guidelines for these peels, control of the penetration depth of TCA is increased, which allows the procedures to be performed with more safety and predictability. With the Blue Peel, wounding is limited to the papillary dermis or immediate reticular dermis. The immediate reticular dermis is a term that indicates reaching but not involving the upper reticular dermis. The peel is performed with a fixed volume of a 15% or 20% concentration of TCA solution, modified by the addition of a prepared volume of additive that contains a nonionic base, glycerin, Complex 272, which slows acid penetration, and a blue dye for uniformity of acid application. A fixed volume of the modified TCA is then applied on a specified 5% of total skin surface. There are clear endpoints, signs that enable the physician to recognize the depth of acid penetration and to stop applying peel solution when the desired depth has been reached. Because of the standardization of the variables, particularly the endpoints, the Blue Peel has a larger safety margin than many other peels. It does not require highly developed peeling skills when performed to the level of the papillary dermis. Postpeel management skills, however, are important.

The Obagi Controlled Depth TCA Peel is an alternative peel with good depth control that is usually used to reach a skin level deeper than the Blue Peel, e.g., the upper or mid dermis.[45,46] Like the Blue Peel, it has the attributes of slower action and depth control, and thus has a larger margin of safety than other peels that reach the dermis. Unlike phenol, which is to be used mostly on fair-skinned patients because it is toxic to melanocytes and bleaches skin permanently, the Obagi Controlled Depth TCA peel can be used on a wide variety of skin types, ranging from very fair to Black. The physician can gain great satisfaction from being able to improve the skin of patients who have been found unsuitable for phenol peeling or CO_2 laser resurfacing because of their skin color. A TCA peel that reaches the upper reticular dermis can have remarkable effects on deep facial wrinkles, scars, and deeply seated pigmentation disorders, but the skill level of the performing physician should be high .

Deeper TCA peels are not to be taken lightly, since acid penetration can be rapid and difficult to control in conventional, nonstandardized TCA peels, leading to undesirably deep dermal penetration followed by complications. This has led to the characterization of TCA peels in concentrations exceeding 35% as erratic, unpredictable, and "too technique-sensitive."[47] Baker and associates have identified the ability to "read the peel" as the key to mastering TCA peels and have found that the rapid penetration of high TCA concentrations make this difficult to do.[48] While deeper TCA peels do require greater caution and a skilled physician, the author believes that TCA can produce a dermal peel with an excellent outcome and a low risk of complications if the peel is standardized to control the associated variables. Chapter 8 presents the Blue Peel in detail and Chapter 9, the Controlled Depth Peel.

ALPHA HYDROXY ACID PEELS

Alpha hydroxy acids (AHAs) have been extolled by manufacturers and the media as products that dramatically improve skin appearance and texture, despite a lack of well-controlled studies. Numerous daily-use skin care products contain AHAs in concentrations of 2% to 10%, and "refresher" or "lunchtime" low-concentration (e.g., 30%) glycolic acid peels are being performed by medical personnel as well as aestheticians for "rejuvenation." These procedures cannot live up to their rejuvenation claims because they remove only stratum corneum for an exfoliation. They can produce smoother skin and improve comedogenic acne, but they have minimal effect on wrinkles or scars and cannot tighten lax skin. Unsubstantiated and inaccurate claims, however, are very prevalent.

Although the mechanism of action is not fully known, glycolic acid is believed to thin the stratum corneum and thicken the stratum granulosum.[49–55] The effects are pH-dependent, and solutions with a pH between 2.8 and 3.5 are the most effective for inducing desquamation. Whether the therapeutic effects are merely a result of pH-induced irritation has not been demonstrated.

AHAs have also been used in concentrations of 50% to 70% for true chemical peeling to the level of the papillary dermis, usually as a glycolic acid peel. A higher concentration or increased length of time the acid is left on the skin results in deeper penetration, but usually these peels do not penetrate to the epidermal/dermal junction, and, if they do, penetration can be uneven. A 70% glycolic acid concentration in contact with the skin for up to 7 minutes may not penetrate into the papillary dermis. Deeper penetration into the dermis, however, can occur if the peel is not monitored or neutralized properly, especially in thin skin. Cases of significant irritation and hypertrophic scarring have been reported. Fifty percent glycolic acid solutions, considered "safer" than the 70%, can also penetrate the dermis if left on the skin long enough.

Glycolic acid agents need to be washed off with large amounts of water to terminate their action when they have penetrated to the desired depth. There are no clear endpoints for ending the peel. After application, the skin appears pink and then progressively more red, indicating penetration of the epidermis. If the solution has penetrated to the epidermal/dermal junction, small gray-white patches will appear, and, with significant dermal involvement, some white frosting may be seen.

Uneven penetration and highly variable results from patient to patient have been reported with glycolic acid peels. Although high concentration (>50%) glycolic acid used repeatedly can stimulate the dermis to form new collagen and increase glycosaminoglycans in the upper dermis, the process has to be repeated a number of times for beneficial effects to be realized. Patients often drop out before completion of the sequence, dissatisfied with the limited improvement and inconvenience. Clinical results have been described as "subtle" and hard to validate scientifically. Surface texture, superficial hyperpigmentation, acne, and xerosis can be expected to improve following a glycolic acid peel. Fine wrinkles may be improved but deeper wrinkles are not.

A clinical study conducted to evaluate short-contact (3 to 6 min) 70% glycolic acid peels used on a monthly basis showed no benefit for the treatment of photodamaged skin.[56] The investigators concluded that the value of glycolic acid "refresher peels" should be questioned as a "value-added" treatment for aging skin, and that topical retinoids and low-concentration TCA peels are a better value for the consumer. Another study, however, of 50% glycolic acid applied for 5 minutes once weekly for 4 weeks, showed mild improvement of some skin photoaging signs.[57] AHA research is currently in its infancy and there is not yet enough scientific evidence to support AHAs as true therapeutic agents.[58]

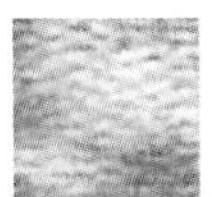

REFERENCES

1. Ancient Egyptian Medicine: The Papyrus Ebers. Bryan CP, trans. Chicago, Ill: Ares Publishers; 1974:158–161.

2. Marmelzat WL. A historical review of chemical rejuvenation of the face. In: Kotler R, ed. *Chemical Rejuvenation of the Face.* St.Louis, Mo: Mosby; 1992:934–938.

3. MacKee GM, Karp FL. The treatment of post-acne scars with phenol. *Br J Dermatol.* 1952;64:456.
4. Ayres S. Dermal changes following application of chemical cauterants to aging skin. *Arch Dermatol.* 1960;82:578.
5. Litton C. Chemical face lifting. *Plast Reconstr Surg.* 1962;29:371.
6. Roberts HL. The chloroacetic acids: a biochemical study. *Brit J Dermatol.* 1926;38:323–391.
7. Monash S. The uses of diluted tricholoroacetic acid in dermatology. *Urol Cutan Rev.* 1945;49:119.
8. Ayres S. Superficial chemosurgery in treating aging skin. *Arch Dermatol.* 1962;82:125.
9. Eller JJ, Wolff S. Skin peeling and scarification. *JAMA.* 1941;116:934–938.
10. Baker TJ, Gordon HL. The ablation of rhytides by chemical means: A preliminary report. *J Fla Med Assoc.* 1961;48:541.
11. Baker TJ. Chemical face peeling and rhytidectomy. *Plast Reconstr Surg.* 1962;29:199.
12. Baker TJ, Gordon HL, Seckinger DL. A second look at chemical face peeling. *Plast Reconstr Surg.* 1966;37:487–493.
13. Baker TJ, Stuzin JM, Baker TM. Histologic effects of photoaging and facial resurfacing. In: *Facial Skin Resurfacing.* St. Louis, Mo: Quality Medical Publishing; 1998:12–28.
14. Wexler MR, Halon DA, Teitelbaum et al. The prevention of cardiac arythmias produced in an animal model by the topical application of a phenol preparation in common use for face peeling. *Plast Reconstr Surg.* 1984;73:595–598.
15. Kligman AM, Baker TJ, Gordon H. Long-term histologic follow-up of phenol face peels. *Plast Reconstr Surg.* 1985;75:652–659.
16. Warner MA, Harper JV. Cardiac dysrhythmias associated with chemical peeling with phenol. *Anesthesiology.* 1985;62:366–367.
17. Stagnone JJ, Orgel MB, Stagnone GJ. Cardiovascular effects of topical 50% trichloroacetic acid and Baker's phenol solution. *J Dermatol Surg Oncol.* 1987;13:999–1002.
18. Lober CW. Chemexfoliation—indications and cautions. *J Am Acad Dermatol.* 1987;17:109–112.
19. Asken S. Unoccluded Baker-Gordon phenol peels—review and update. *J Dermatol Surg Oncol.* 1989;15:998–1008.
20. Alt TH. Occluded Baker-Gordon chemical peel: review and update. *J Dermatol Surg Oncol.* 1989;15:980–993.
21. Klein DR, Little JH. Laryngeal edema as a complication of chemical peel. *Plast Reconstr Surg.* 1983;71:419–420.
22. Beeson WH. Chemical peeling: a facial plastic surgeon's perspective. *Dermatol Surg.* 1995;21:389–391.
23. Litton C, Trinidad G. Complications of chemical face peeling as evaluated by a questionnaire. *Plast Reconstr Surg.* 1981;67:738–44.
24. Baker TJ, Stuzin JM, Baker TM. Histologic effects of photoaging and facial resurfacing. In: *Phenol Peels.* St. Louis, Mo: Quality Medical Publishing; 1998:118–143.

25. Brody HJ. Complications of chemical peeling: a variation of superficial chemosurgery. *J Dermatol Surg Oncol.* 1989;15:1010–1019.

26. Hopping SB. Chemical peeling in 1996: What have we learned? *Int J Aesthetic Restor Surg.* 1996;4:73–80.

27. Stegman SJ. A study of dermabrasion and chemical peels in an animal model. *J Dermatol Surg Oncol.* 1980;6:490–497.

28. Stegman SJ. A comparative histologic study of the effects of three peeling agents and dermabrasion on normal and sundamaged skin. *Aesthetic Plast Surg.* 1982;6:123–135.

29. Brodland DG, Cillimore KC, Roenigk RK. Depths of chemexfoliation induced by various concentrations and application techniques of trichloroacetic acid in a porcine model. *J Dermatol Surg Oncol.* 1989;15: 967–971.

30. Resnick SS, Lewis LA, Cohen BH. Trichloroacetic acid peeling. *Cutis.* 1976;17:127–129.

31. Resnik SS, Lewis LA. The cosmetic uses of trichloroacetic acid peeling in dermatology. *South Med J.* 1973;66:225.

32. Brodland DG, Roenigk RK. Trichloroacetic acid chemexfoliation (chemical peel) for extensive premalignant actinic damage of the face and scalp. *Mayo Clin Proc.* 1988;63:887.

33. Brody HJ. *Chemical Peeling and Resurfacing.* 2nd ed. St. Louis, Mo: CV Mosby; 1997:109–136.

34. Collins P. Trichloroacetic acid peel revisited. *J Derm Surg Oncol.* 1989; 15:933–940.

35. Brody HJ, Hailey CW. Medium depth chemical peeling of the skin: a variation of superficial chemosurgery. *J Dermatol Surg Oncol.* 1986;12: 1268–1272.

36. Brody HJ. Variations and comparisons in medium-depth chemical peeling. *J Derm Surg Oncol.* 1989;15:953–963.

37. Monheit G. The Jessner's + TCA peel: a medium depth chemical peel. *J Dermatol Surg Oncol.* 1989;15:945–952.

38. Monheit GD. The Jessner's-trichloroacetic acid peel: an enhanced medium-depth chemical peel. *Cosmet Dermatol.* 1995;13:277–283.

39. Fulton JE. Step-by-step skin rejuvenation. *Am J Cosmet Surg.* 1990;7:199–205.

40. Coleman WP, Futrell JM. The glycolic acid-trichloroacetic acid peel. *J Dermatol Surg Oncol.* 1994;20:76–80.

41. Fulton, JE. Paper presented at American Academy of Aesthetic and Restorative Surgery, World Congress, Los Angeles, 1997.

42. Dinner MI, Artz JF. Chemical peel—what's in the formula? *Plast Reconstr Surg.* 1994;94:406–407.

43. Laub DR. Polysorbate as an adjunctive chemical in the trichloroacetic acid peel [letter]. *Plast Reconstr Surg.* 1995;95:425.

44. Collins PS. Trichloroacetic acid revisited. *J Dermatol Surg Oncol.* 1989;15:933–940.

45. Johnson JB, Ichinose H, Obagi ZE, Laub, DR. Obagi's modified trichloroacetic acid (TCA)-controlled variable depth peel: a study of clinical signs correlating with histological findings. *Ann Plast Surg.* 1996;36:225–237.

46. Obagi ZO, Sawaf MM, Johnson JB, et al. The controlled depth trichloroacetic acid peel: methodology, outcome, and complication rate. *Int J Aesthetic Restor Surg.* 1996;4:81–94.

47. Duffy D. Alpha hydroxy acids/trichloroaceitc acids risk/benefit strategies: a photographic review. *Dermatol Surg.* 1998;24:181–189.

48. Baker TJ, Stuzin JM, Baker TM. *Facial Skin Resurfacing.* St. Louis, Mo: Quality Medical Publishing; 1998:88.

49. Van Scott EJ, Yu RJ. Alpha hydroxy acids: therapeutic potentials. *Can J Dermatol.* 1989;1:108–112.

50. Matarasso ST, Salman SM, Glogau RG, et al. The role of chemical peeling in the treatment of photodamaged skin. *J Dermatol Surg Oncol.* 1990;16:945–954.

51. Moy LS, Murad H, Moy RL. Glycolic acid peels for the treatment of wrinkles and photoaging. *J Dermatol Surg Oncol.* 1993;19:243–246.

52. Moy LS, Murad H, Moy RL. Glycolic acid therapy: evaluation of efficacy and techniques in treatment of photodamage lesions. *Am J Cosmet Surg.* 1993;10:1.

53. Murad H, Shamban AT, Premo PS. The use of glycolic acid as a peeling agent. *Dermatol Clin.* 1995;13:285–307.

54. Daniello NJ. Glycolic acid controversies. *Int J Aesthetic Restor Surg.* 1996;4:113–116.

55. Draelos ZD. Dermatologic considerations of AHAs. *Cosmet Dermatol.* 1997;10:14–18.

56. Piacquadio D, Dobry M, Hunt S, et al. Short contact glycolic acid peels as a treatment for photodamaged skin: a pilot study. *Dermatol Surg.* 1996;22:449–452.

57. Newman NN, Newman A, Moy LS, et al. Clinical improvement of photoaged skin with 50% glycolic acid. *Dermatol Surg.* 1996;22:455–460.

58. Brody H, Coleman WP, Piacquadio D, et al. Round table discussion of alpha hydroxy acids. *Dermatol Surg.* 1996;22:475–477.

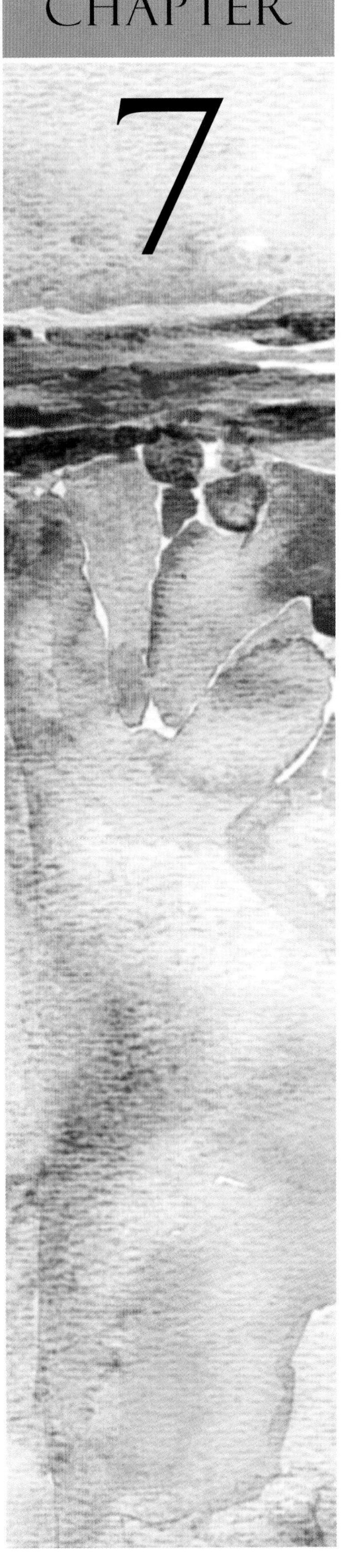

THE TREATMENT PLAN FOR REJUVENATION

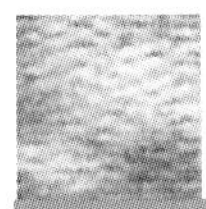

SKIN REJUVENATION: OVERVIEW

DEFINITION OF SKIN REJUVENATION

Skin rejuvenation is a term that has different meanings for different people. To physicians, rejuvenation usually means making skin look younger by means of a procedure. To cosmetics companies and cosmetolologists, however, it means the use of topical products. The media have also joined in, usually disseminating inaccurate, exaggerated, and out-of-context information on the benefits of the latest miracle cream or high-tech treatment. Clearly, skin rejuvenation needs a comprehensive, standard definition to make it easier for physicians to communicate with each other, the media, and the public.

TABLE 7.1	
PROCEDURES DEPTH DEFINITIONS	
Term for Depth	***Skin Level***
Exfoliation	Epidermis above basal layer
Light	Papillary dermis
Light-medium	Immediate reticular dermis (IRD)
Medium	Upper reticular dermis
Deep	Mid dermis

To me, skin rejuvenation is neither a cream program nor a particular procedure. It is instead a *comprehensive* treatment plan that involves the use of creams to regulate skin function and may involve one or more procedures. The rejuvenation program should be controlled by the physician, not the patient, although the patient may have valuable input. The choice of treatment program and the depth of the procedure most suitable for the patient's skin type must be controlled by the physician.

The area of skin rejuvenation also needs uniformity in language and terminology so that treatment protocols and procedures and their depth can be discussed without misunderstanding or confusion. Table 7-1 presents terminology for procedure depth.

Box 7-1

Skin rejuvenation is the art of transforming skin to its most natural and youthful state through topical agents that regulate skin function. It may or may not involve a procedure. The goal is to maintain the transformation indefinitely.

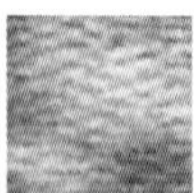

PATIENT SELECTION

In all aesthetic procedures, proper patient selection is a crucial component of a successful outcome. Prospective skin rejuvenation patients often come to the physician with a "consumer" attitude. They want to look younger and better and are willing to put forth the associated out-of-pocket expenses for such improvement. As consumers, however, they often "shop" for a physician, expecting a predictable postprocedure course, an excellent

Box 7-2

Patients to Exclude

- **Those who do not keep appointments**
- **Those who show poor compliance during the skin conditioning program**
- **Those who have high and unreasonable expectations**
- **Those who blame every previous physician for their problems**
- **Those who believe their appearance is responsible for a failed marriage or poor social life**
- **Those who are not willing to allow the necessary amount of time for healing recovery to occur after the procedure**
- **Those who are depressed or undergoing an emotional crisis**

outcome, and minimal disruption in their busy lives during recovery. Because there is considerable variation in individual expectations, demands, and level of understanding of preprocedure skin conditioning and procedures, the physician must make an effort to ensure that every patient is fully informed and has realistic expectations.

Patients seeking better skin may ask for one thing from the physician, without knowing that they really want another. Their expectations may appear reasonable and realistic preoperatively, and the unrealistic expectations may only come to light postoperatively. The physician must attempt to detect such problem patients at the initial consultation to avoid time-consuming postprocedure complaints and possible lawsuits. Finding a tactful way to exclude patients who appear to have inappropriate motivation and expectations will in the end provide invaluable peace of mind.

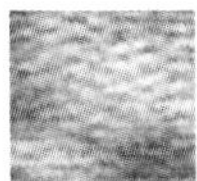

THE TREATMENT PLAN FOR SKIN REJUVENATION

For the sake of simplicity, I have standardized the process of skin rejuvenation by presenting it in six parts, proceeding from the time the patient presents him or herself to the physician to the time the patient begins the maintenance program. The six steps of the treatment plan are shown in Box 7-3.

Box 7-3

THE TREATMENT PLAN FOR SKIN REJUVENATION

1. **Classify the skin.**
2. **Make the diagnosis.**
3. **Set the objective and begin the process of Skin Conditioning or Skin Health Restoration.**
4. **Choose the procedure (if needed) based on the dominant mechanism of action/ideal depth.**
5. **Have a plan for expediting recovery and treating any possible complications.**
6. **Establish a maintenance program.**

SKIN CLASSIFICATION

Skin classification (discussed in depth in Chapter 4) involves consideration of factors that influence Skin Conditioning and Skin Health Restoration program and procedure selection, including the patient's skin color, thickness, oiliness, laxity, and fragility. For example, thick skin can tolerate invasive procedures, while, in thin skin, depth should not exceed the papillary dermis or immediate reticular dermis; in fragile skin, the papillary dermis; and in dark skin (Original type), the immediate reticular dermis in order to avoid any possibility of hypopigmentation. Skin laxity can be reversed by procedures reaching the level of the immediate reticular dermis (tightening procedure), but skin that shows muscle laxity needs incisional surgery as well as a tightening procedure for best results. Classifying skin according to degree of oiliness is also important because sebum in oily skin decreases the effects of the conditioning program before and after the procedure and consequently diminishes the chances of an optimal outcome.

When skin is properly classified, an effective skin rejuvenation program can be developed that works for anyone. Unlike CO_2 laser resurfacing, phenol peeling, or dermabrasion, which usually produce best results in White skin, the treatment plan presented in this book will address rejuvenating all types of skin. Whatever the patient's skin type, a treatment plan can be devised that restores skin to a healthier and more youthful look without changing the texture or natural color.

THE DIAGNOSIS

The diagnosis should be made based on 1) the nature of the condition, i.e., inflammatory, functional, textural and 2) the depth of the condition, i.e., epidermal, dermal, or subcutaneous. The diagnosis will have a significant effect on the time needed to complete the rejuvenation program. For example, scars and wrinkles can be corrected rapidly, while the correction of melasma or dermal melanosis usually takes a long time and may involve multiple approaches and procedures.

Inflammatory skin conditions, such as acne vulgaris, acne rosacea, seborrheic dermatitis, folliculitis, etc., can have a negative influence on the healing stage after a procedure. These conditions should be treated before carrying out the procedure. Functional disorders, such as melasma, excessive skin oiliness, or skin sensitivity, should also be treated before the procedure. Furthermore, patients with these conditions should be told about their required participation in pre- and postpeel care, e.g., the need for multiple treatments for melasma, long-term treatment for oiliness, restoration of tolerance for skin sensitivity, etc. Textural skin changes, such as solar elastosis, disseminated sebaceous gland hyperplasia, and rhynophyma, may require different types of procedures, combined procedures, and, often, multiple procedures for the best results.

Depth of the Condition

The depth of the diagnosed condition will affect the selection of a procedure to obtain the desired mechanism of action (Figure 7-1). Conditions

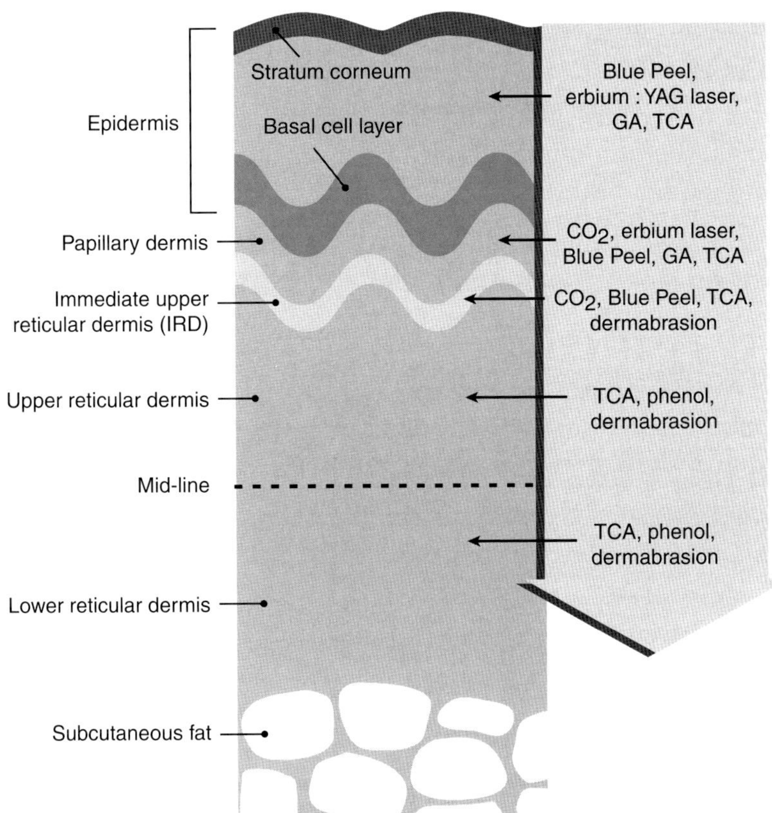

FIGURE 7-1. *The layers of the skin and the procedures that can reach that depth. (GA = glycolic acid, TCA = trichloroacetic acid)*

limited to the epidermis will respond well to any exfoliative process, while conditions at the dermal level can be improved with tightening or leveling. Subcutaneous conditions respond best to surgery, filling procedures (fat, collagen), Botox, and other mechanisms.

TREATMENT PLAN GUIDELINES

After classifying the skin and making the diagnosis, the physician should form a treatment plan and present it to the patient as a treatment program. This puts emphasis on the complexity and long-term aspects of the program and gives the physician more control over the process. The guidelines for the program are shown in Box 7-4.

Box 7-4

PROGRAM GUIDELINES FOR THE PHYSICIAN

1. **Keep the objective in mind—to restore healthy skin while treating existing skin problems.**
2. **Communicate with the patient. Explain the program, answer questions, mention the chances that the program will not succeed and the potential for complications. Discuss available alternative treatments.**
3. **If a procedure is needed, explain the most suitable procedure, the number of times it may need to be performed, and the associated healing time.**
4. **Never perform a procedure without first preparing the skin with proper skin conditioning.**
5. **Keep control of patient compliance. Inform the patient that you will terminate the program for noncompliance.**
6. **Emphasize the need for following a maintenance program after completion of the program.**

CHOOSING THE PROCEDURE

Currently, physicians choose light, medium, or deep procedures for their patients without truly knowing (or agreeing among each other) what these terms imply. They also consider only skin color in their choice of a procedure and ignore important factors such as skin thickness, laxity, and fragility. Results of procedures are judged on the degree of correction achieved in, for example, wrinkles or scars, and factors such as overall skin quality or function after the procedure are not considered. Undesirable results are labeled as complications. Furthermore, with no guidelines in procedure selection, physicians usually select a procedure based on their personal expertise and the popularity and profitability of the procedure, which may not correlate with what is the best procedure for the particular patient. Exfoliations are being performed to correct wrinkles and scars and medium-deep procedures are being performed for conditions that would respond to a lighter procedure. In many cases, procedures are more invasive than is indicated.

Procedure Mechanism of Action

A procedure produces one or more of the following effects: 1) exfoliation, 2) tightening, 3) leveling, 4) matrix build-up, 5) filling or replacement, and 6) immobilization. The ideal procedure improves skin appearance while maintaining its normal color and natural look. It is invasive only to the extent that is necessary to achieve the desired effect. To come as close as possible to the ideal, a procedure should be selected based on its dominant mechanism of action (Tables 7-2, 7-3), which is related mostly to it depth. For example, skin roughness, comedones, or pigmentation problems limited to the epidermis need only *exfoliation* as a mechanism of action, which

TABLE 7.2

MECHANISM OF ACTION OF PROCEDURES

Dominant Mechanism of Action	*Depth*	*Procedure*
Exfoliation	Epidermis	30% to 70% AHAs; 15% Blue Peel; microdermabrasion (power peel)
Skin tightening	Papillary dermis, immediate reticular dermis (IRD)[1]	Blue Peel; CO_2 and erbium laser resurfacing
Muscle tightening	Muscle	Incisional surgery (i.e., facelift)
Leveling	Upper reticular dermis; mid dermis	CO_2 laser resurfacing medium to deep chemical peels; Obagi Controlled Depth peel, dermabrasion
Matrix build-up	Epidermis, papillary dermis	Long-term stimulation with tretinoin, phytic acid, and AHAs
Filling	Dermis, subcutaneous layer	Collagen, fat, Gortex
Immobilization	Muscle	Botox injection; incisional surgery

[1]The IRD is a clinical term that indicates reaching but not involving the upper reticular dermis (Chapter 8).

TABLE 7.3

DOMINANT AND WEAK MECHANISMS OF ACTION OF PROCEDURES

Procedure	*Skin Zone*	*Leveling Action*	*Tightening Action*
CO_2 laser	Upper reticular dermis	Strong	Weak
Conventional TCA peel	Papillary dermis Immediate reticular dermis	Weak Strong	Strong Strong
Phenol Peel	Mid dermis or below	Strong	Weak
Obagi Blue Peel	Papillary dermis or immediate reticular dermis	Weak	Strong
Obagi Controlled Depth Peel	Upper to mid reticular dermis	Strong	Strong
Dermabrasion	Upper to mid reticular dermis	Strong	Weak
70% glycolic acid	Epidermis Papillary dermis	None None	None Weak

can be obtained with an AHA peel or 1 or 2 coats of a 15% Blue Peel, microdermabrasion (power peel), fine to medium stretchable wrinkles, stretchable scars, and lax skin need a *tightening* mechanism, which can be achieved with a Blue Peel, a TCA peel to the papillary dermis or the IRD or the erbium laser. Deep, nonstretchable wrinkles and deep, nonstretchable scars need *leveling*, for which CO_2 laser resurfacing, dermabrasion, or a chemical peel to the mid dermis may be ideal. A combination of procedures may be needed for best results and to to avoid unnecessary depth.

Selecting a procedure based on its mechanism of action ensures that the procedure reaches only to the depth that is necessary to improve the patient's condition. The correct mechanism of action avoids unnecessary depth of penetration that can cause damage to adnexal structures, melanocytes, and fibroblasts and possible complications (Table 7-4). Depth is also important in regard to a patient's skin type according to the Obagi classification system because there are depth limitations for certain skin types. This is discussed in greater detail below.

Box 7-5

When the correct procedure mechanism of action is chosen, penetration is only to the depth needed to achieve the desired results and invasiveness is minimized.

TABLE 7.4

REACTIONS AND COMPLICATIONS ASSOCIATED WITH DOMINANT MECHANISMS OF ACTION

Dominant Mechanism of Action	*Complication*			
	Hyperpigmentation	*Hypopigmentation*	*Milia*	*Scarring*
Leveling	Common	Possible	Common	Possible
Tightening	Possible	Rare	Possible	Rare
Exfoliation	Rare	No	Rare	No

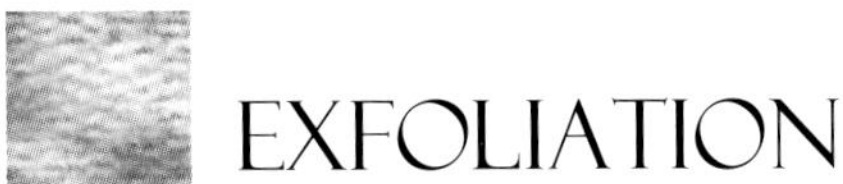

EXFOLIATION

NATURAL EXFOLIATION

The process of exfoliation can be classified as natural, true, or false exfoliation. Natural exfoliation is the daily shedding of nonviable cells from the stratum corneum, which renews the epidermis and allows it to maintain the barrier function. The process is slowed down through aging, application of moisturizers, and application of oil-based cosmetics. The process can be accelerated by rubbing, shaving, and stripping and through diseases such as psoriasis, seborrheic dermatitis, hypertrophic actinic keratosis, and others. Partial corneocyte separation gives skin the rough texture that is interpreted as dryness and leads to the habitual use of moisturizers. This practice reduces the rate of mitosis and leads to reduced natural exfoliation, a weakened barrier function, and a thinner, more sensitive epidermis. Defects in the keratinization process, as seen in acne, increase the cohesiveness of keratinocytes and lead to the clogging of pores and a sallow skin appearance.

TRUE EXFOLIATION

With certain concentrations and exposure times on the skin, alpha hydroxy acids, beta hydroxy acids, and kojic acid disrupt the bonds between corneocytes and, to some extent, between keratinocytes. Alpha hydroxy acids lead to exfoliation of individual cells ("school of fish" effect), while beta hydroxy acids melt the cells through their keratolytic action.

FALSE EXFOLIATION

Tretinoin, benzoyl peroxide, and other agents may cause temporary exfoliation of the stratum corneum through a dehydrating effect. With these agents, groups of cells are shed (coarse exfoliation), but this stops after a few weeks of use. Thus, they are false exfoliators. False exfoliation can be produced mechanically by means of devices such as sandpaper, "power" peels, scraping with a blade, and stripping with adhesive tape.

EXFOLIATION: MECHANISM OF ACTION

Exfoliating procedures remove parts of the epidermis above the basal layer (Figure 7-2). They are beneficial for the temporary correction of epidermal problems but have no effect on dermal problems, such as wrinkles or scars, regardless of how many times they are repeated. Healing is rapid (3 to 6 days) after an exfoliation procedure.

EXFOLIATION PROCEDURES

Exfoliation peels (e.g., 30% to 70% glycolic acid peel, 1 to 2 coats of 15% Blue Peel, salicylic acid peel, Power Peel, erbium laser resurfacing) in a physician's office are undertaken to improve epidermal conditions such as roughness, clogged pores, comedones, and superficial hyperpigmentation. Although such exfoliation peels can bring healthy new keratinocytes to the epidermis, exfoliation peels have no beneficial effect on wrinkles, skin laxity, or other dermal conditions.

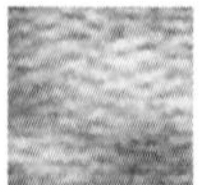

SKIN TIGHTENING

The term "skin tightening" resulted from the author's observation that patients who underwent a Blue Peel or Designed Blue Peel demonstrated reduced skin laxity and increased skin tightness. Tightening is obtained by procedures that penetrate to the depth of the papillary dermis or to the

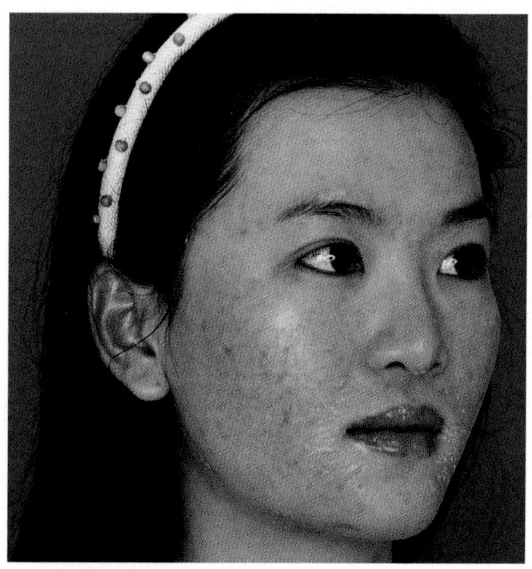

FIGURE 7-2. *Patient showing vigorous exfoliation during an aggressive Skin Health Restoration program (5 weeks of correction and stimulation with tretinoin, AHA, hydroquinone).*

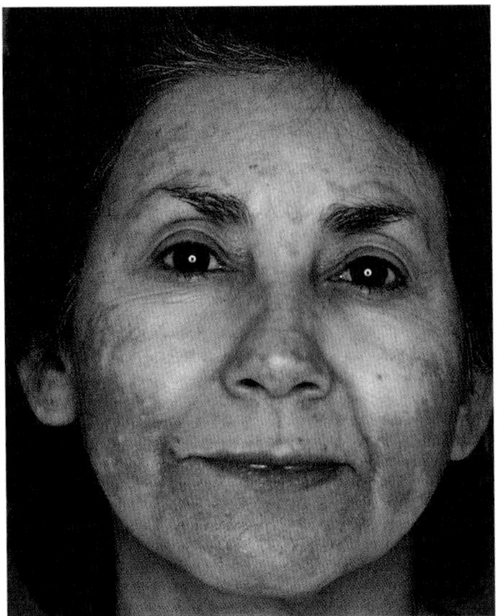

a

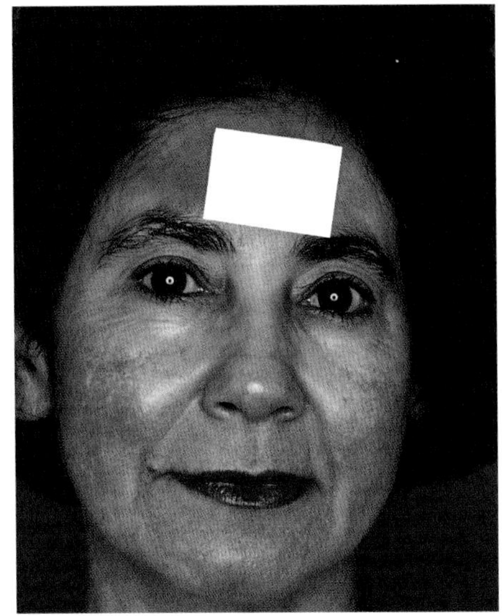

b

FIGURE 7-3. *(a) Before—Patient had epidermal melasma and laxity. Treatment consisted of Skin Health Restoration with emphasis on stimulation for one year. (b) After—1 Year. The benefits of long-term stimulation are evident. Note the increased tightness and clearing of hyperpigmentation without any procedure being performed.*

IRD; these procedures are ideal for treating problems in the epidermis and the papillary dermis (wrinkles, scars, large pores, dermal melasma, and others). Tightening procedures are light, noninvasive procedures that heal quickly (7 to 10 days) with almost no occurrences of hypopigmentation or scarring. Most of the adnexal structures remain intact, and skin texture remains normal. These procedures can be performed on all skin types and on facial as well as nonfacial skin. Tightening procedures maintain natural skin color and do not have the risk of hypopigmentation because penetration to the level of the IRD does not reduce the number of melanocytes. Early stages of skin laxity can be corrected with a Skin Health Restoration topical treatment program or with a tightening procedure (Figures 7-3—7-5).

MECHANISM OF ACTION: TIGHTENING

Skin tightness is related to the amount and quality of elastin in the dermis and, to a lesser extent, to the amount and quality of collagen. The opposite of tightness is laxity, which is characterized by changes in the quality and quantity of elastin and collagen, as seen in chronological aging and photoaging. Laxity can be reversed and tightness restored through the regeneration of new collagen and elastin that follows tightening procedures.

TIGHTENING INDICATIONS

Generally fine to medium stretchable wrinkles, photodamage, and upper reticular dermis stretchable scars can benefit from procedures that have

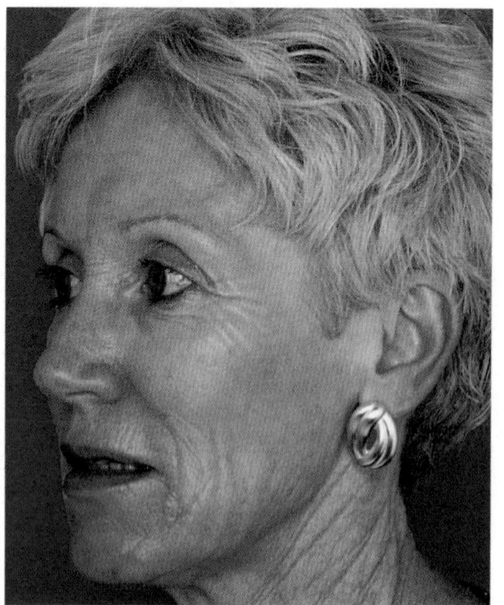

a

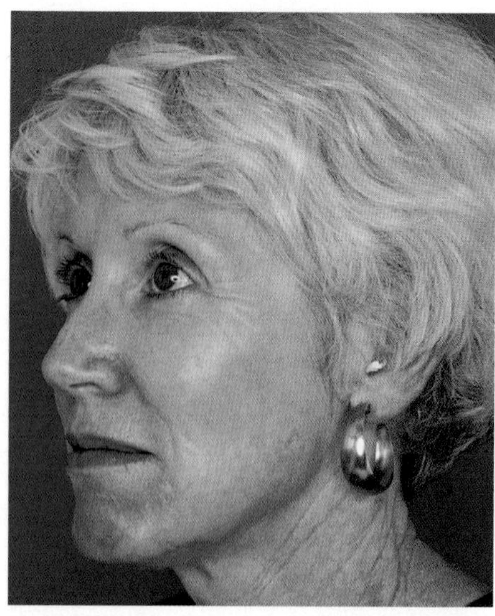

b

FIGURE 7-4. *Tightening after Blue Peel procedure. (a) Before—Patient had thin skin with laxity. Skin Health Restoration for 5 months, during which time a Blue Peel with Design (to immediate reticular dermis) was performed. (b) After—1 year. Note the increased tightness of skin.*

tightening as a dominant mechanism of action, such as the Blue Peel. For a greater tightening effect, the Designed Blue Peel or more than one Blue Peel can be performed. While CO_2 laser resurfacing and dermabrasion can be performed to the level of the papillary dermis, these procedures tend to be more invasive, require greater physician skill for depth uniformity, and have more potential for complications. They are more suitable for leveling

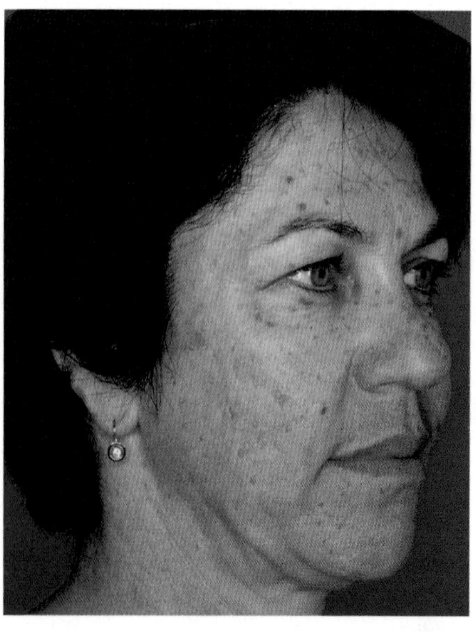

a

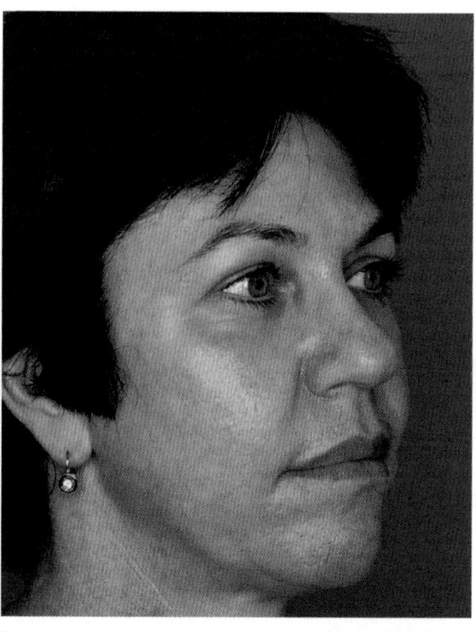

b

FIGURE 7-5. *Tightening after Blue Peel procedure. (a) Before—Patient had freckles, lentigines, sun damage, laxity. (b) After—Five months of Skin Health Restoration and two Blue Peels with Design were performed. Note the increased tightness of skin.*

purposes (see below for definition). Tightening is ideal for patients with thin skin and few adnexal structures. Procedures with leveling as a mechanism of action would penetrate too deeply and have a higher risk of causing hypopigmentation, changes in skin texture, and scarring. Muscle and skin laxity need surgical correction, such as a face lift, as well as a tightening procedure to address the skin laxity.

THE SKIN STRETCHING TEST

The skin stretching test was devised to help the physician determine whether the patient's skin condition will respond to a tightening procedure. In this test, the physician gently stretches the skin with one hand, without pressure or pulling of underlying structures. If the wrinkle or scar diasppears or improves more than 50% with such stretching, a tightening procedure such as the Blue Peel will improve the condition, although there is a possibility that 2 to 3 peels may be needed. If there is less or no improvement, a leveling procedure would be a better choice.

The test can also help in determining whether a pigmentation disorder is epidermal or dermal. If the pigmented lesion becomes lighter with the stretching test, it is epidermal. If it does not, the lesion lies in the dermis and a procedure such as the Blue Peel or pigment laser must be performed. Pigmentation disorders that can be tested with the stretching test include melasma, dermal melanosis, Becker's nevus, nevus spilous, café-au-lait spots, and others.

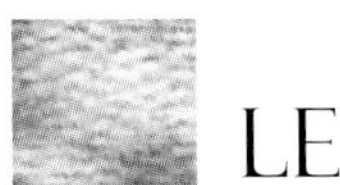

LEVELING

Leveling smooths down an uneven skin surface and is beneficial for treating deep wrinkles and scars. Procedures that reach the IRD can produce some leveling, but the best results are obtained with procedures that reach the upper or mid dermis. However, since no reliable depth signs are available for leveling below the IRD, a safe and effective outcome depends on the skill of the surgeon. The deeper the leveling, the more injury is inflicted on the skin, including destruction of adnexal structures, permanent skin textural changes (thinning, decreased color, demarcation lines, and scarring), and increased skin sensitivity. Dark skin and skin of the Deviated type generally are unsuitable because permanent color changes often occur. Healing time is longer, and home care is more troublesome after leveling procedures.

LEVELING INDICATIONS

If a scar or wrinkle remains after gentle stretching, it lies below the IRD level and is best treated with a procedure that has leveling as a dominant mechanism of action and can reach the upper to lower reticular dermis. These include CO_2 laser resurfacing, dermabrasion, and medium to deep chemical peels. The trade-offs for penetration below the IRD to reduce deep wrinkles and scars are hypopigmentation and increased incidence of keloid formation and hyperpigmentation. The patient should be told about the potential risks and sign a specific consent form before undergoing such a procedure.

SELECTING A LEVELING PROCEDURE

The factors inherent in leveling procedures, such as selecting the suitable procedure, determining depth, and the effect of skin type, make it difficult to routinely obtain good results. Physicians should attempt to master a leveling procedure that they can best control. Special attention should be given to the patient's skin type (thickness, fragility, color) in selecting a procedure. The maximum safe depth for thin skin is the upper reticular dermis, but for very thin skin the IRD is the maximum. A history of keloid formation or poor healing, revealed by the presence of scars, suggests skin fragility, and the depth should not exceed the papillary dermis for these patients. The safest level for patients with dark or Deviated type skin is the IRD because these patients are susceptible to color changes; deeper procedures will sacrifice color for smoothness.

Leveling procedures that reach the mid dermis (phenol peel, dermabrasion, medium-depth peel) cannot be repeated with safety in every skin type and have a high risk of complications in thin skin. It is important to note that depth determines the risk of poor results or complications, and that leveling procedures that reach the same depth have the same risks.

As a leveling modality, the benefits of CO_2 laser resurfacing need to be balanced against the downsides. The benefits include control of depth through joules setting and number of passes, clear endpoints, and ease of learning the technique. The downsides include thermal damage to the skin, prolonged erythema, the occurrence of PIH, and the inability to correct poorly hydrated tissue that is characteristic of fibrotic scars and wrinkles. Dermabrasion or a medium-deep TCA peel are better choices for fibrotic scars and wrinkles. Dark skin, nonfacial skin, and thick skin are not suitable for laser resurfacing. In thick skin, CO_2 laser resurfacing does not produce consistently good results because charring may occur as water evaporates, and numerous passes can produce detrimental thermal effects. Also, physicians often have a false sense of safety in performing laser resurfacing procedures that can lead to deep penetration and subsequent skin burns, depigmentation, and scars if skin type is not selected properly.

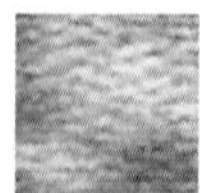

COMBINATION APPROACH

Combined procedures offer multiple mechanisms of action and penetration depths and help to avoid the risks of leveling depth on the entire face. A combination of procedures is the safest and most effective approach for correcting specific skin problems, treating nonfacial in conjunction with facial skin, and treating skin that is not uniformly thick. For example, ex-

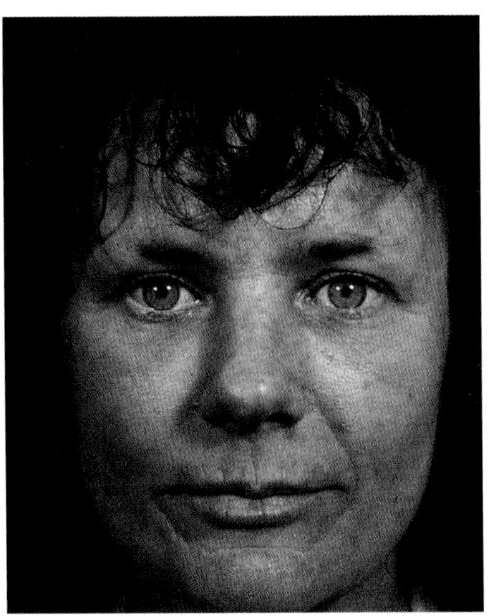

a

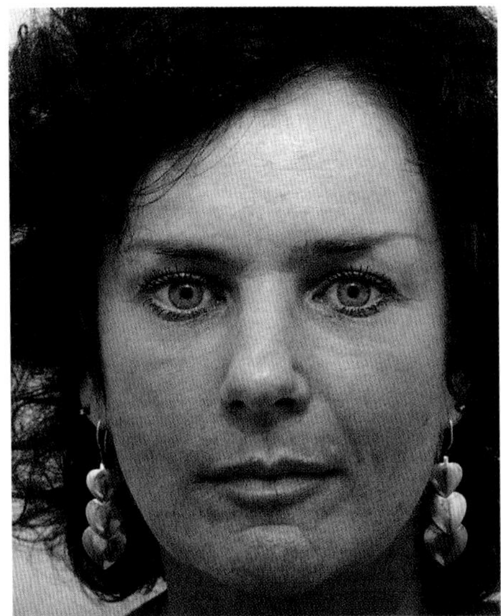

b

FIGURE 7-6. *(a) Before—Patient had actinic keratoses, large pores, deep perioral rhytids, and laxity. During 5 months of Skin Health Restoration, an IRD level Blue Peel on the face and upper lip and a papillary dermis peel on the lids were performed. (b) After—one year later.*

foliation can be performed in undamaged areas, tightening to the level of the papillary dermis or IRD in areas where damage is present but is not deep in the dermis, and leveling for deeper scars and wrinkles. Feathering is then performed to make a uniform and smooth transition between the differently treated areas and to avoid demarcation lines. This combined approach minimizes patient exposure to deep penetration while maximizing the chances for clinical improvement. Figures 7-6 to 7-11 show patients who have benefited from a combination of procedures producing mild leveling and maximum tightening.

Box 7-6

Skin laxity is not corrected by surgery alone; the best results follow a combined procedure that addresses the muscle laxity surgically and the skin laxity by a nonsurgical tightening procedure.

Box 7-7

After a leveling procedure, skin has fewer adnexal structures and melanocytes and is usually permanently thinner. These changes make it more difficult for a physician to perform a second leveling procedure safely in the future, especially in thin skin.

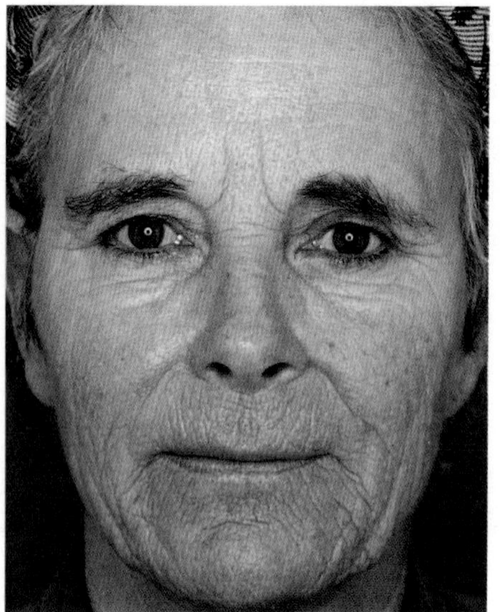

a

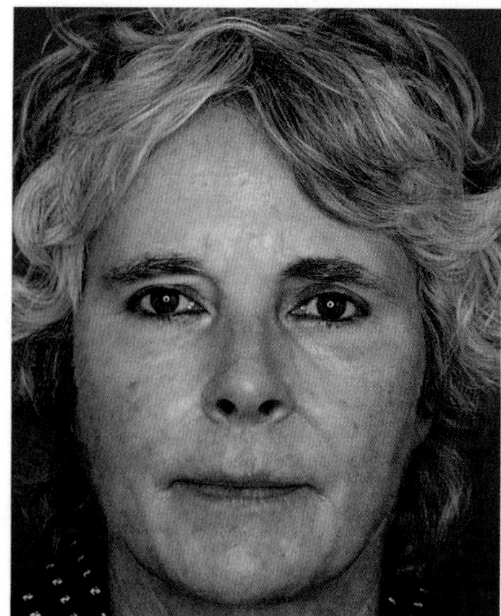

b

FIGURE 7-7. *(a) Before—Patient had photoaging, solar elastosis, deep perioral and periocular rhytids. This patient would not benefit from a standard Blue Peel or a facelift; leveling to the mid dermis was needed. Treatment consisted of 5 months of Skin Health Restoration during which time 1 Controlled Medium-Depth TCA Peel was performed. Healing took 14 days. (b) After—One year later.*

Box 7-8

The exfoliation zone—epidermis above the basal layer
The tightening zone—papillary dermis and IRD
The leveling zone—upper reticular to mid dermis

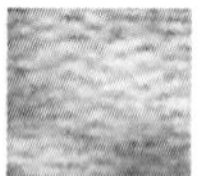

ERBIUM:YAG LASER RESURFACING

The recent introduction of erbium:YAG lasers was expected to be the solution to safe skin resurfacing, safer than the CO_2 laser or chemical peeling because it ablates only 20 to 30 μm of tissue in each pass. This laser has been promoted for treating epidermal lesions from pigmented seborrheic keratitis, lentigo, and solar damage as well as dermal lesions such as wrinkles and scars, and for resurfacing of nonfacial skin such as that on the neck, hands, and arms. Anecdotal reports and those from scientific meetings and publications suggest that it is too soon to make the final judgment as to the value of this device; while it produces fine results, simpler and less costly procedures will be sufficient (exfoliation, Blue Peel) for epidermal and papillary-level skin problems. As for deeper wrinkles and scars,

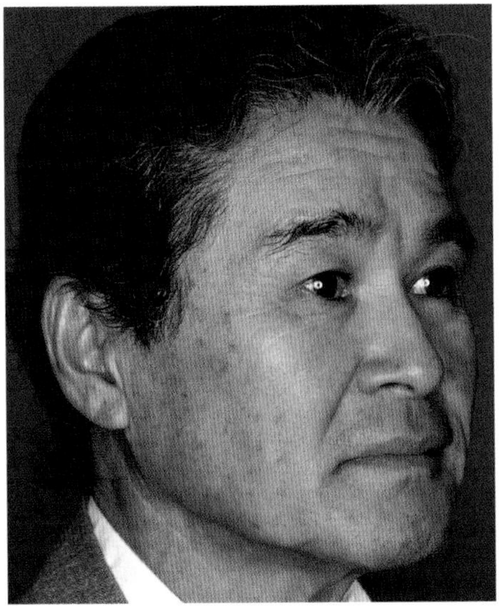

a

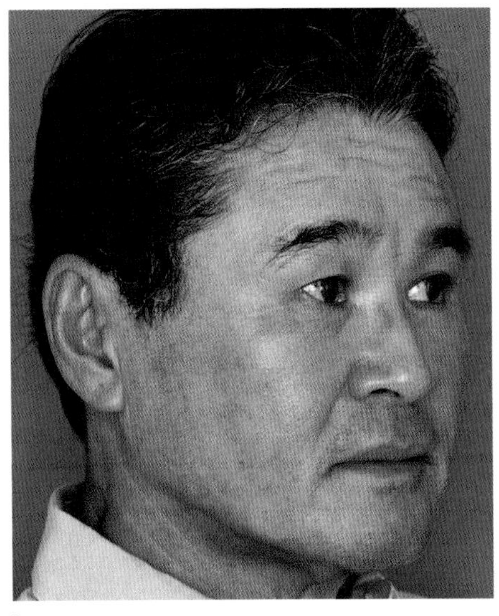

b

FIGURE 7-8. *(a) Before—Patient had lentigo and photodamage. Treatment consisted of 5 months of Skin Health Restoration, during which time 1 Peel to the immediate reticular dermis was performed. (b) After—Eight months later.*

CO_2 laser resurfacing may be more suitable than erbium:YAG laser, which provides no clear endpoints and often follows a trial-and-error approach. Furthermore, as in all leveling procedures; erbium laser can cause severe and recalcitrant pigmentary problems in dark skin.

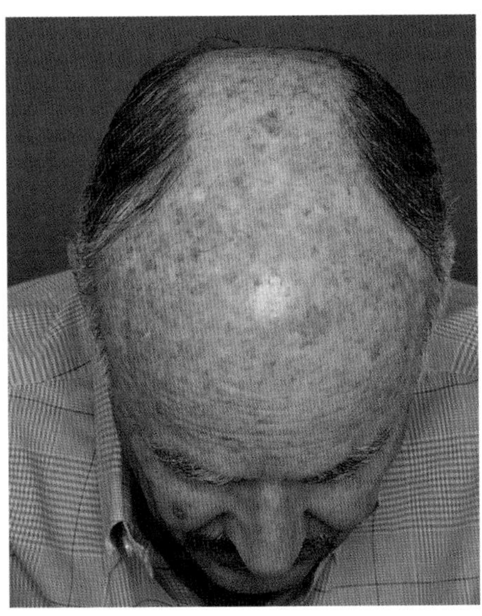

a

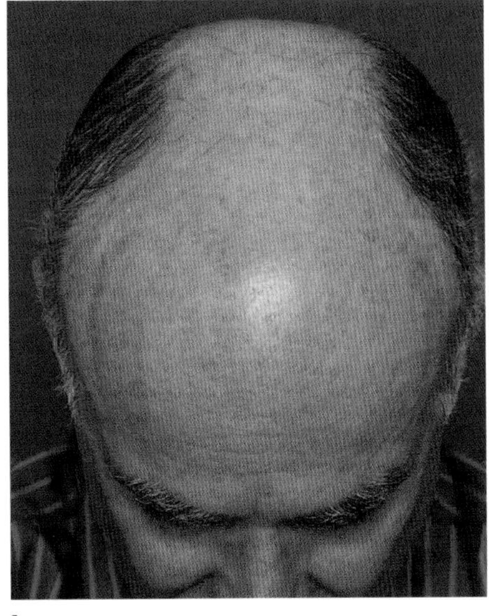

b

FIGURE 7-9. *(a) Before—Patient had actinic keratoses with a history of basal cell carcinomas; one can be seen on the right cheek. Treatment consisted of excision of the carcinoma and 5 months of Skin Health Restoration followed by maintenance. One Blue Peel with Design to the immediate reticular dermis was performed during this time. (b) After—One year later.*

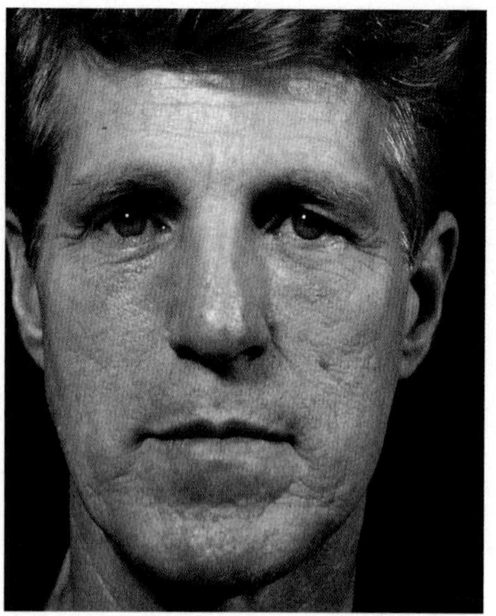

a

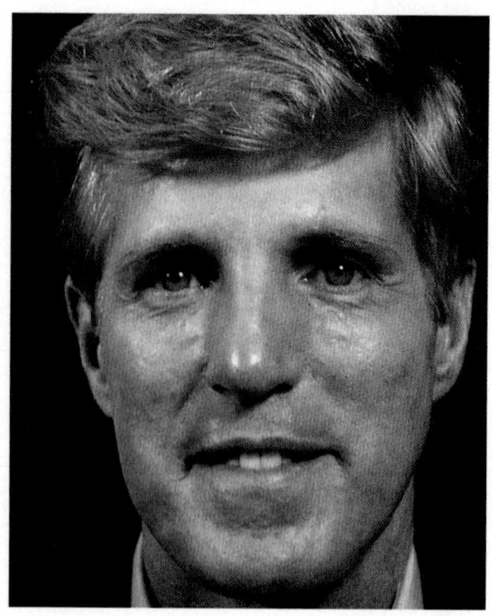

b

FIGURE 7-10. *(a) Before—Patient with chronological aging, large pores, skin laxity. Treatment consisted of 5 months of Skin Health Restoration, followed by maintenance, during which time 1 Controlled Medium-Depth Peel to the upper reticular dermis was performed. (b) After—One year later.*

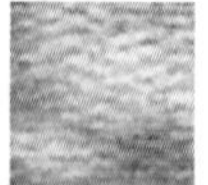

EXPEDITING RECOVERY

Proper management after procedures, including prompt treatment of anticipated reactions such as PIH, erythema, milia, and skin sensitivity, shortens the recovery time. The plan for expediting recovery after the procedure should be explained to the patient before the procedure is performed. This includes skin reconditioning using the concepts of correction, stimulation, bleaching, and blending that help to treat anticipated reactions and restore skin tolerance. The reconditioning processes should start immediately after re-epithelialization, as tolerated, and should continue for at least 6 weeks.

Topical tretinoin 0.05% to 0.1% is the most important agent used during the recovery period and should be started at the highest frequency tolerated by the patient and gradually increased to use once daily. AHA 2% to 4% can be used together with the tretinoin to increase its penetration. AHA should not be used alone without tretinoin for 3 weeks after laser resurfacing and for 1 week after a chemical peel to allow the stratum corneum to mature. AHA concentration can be increased to 10% if it is tolerated. Bleaching and blending should be started as soon as possible, before the appearance of PIH, to stabilize skin color. Treated areas should be blended with untreated areas to reduce demarcation lines. The benefits that can be expected from postprocedure skin conditioning are shown in Box 7-9.

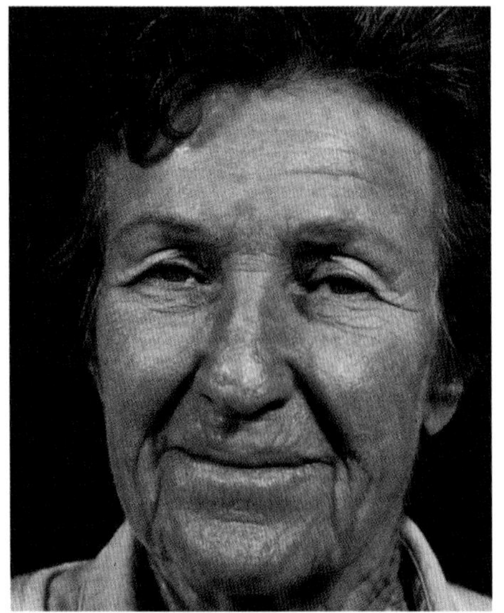
a

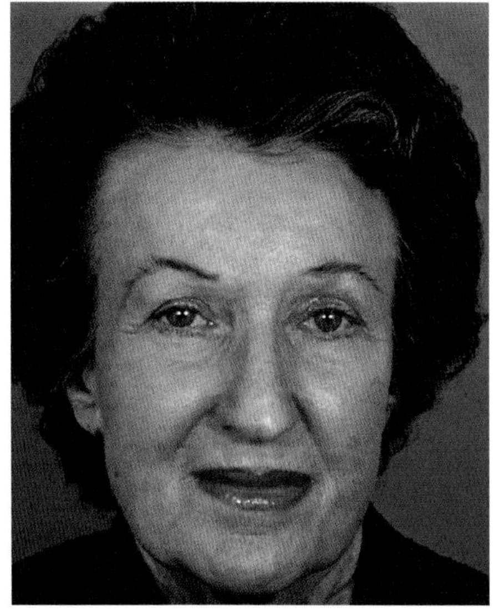
b

FIGURE 7-11. *(a) Before—Patient with chronological and photoaging, with muscle and skin laxity, and dermatochalasis on the upper eyelids. Patient did not want facelift surgery. Treatment consisted of 5 months of Skin Health Restoration, during which time 1 Controlled Medium-Depth Peel to the upper reticular dermis on the face only was performed. Skin and muscle laxity remains on the neck, which had no treatment. (b) After—One year later.*

Box 7-9

BENEFITS OF POSTPROCEDURE SKIN CONDITIONING

- **Prevention of milia, postinflammatory hyperpigmentation (PIH)**
- **Shortening of the period of erythema, especially after CO_2 laser resurfacing**
- **Improved procedure results**
- **Restoration of proper skin tolerance and reduction of skin sensitivity**
- **Longer lasting results of the procedure if long-term maintenance conditioning is performed**

MAINTENANCE AND PREVENTION

The maintenance program for extending the benefits of the skin rejuvenation procedure should be explained to the patient before the procedure is performed. The recommended maintenance plan consists of at least twice-weekly stimulation and correction (see Chapter 5) and prevention of further deterioration and damage through use of sunscreens and care in sun exposure. Moisturizer use is permitted when the skin feels dry. The combination of the maintenance program and prevention can help skin to stay in a healthy state, maintain the results of the procedure, and minimize the need for further procedures. Theoretically, persons who follow an effective skin health restoration program and undergo skin tightening with a procedure such as the Blue Peel every 1 to 2 years, or when skin laxity begins to appear, can have younger, vibrant, and healthy skin indefinitely.

CHAPTER

8

THE BLUE PEEL

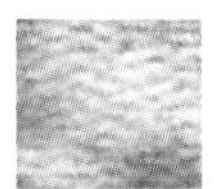

THE TCA-BASED BLUE PEEL

OVERVIEW

The Blue Peel is a highly controlled, trichloroacetic acid (TCA)-based skin rejuvenation procedure created with the goal of eliminating the variables associated with TCA peels that contribute to uneven results. This was accomplished by standardizing most variables of TCA peels, as shown in Box 8-1. The standard Blue Peel is intended to reach the papillary dermis, while the Design Blue Peel (greater depth in certain areas) is intended to reach the immediate reticular dermis (IRD).

Cosmetic and medical skin conditions located as superficially as the stratum corneum or as deeply as the IRD can be corrected. Skin tight-

Box 8-1

VARIABLES STANDARDIZED IN THE BLUE PEEL

- Concentration: Fixed at 15% or 20% TCA
- Volume: Fixed at 4–6 ml
- Solution color: Adding blue color guide
- Application: Coat system
- Size of surface area: 5% of body surface
- Depth control: All of the above + clear endpoints
- Skin response:
  - Skin conditioning
  - Identifying thins vs. thick skin

ening, the clinical term for correction of skin problems located in the papillary dermis or IRD, is the primary clinical objective of the Blue Peel. Skin leveling (smoothing down), the term for correction of skin problems located below the IRD, is not the objective (Table 8-1). Tightening effects from the Blue Peel are very good, but the leveling effects are limited; more leveling effects can be obtained by performing 2 to 3 procedures. The Blue Peel is easy to learn and perform, and there are almost no contraindications to its use. A physician with little previous experience can perform the procedure and obtain good results in all types of skin and all race and ethnic group variations if he or she has proper training, strictly follows the peel guidelines, and provides proper follow-up. It is important to note that the Blue Peel should not be used for a medium-depth peel.

The Blue Peel modality, with its fixed (15% or 20%) concentration of TCA combined with the Blue Peel base, leads to slower skin penetration

TABLE 8.1

TIGHTENING AND LEVELING DEFINITIONS

Mechanism of Action	*Skin Level*	*Clinical Indication*	*Comment*
Skin tightening	Papillary dermis or immediate reticular dermis (IRD)	Stretchable scars or wrinkles,[1] photodamage	A gradual, noninvasive effect that improves skin laxity but does not change skin texture
Skin leveling	Upper to mid dermis	Nonstretchable scars or wrinkles	A more invasive effect that changes the skin's normal texture to varying degrees

[1]Stretchable scars or wrinkles—those that disappear with light stretching of the skin

Box 8-2

THE IMMEDIATE RETICULAR DERMIS (IRD)

- **A clinical term that indicates reaching but not involving the upper reticular dermis.**
- **Is the maxium depth for the Designed Blue Peel (standard Blue Peel depth is the papillary dermis).**

and slower frost formation relative to plain TCA. This gives the physician time to observe the depth signs (development of the endpoints) and increases the safety margin. The guesswork and prevailing approach of "learn by watching others" or "learn from your mistakes" of other chemical peels is eliminated with the Blue Peel approach. The Blue Peel has no systemic toxicity, takes little time to perform, and can be tolerated without sedation or nerve blocks by many patients. Patients' skin heals rapidly (compared with CO_2 laser resurfacing or deeper TCA peels), and patients have little or no pain during healing. The advantages of the Blue Peel procedure are shown in Box 8-3.

Box 8-3

ADVANTAGES OF THE BLUE PEEL PROCEDURE

1. **Improvement of a wide range of cosmetic/medical skin problems**
2. **Excellent, gradual skin tigthening; mild and gradual skin leveling**
3. **Suitable for all skin types**
4. **Produces consistent results**
5. **Standardized to control peel variables (concentration, volume, size of surface area, number of coats)**
6. **Easy recognition of endpoints to control penetration depth and minimize complications/side effects**
7. **Suitable for facial and nonfacial skin**
8. **A "design" modification can be performed to increase the intended depth in certain areas**
9. **Short recovery period**
10. **Easy procedure for the physician to learn and perform**

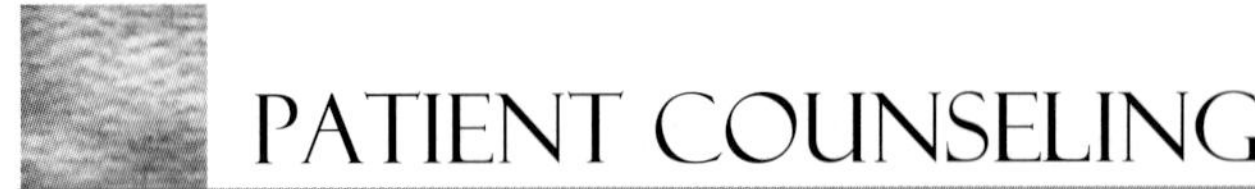

PATIENT COUNSELING

A prepeel office visit should be scheduled (Table 8-2) for patient discussions and consent, as well as postpeel appointments every 3 to 4 days, if possible.

Box 8-4

INFORMATION FOR THE PATIENT ABOUT THE BLUE PEEL

- **The Blue Peel is a light chemical peel. If a medium-depth peel is desired, a peel with a higher concentration of TCA may be more suitable.**
- **The Blue Peel is designed to provide gradual skin improvement and correction of certain skin problems. Compared with deeper procedures, this gradual approach is safer, has a lesser risk of complications, gives a faster recovery, and maintains normal skin texture.**
- **For maximum improvement of wrinkles, surface scars, and dermal pigmentation, more than one peel may be needed. Wrinkles and scars that disappear with gentle stretching usually respond to the peel better than nonstretchable ones.**
- **Most of the blue color will wash off with a special cleanser after the peel. If you want to remove all of the color immediately, you must wash vigorously a number of times during the first hour after the peel. After 1 hour, washing must be gentle.**

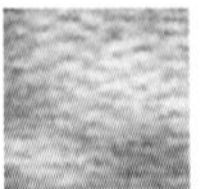

CHEMICAL PEEL VARIABLES

The many factors that can influence the results obtainable with a TCA peel (which have been standardized in the Blue Peel modality) are skin thickness, quality of the skin prior to the peel, acid concentration, solution volume, size of surface area peeled, and depth of penetration. Skin thickness should be determined before the peel, and skin quality should be improved through a precise Skin Conditioning program.

TABLE 8.2	
PREPEEL OFFICE CONSULTATION	
Explanation of procedure and instructions	■ Explain the procedure and healing to the patient (See Box 8-3 for details). ■ Give instructions for the day of the peel. ■ Remind patient to discontinue Skin Conditioning 3 to 4 days before the peel. ■ Discuss use of sedation. If sedation is to be used, remind patient about fasting and the need for a companion to drive her/him home.
Herpes simplex	Treat patients with a history of Herpes simplex infection prophylactically with 400 mg of acyclovir (Zovirax) 3 times daily or 500 mg of valcyclovir (Valtrex) twice daily, beginning the day before the peel and continuing for 7 to 10 days after the peel.
Healing and recovery stages	Discuss with patient.
Potential for complications	Discuss with patient potential for PIH, erythema, infection, scars, and keloids.
Number of procedures needed	Discuss possible need for more than one procedure.
Consent form	Several days before the procedure, have the patient read and sign a consent that presents a realistic picture of othe benefits, risks, and potential complications. Be sure the patient understands what she/he is signing.

CONCENTRATION

In developing the Blue Peel, the author recognized that the concentration of TCA alone does not determine skin penetration depth (as it does with phenol or AHA peels) but only determines the speed at which the acid penetrates the skin.[1,2] For any concentration, the volume applied is important. This conclusion is in contrast to Brody[3] who classifies 10% to 35% TCA as concentrations that reach a superficial depth and 35% TCA combined with other wounding agents or 50% TCA alone as concentrations that reach a medium depth.

Depending on its concentration, TCA can have therapeutic effects that are followed by proper healing or caustic effects that lead to improper healing. Therapeutic effects are a result of controlled concentration and penetration depth so that a sufficient number of dermal adnexal structures and fibroblasts are preserved for reepithelialization and dermal regeneration. Caustic effects, on the other hand, damage the dermal adnexal structures to the extent that hypopigmentation, fibrosis, scarring, or prolonged skin sensitivity occur. These effects are similar to those seen following second- and third-degree burns. Concentrations of TCA exceeding 45% are asso-

Box 8-5

Given the same volume, the higher the concentration of TCA, the faster and deeper the penetration.

ciated with caustic effects, although 30% to 40% TCA can produce the same effects in thin, fragile skin (Figure 8-1).

Concentrations higher than 25% easily overcome the initial neutralizing ability of the epidermis and papillary dermis and reach the lower reticular dermis in a short time (with less solution volume needed), while lower concentration can reach the same depth but do so more slowly (with more solution volume needed). Thus, by manipulating volume and number of applications, any concentration of TCA can be made to penetrate to any depth.

Concentrations of 15% and 20% TCA were carefully chosen for the Blue Peel because these concentrations penetrate slower and skin is able to neutralize the acid efficently at the papillary dermis level. Furthermore, TCA in these concentrations will not penetrate deeply unless a large volume is applied for a long period of time, which would be difficult to do since the peel parameters are set in a form that controls all variables.

VOLUME AND SURFACE AREA

The Blue Peel utilizes a fixed-volume formula for 1 coat of TCA solution. A coat is complete when the entire fixed amount has been evenly applied

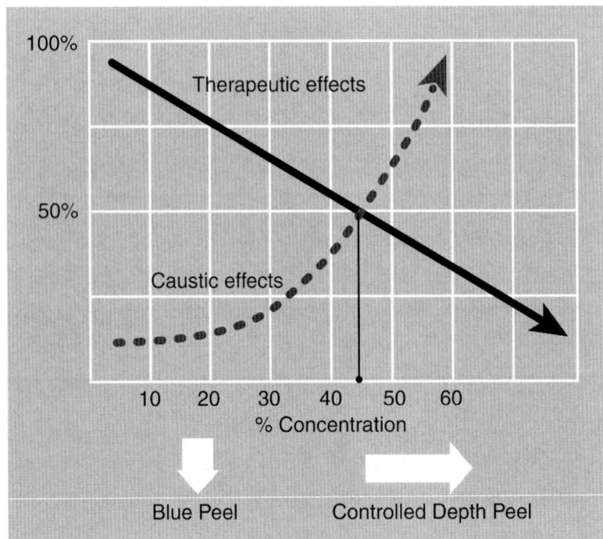

FIGURE 8-1. **Therapeutic and caustic effects of TCA.** *At concentrations below 25%, the therapeutic effects of TCA dominate the caustic effects. At 45%, caustic effects can dominate, penetration can be too deep, and the regenerating ability of the dermis can be destroyed.*

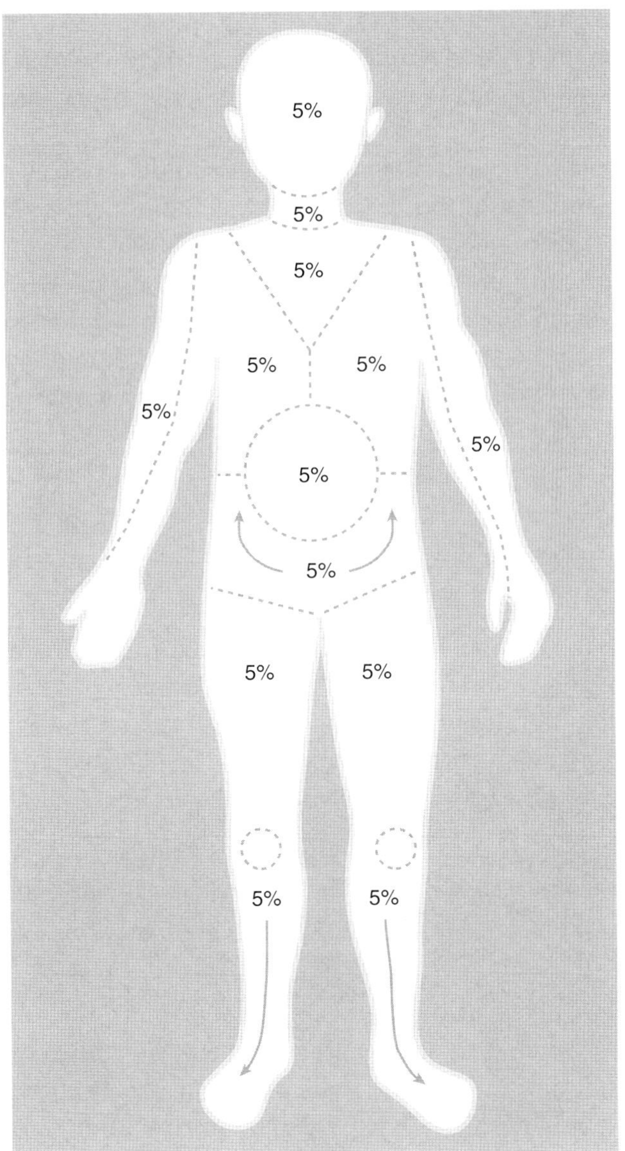

FIGURE 8-2. **Areas of the skin surface expressed as percentage of entire skin surface.** *The skin of the human body can be divided into areas of approximately 5% each. The 4 cc of 15% prepared Blue Peel solution or 6 cc of the 20% are sufficient to prepare 1 coat to treat 1 of these 5% areas. For increased depth, more than 1 coat is needed.*

to the surface area being treated, which must comprise 5% of the surface area of the body's skin. This is most often the face, although the same applies to any 5% area of the body (Figure 8-2). Multiple applications may be needed to use up all of the fixed coat volume for a single coat.

For the 15% Blue Peel coat system, 1 coat is made up of a fresh mixture of 2 cc of 30% TCA combined with 2 cc of the blue base, yielding a 4 cc volume, which is used to cover the entire face evenly from the hairline to the jawline. For the 20% Blue Peel coat system, the volume for 1 coat consists of 4 cc of 30% TCA combined with 2 cc of the blue base, yielding a 6 cc volume. With both the 15% and 20% Blue Peel coat systems, multiple applications may be needed to use up all of the prepared volume. It must be emphasized that these are multiple applications and *not multiple coats*.

Multiple coats are used to reach the desired depth of TCA penetration into the skin. One coat of the 15% prepared solution will exfoliate the stratum corneum, while 4 coats will peel the skin to the level of the papillary dermis in skin with medium thickness. With the 20% solution, 1 coat exfoliates the epidermis below the stratum corneum and above the basal layer, and 2 coats reach the papillary dermis in skin of medium thickness. In thin skin, fewer coats may be sufficient to reach the papillary dermis, while in thick skin, additional coats may be needed.

SKIN THICKNESS

Skin thickness is an important variable in selecting the depth of a skin rejuvenation procedure and must be determined prior to performing any procedure including the Blue Peel. Thick skin requires more coats of the Blue Peel solution to reach a certain depth, while thin skin requires fewer coats of the same solution to reach the same depth.

SKIN QUALITY

The aim in TCA peeling of facial skin is to obtain an even frost. Frosting is affected by skin quality factors such as stratum corneum thickness, skin conditioning, and the hydration and compactness level of the skin. Certain skin areas will frost well, other areas may not frost easily or not frost at all. While even frosting is desirable in facial skin, uneven frosting is quite common in nonfacial skin due to skin quality changes in certain anatomical areas. Here uneven frosting does not indicate uneven depth. An example is in peeling of the hands, where, despite equal painting of all areas, the dorsum frosts long before the knuckles and distal periungual areas, which are more compact and have a thicker stratum corneum. The same is true for the skin of the ankles, knees, and elbows.

Box 8-6

Why Blue? The color blue was found to be best for revealing the presence of other, associated colors, such as the white of the frost and the pink of the "Pink sign."

PREPARATION FOR THE BLUE PEEL

SELECTION OF DEPTH

Different levels of penetration depth can be obtained with a Blue Peel, ranging from exfoliation of the epidermis to a true peel reaching the papillary dermis or the IRD. The depth selected should be determined by the clinical condition being treated. Epidermal conditions, such as actinic keratoses, superficial pigmentary problems, acne, skin roughness, or sallowness, can be improved from a peel to the exfoliation level (light exfoliation to the stratum corneum, heavy exfoliation down to the basal layer), which can be repeated every 2 to 4 weeks, if desired. Exfoliation does not thin the skin and may actually thicken the epidermis. However, the effect on wrinkles, scars, large pores, and skin laxity is minimal or nonexistent.

The standard Blue Peel, which penetrates to the papillary dermis, has a beneficial effect on both epidermal and dermal conditions, including dermal melasma, actinic keratoses, general skin laxity, stretchable wrinkles, early solar elastosis, and large pores. Peeling to the papillary dermis increases skin tightness, does not thin the skin, and does not change skin color. The standard Blue Peel can be repeated every 6 to 8 weeks, as needed for treating severe dermal melasma and melanosis.

The Designed Blue Peel involves performing the standard Blue Peel, and then, in addition, applying more coats to certain areas to increase the penetration depth to involve the entire papillary dermis, but not the upper reticular dermis. This level has been designated as the IRD and is the maximum depth recommended for the Blue Peel. Clinically the Designed Peel provides more leveling action for correcting skin laxity and stretchable wrinkles and scars than the standard Blue Peel.

The skin conditions that can be improved with a Blue Peel are shown in Table 8-3 and Figures 8-3 to 8-7. The coat system guidelines for specific skin conditions are shown in Table 8-4. Physicians should be properly trained before undertaking a Blue Peel, and the patient's skin must be properly conditioned (see Chapter 5). The author has found that use of isotretinoin (Accutane) does not need to be discontinued prior to a Blue Peel that is limited to the papillary dermis.

SELECTION OF THE 15% OR 20% CONCENTRATION

With the 15% solution, 1 coat alone exfoliates the stratum corneum, 2 coats exfoliate the epidermis above the basal layer, and 3 coats peel the basal layer in thick skin and may reach the papillary dermis in thin skin. With the 20% solution, 1 coat exfoliates the epidermis to the basal layer in medium-thick skin and may reach the papillary dermis in thin skin. Two coats of 20% penetrate to the papillary dermis in all but thick skin, which may require a third coat (Figure 8-8).

TABLE 8.3

CLINICAL CONDITIONS TREATABLE WITH THE BLUE PEEL

Clinical Condition	*Procedure*
Fine and medium-deep, stretchable wrinkles[1]	Standard Blue Peel (for tightening) or Designed Blue Peel (for maximum tightening)
Epidermal and dermal hyperpigmentation or uneven patches of hypo/hyperpigmentation	Standard Blue Peel
Stretchable scars[1]	Designed Blue Peel (for tightening and leveling)
Acne, comedones, flat warts	Exfoliation
Large pores	Standard Blue Peel (for tightenng)
Skin laxity	Standard Blue Peel (for tightening) or Designed Blue Peel (for maximum tightening)
Actinic keratoses and other premalignant lesions	Standard Blue Peel

[1]Stretchable scars or wrinkles—those that disappear with light stretching of the skin.

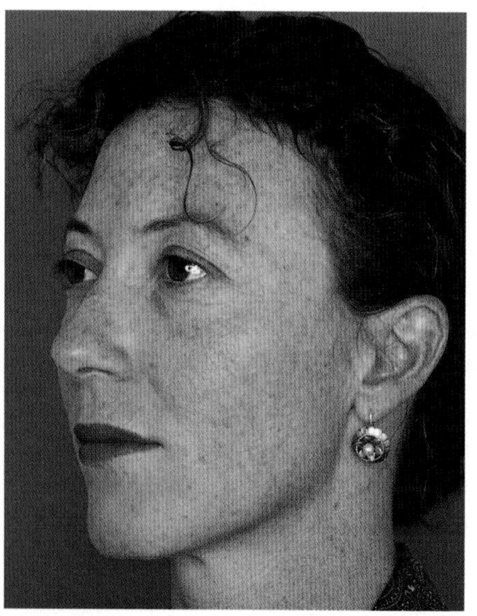

a

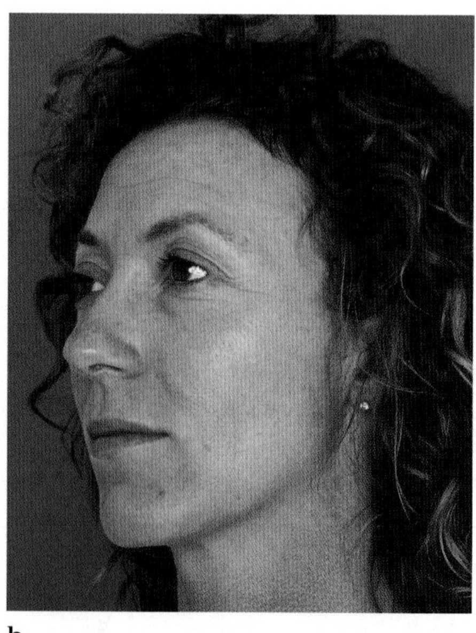

b

FIGURE 8-3. *(a) Before—Patient with freckles that in the past had not responded to different modalities. Treatment consisted of 5 months of creams for correction and stimulation, with emphasis on bleaching and blending, a Blue Peel, followed by maintenance. (b) After—1 year.*

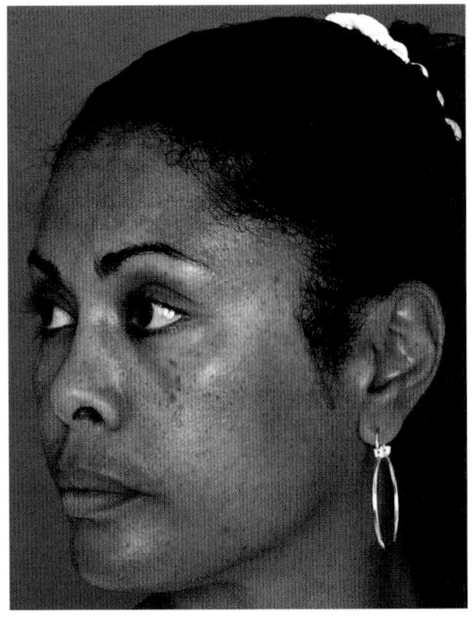

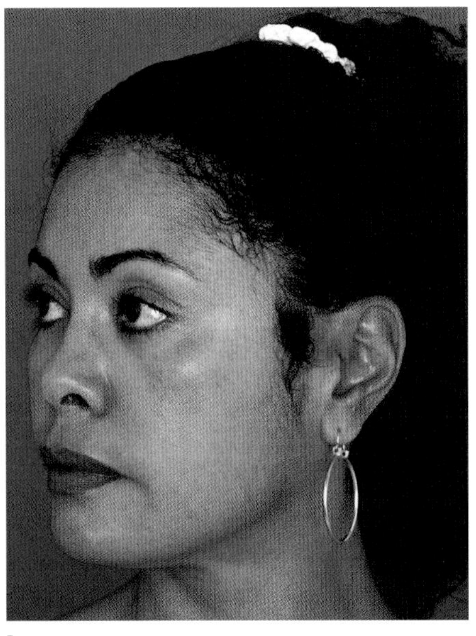

a b

FIGURE 8-4. *(a) Before—Patient, an ethnic mix of Black (AA) and Asian, with acne, hyperpigmentation, dermatitis papulosa nigra. Treatment consisted of Skin Health Restoration for correction and stimulation, with emphasis on bleaching and blending, during which Blue Peel was performed. Nd:YAG-532 laser treatment and hyphercation were also administered to treat the dermatosis before the Blue Peel. (b) After—1 year.*

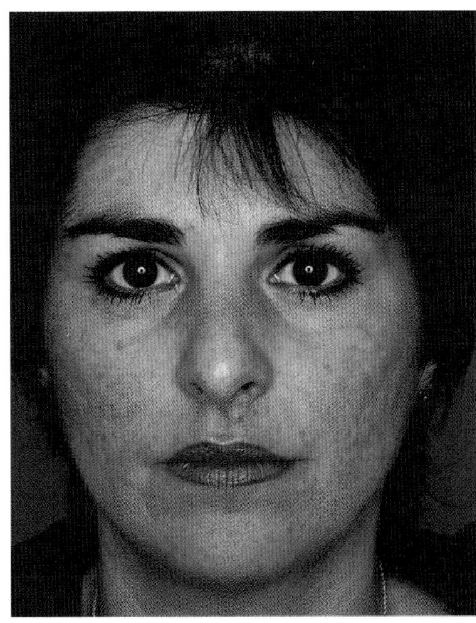

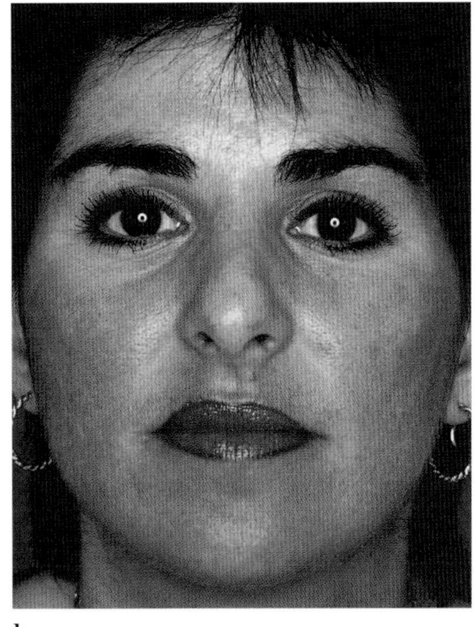

a b

FIGURE 8-5. *(a) Before—Patient, brunette, with acne, scarring, and uneven pigmentation. Treatment consisted of correction and stimulation through the Skin Health Restoration program. Two Blue Peels with Design were performed 2 months apart. (b) After—1 year.*

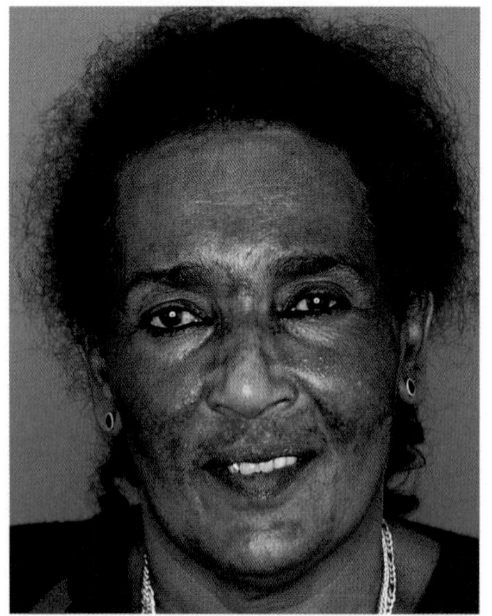

a

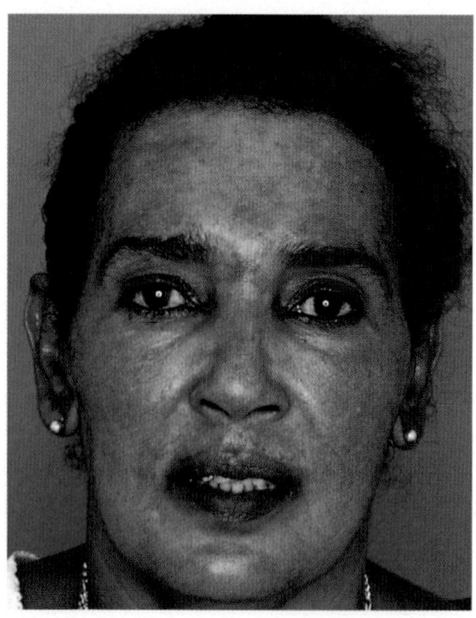

b

FIGURE 8-6. *(a) Before—Patient, Black (AA), with severe epidermal and dermal melasma and suspected ochronosis. Previous treatment with bleaches, Kligman formula, kojic acid, and AHA peels were not effective. Treatment consisted of 6 weeks of very aggressive bleaching and blending and 1 Blue Peel during treatment. (b) After—1 year. Multiple Blue Peels are planned for this patient (living overseas).*

In comparison with glycolic acid peels, two coats of a 15% Blue Peel solution generally have an exfoliative effect equal to 70% glycolic acid left on for 3 to 5 minutes, with the Blue Peel producing more even exfoliation and less irritation. Table 8-5 shows a comparison of the features

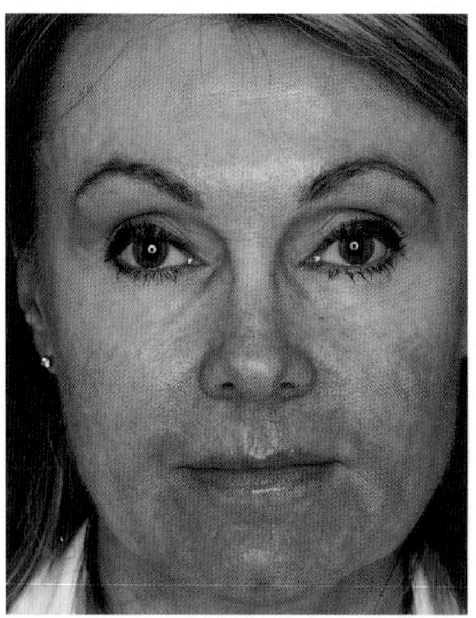

a

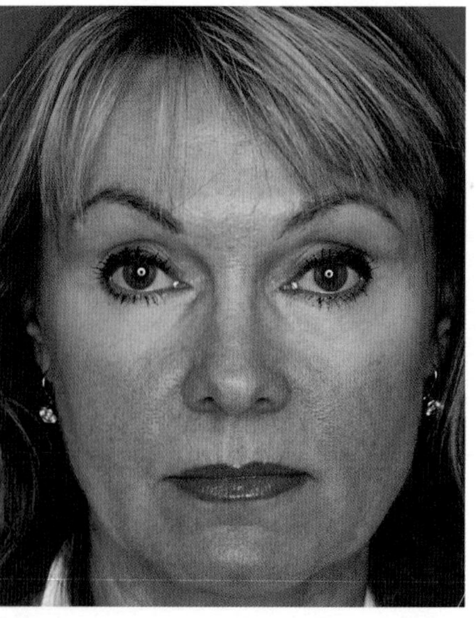

b

FIGURE 8-7. *(a) Before—Patient, White, with acne rosacea and large pores. Treatment consisted of 8 months of an aggressive program of Skin Health Restoration and a Blue Peel, 2 coats of 20%, to the papillary dermis. (b) After—1 year.*

TABLE 8.4					
THE BLUE PEEL COAT SYSTEM FOR SPECIFIC CONDITIONS					
	15% Coat System Depth and Number of Coats		***20% Coat System Depth and Number of Coats***		
Treatment Goal	***Thin Skin***	***Thick Skin***	***Thin Skin***	***Thick Skin***	***Comments***
Enhance Skin Health Restoration	1 to 2 coats for light to deep exfoliation	1 to 2 coats for light to deep exfoliation	Not recommended	1 coat for light to deep exfoliation	15% preferred for exfoliation
Treat comedones, active acne	1 to 2 coats for light to deep exfoliation	1 to 2 coats for light to deep exfoliation	Not recommended	1 coat	Can also perform comedone extraction surgery
Freshen skin	1 coat for exfoliation	1 coat for exfoliation	Not recommended	1 coat	Can be repeated if desired
Brown spots, actinic keratoses, epidermal melasma, skin roughness	2 to 3 coats for a deep exfoliation or a papillary dermis peel	3 to 4 coats	1 coat	2 coats	Two to 3 peels may be needed; wait 6 weeks between peels
Large pores	2 to 3 coats for a papillary dermis peel	3 to 4 coats	1 coat	2 coats	Can be repeated every 6 to 8 weeks in the first year; then once yearly
Skin laxity, fine lines, stretchable wrinkles and scars	3 to 4 coats for a papillary dermis or IRD peel	4 to 5 coats	1 to 2 coats	2 to 3 coats	Can use 1 coat of 20% followed by 1 coat of 15% for thin skin and 2 coats of 20% followed by 1 coat of 15% for thick skin
Peeling nonfacial skin	1 coat for exfoliation, 2 coats for Standard Blue Peel	1 coat for exfoliation, 2 coats for a papillary dermis peel	1 coat 15%	1 coat 20% for a papillary dermis peel	Obtain even blue color, do not expect an even frost

of a 15% to 20% Blue Peel with the features of a 20% to 70% glycolic acid peel.

COMPONENTS OF THE BLUE PEEL BASE

The base of the Blue Peel was formulated with two principal goals: 1) to obtain a mixture of oil, water, and TCA that penetrates more slowly into the skin and 2) to provide a guide that facilitates even application of the mixture to the skin. The components include glycerin (the oil), plant

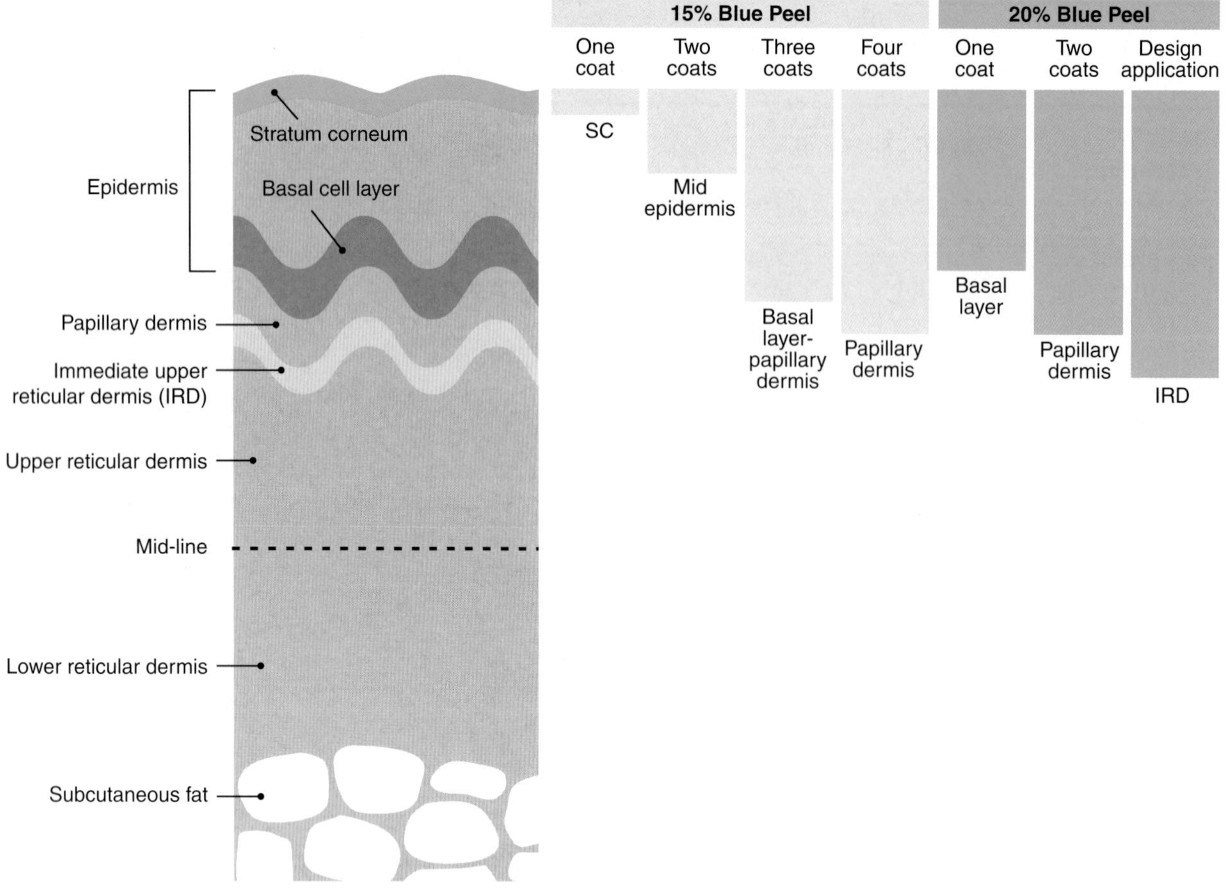

FIGURE 8-8. *Layers of the skin and the depth of penetration of each coat of the 15% Blue Peel, the 20% Blue Peel, and the Blue Peel with Design.*

saponins such as Complex 272, the blue color (FD&C Blue #1), and a nonionic base (Table 8-6). The saponins act as a wetting and surface tension-reducing agent that allows TCA to mix homogenously with the glycerin. The blue color does not penetrate below the stratum corneum and facilitates equal and even coverage. It also helps in preventing accidental deeper

Box 8-7

PROPERTIES OF MODIFIED TRICHLOROACETIC ACID (TCA) IN THE BLUE PEEL MIXTURE

- **Penetrates more slowly than unmodified TCA. Clinical depth signs therefore develop more slowly, allowing time for recognition**
- **Is neutralized by the skin more effectively**
- **Intensity and duration of burning sensation are decreased**
- **Is less irritating to the skin**

TABLE 8.5

COMPARISON OF GLYCOLIC ACID PEEL WITH THE BLUE PEEL

Feature	*Glycolic Acid Peel*	*Blue Peel*
Concentration	20% to 70%	15% or 20%
Need for neutralization	Yes	No, self-neutralizing
Suitable skin types	All	All
Depth control	Variable	Good
Occurrence of irritation	Common	Rare
Occurrence of post-inflammatory hyperpigmentation (PIH)	Possible	Possible
Guide for even application of peel solution	None	Blue color
Endpoint	Arbitrary (time of contact with skin)	Blue color evenness and intensity, frost quality, pink background sign, epidermal sliding
Number of peels required	Usually 3 to >10	1 to 3
Skin tightening effect	Weak	Excellent
Skin leveling effect	None	Mild

TABLE 8.6

MAJOR COMPONENTS OF THE BLUE PEEL BASE

Blue Base Component	*Description*
Glycerin	An oily substance that, when added to TCA/water mixture, slows down TCA penetration and allows more even application
Plant saponins such as Complex 272	A water-soluble, botanically derived saponin product in the form of a colloidal glycoside with a corticosteroid structure. It reduces the surface tension between TCA, glycerin, and water to create a homogenous mixture
FD&C Blue #1	A blue dye that acts as an indicator for the even application of the prepared Blue Peel solution.
Nonionic base	Gives the mixture a thicker consistency and lubricating properties that facilitate even application

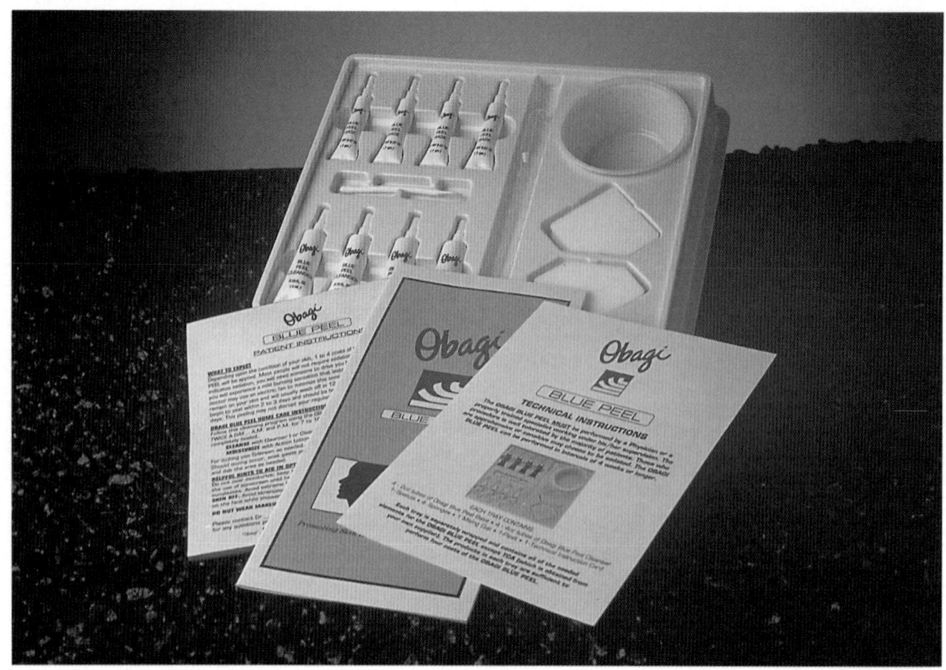

FIGURE 8-9. *The Blue Peel tray containing four 2-cc tubes of Blue Peel base, one mixing cup, one pipette, one spatula, four sponges, and four 4-cc tubes of Blue Peel cleanser. Four trays are included in each Blue Peel kit. One tray, together with the TCA obtained from a supplier, contains the ingredients necessary for preparing the solution mix for 4 coats of 15% TCA or 20% TCA.*

than desired penetration with the risk of scarring as seen when using a colorless solution on nonfacial skin as a result of overpainting certain areas that do not frost easily. The Blue Peel tray is shown in Figure 8-9.

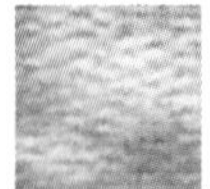

PERFORMING THE BLUE PEEL

SEDATION

The Blue Peel is not systemically toxic and is tolerated by most patients. The 15% concentration can often be applied without patient sedation. For sensitive, apprehensive patients, conscious sedation can be offered. Sedation with EMLA or other topical agent is not recommended because it can cause uneven penetration. Adhere to local laws as they apply to sedation in an office setting. Be sure to tell patients who are having sedation that they will need someone to drive them home.

SELECTION OF 15% OR 20% CONCENTRATION

The 15% and 20% Blue Peels are distinguished from plain 15% to 20% TCA preparations in that they allow TCA to act more slowly on the skin (smaller amount penetrating at any given time), they penetrate more evenly, and they cause less irritation. The 15% coat system is recommended for 1) the physician with minimal peeling experience, 2) patients with dry, thin, or sensitive skin, and 3) nonfacial skin. It is more suitable than the 20% concentration for patients with a low tolerance for the temporary (1 to 2 minutes) burning sensation that occurs during the peel.

Three to 4 coats of the 15% solution are the standard for treating the face, and 2 to 3 coats when treating nonfacial skin. The exceptions are patients with very thin skin who may get an even frost with pink on the face with 2 to 3 coats, and patients with very thick skin who may need 5 or 6 coats for such a frost.

The 20% coat system is to be used by the physician who has experience in chemical peeling. It is recommended for patients 1) with thick skin, 2) who can tolerate the more intense, temporary burning sensation during the peel, 3) who are receiving sedation, and 4) who are having combined procedures (Blue Peel as well as other aesthetic surgery or laser resurfacing). Two coats are the average with the 20% concentration. However, one 20% coat with or without another 15% coat may suffice for very thin skin, while a third coat may be needed for thick skin. The 20% solution allows the procedure to be completed faster and also uses less blue base.

SOLUTION PREPARATION

A 15% or 20% Blue Peel mixture must be freshly prepared (Table 8-7) prior to the application of each coat to ensure the correct concentration. Any unused portion of the mixture should be discarded because evaporation may have made the solution more concentrated. The entire 4 to 6 cc should be used to accomplish one coat that covers the entire face evenly multiple times from the hairline to the jawline. Follow the same procedure for preparation of additional coats.

TABLE 8.7

BLUE PEEL SOLUTION PREPARATION FOR ONE COAT

Component	*15% Blue Peel Coat System*	*20% Blue Peel Coat System*
30% TCA	2 cc (use pipette provided to measure)	4 cc (use pipette provided to measure)
Blue base	2 cc (use premeasured tube provided)	2 cc (use premeasured tube provided)
Total volume	4 cc (use all for one coat)	6 cc (use all for one coat)

Note: Discard any unused portion of the mixture after coat application. Solution that is left to stand may evaporate and become more concentrated.

APPLICATION OF BLUE PEEL SOLUTION (15% OR 20%)

Ask the patient to arrive without facial make-up and to remove any jewelry. Position the patient comfortably in a chair and place a roll under the neck to extend the neck. A room lit by daylight fluorescent lighting is best for color observation. Spot lighting is not helpful. A small, hand-held electric fan should be available beside the patient's chair for cooling the patient's face during the peel. The fan can be held by the patient or by the doctor's assistant. Also, have a bottle of normal saline at hand for flushing the eyes if the acid accidentally gets into the eyes. I do not advise placing shields in the patient's eyes. Have cotton swabs available for application of solution to the eyelids and "ice-pick" scars.

Prior to application of the peel solution, degrease the patient's face with alcohol or acetone. Dip, but do not saturate, a corner of the sponge provided in the Blue Peel tray into the freshly prepared solution. Apply with short, gentle strokes in all directions using light pressure. Apply 2 to 5 strokes to an area and then move to another area at a steady speed and rhythm. Many physicians prefer to begin with the chin, proceeding clockwise to the area around the mouth, nose, cheeks, and forehead. Proceed clockwise or counterclockwise, but do not return to an already treated area until the solution has been evenly applied to the face. Do not skip application to any area.

Treatment of eyelids helps to eliminate wrinkles and tighten the lids for better cosmetic results. Coat the eyelids with solution as you coat the rest of the face. Keep the patient's eyes open while coating the lower lids by lifting and holding the upper lid against the eyebrow bone with your thumb. This can also be done by your assistant. Apply the solution to the lower lid by stroking sideways. Extend the application beyond the lateral canthi, inward toward the nasal canthus, upward toward the eylashes, and downward to the infraorbital rim. Coat the upper eyelids with the patient's eyes closed and apply the solution downward and sideways to prevent opening the eye. Do not allow the solution to drip or run onto the skin, and, most important, do not allow the solution to get into the patient's eyes. Apply the solution without pressure. In addition, refine the eyelid application at the end of the procedure with a cotton swab applicator dipped in the solution. To accurately reach the endpoints, use all of the suggested solution coat volume.

Treat the upper and lower lip areas down to the chin in the usual fashion. If a Designed Blue Peel is desired, remember that the maximum depth is the IRD. Unnecessary depth must be avoided in this area because scarring can occur, especially in the upper lip area where the dermis is thin and there is little subcutaneous fat between the dermis and the underlying muscle. For further correction in this area, it is preferable to repeat the peel 6 to 8 weeks later instead of attempting deeper correction through a single peel.

Adherence to the maximum depth rule—no deeper than the papillary dermis or immediate reticular dermis—is very important. If a deeper peel is desired, a medium-depth peel with 30% to 40% TCA, such as the Obagi Controlled Depth Peel, or CO_2 laser resurfacing, can be performed instead.

A mild burning sensation develops as the solution is applied that will start to subside in 2 to 3 minutes and is tolerated by most patients. When the sensation increases, stop application for 2 minutes. Bringing the handheld fan close to the patient's face is very helpful in cooling the skin and reducing discomfort during this period. This can be repeated as often as necessary. Wait 2 minutes between coats to allow the frost to develop and the burning sensation to subside. Apply subsequent coats in the same manner as described for the initial coat.

Feathering

To prevent sharp demarcation lines, feather out at the chin and jaw line. To feather, apply solution 1 to 2 inches beyond the peeled areas using progressively lighter pressure and progressively shorter intervals of acid contact with the skin. Wipe the applied solution with a tissue after contact with the skin. Feathering should achieve a decreasing peel depth, progressing from the IRD to the papillary dermis to a deep exfoliation to end with a very light exfoliation, 1 to 2 inches away from the main peeled area.

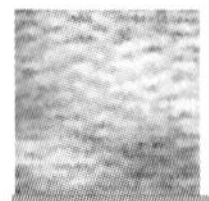

ENDPOINTS

Endpoints are skin changes that indicate the depth of penetration of the acid solution and allow the physician to stop adding further coats of solution or to continue until the desired depth has been reached. Monitoring of the endpoints produces consistent results and reduces the risk of complications. The relationship of Blue Peel endpoints with depth is shown in Table 8-8 on page 169. Standard TCA peels that use plain or augmented TCA do not have such clear endpoints and thus have unpredictable results and a higher risk of complications.

Despite my recent publication documenting the presence of reproducible changes in the appearance of the skin correlating to depth of acid penetration in chemical peels (depth signs), certain authors remain doubtful about the existence of these clinically based signs of depth of a chemical peel. There is no question in my mind that recognition of the development of depth signs requires careful clinical observation and experience. One only hopes that the inability of these authors to recognize the development of depth signs relates to inexperience and not to an attempt to hold on to old dogma or to promote their methods of peels. I am happy at any time to teach my method of depth control based on development of depth signs to anyone interested in performing a safer and more controlled chemical peel.

The progression of endpoints in the Blue Peel are 1) even blue color with no frost, 2) deeper blue with a nonorganized frost, 3) deeper blue with organized, sheet-like frost with pink background and epidermal sliding, and 4) deeper blue with organized, sheet-like frost with no pink background and no epidermal sliding.

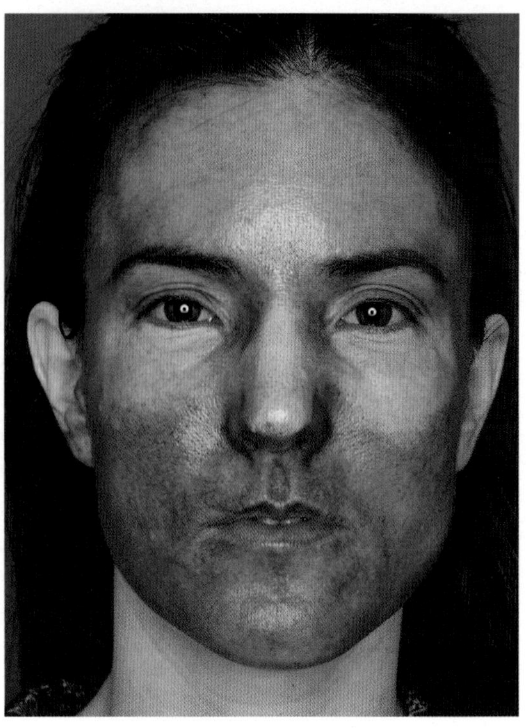

FIGURE 8-10. *Patient showing all levels of frost at the same time (for teaching purposes). 1) Forehead, which received 1 coat of 15% Blue Peel, shows light blue color and no frost; 2) perioral and lower cheeks, which received 2 coats of 15% Blue Peel, show deeper blue and only a light cloud (not an organized frost); 3) nose, upper cheeks, and lower eyelids, which received 4 coats of 15% Blue Peel, show an organized frost with pink. This was a teaching demonstration, and the patient's peel was subsequently evened out.*

FROSTING AND PINK BACKGROUND

Frost appears on the skin as a result of coagulation of epidermal and dermal proteins by the action of TCA. If the penetration is limited to the epidermal layer (exfoliation), the skin shows an even blue appearance and an initial frost that is not organized and looks like a cloud or fog, or there is no frost at all. Following the application of more coats and deeper penetration of the acid, the blue becomes darker. The nonorganized cloud-like frost starts to organize and appears as a sheet. This will appear earlier in thin skin. When the papillary dermis has been reached, the frost will look like a thin, transparent, organized sheet with a pink background. Frosting of the papillary dermis should last for 5 to 10 minutes before total defrosting, which indicates that the proper depth was reached. When the IRD has been reached, the frost will be a solid white sheet without a pink background. This indicates that no further solution should be applied (Figures 8-10, 8-11).

The author has named the pink background to the frost during a peel the "pink sign." When TCA has begun to penetrate the papillary dermis, the frost has a pink background due to the intact blood vessels and the continuous blood flow in the capillary loops of the papillary dermis (Figure 8-12). When the TCA has penetrated to the IRD and occluded or caused vasospasm in the capillary loops of the papillary derrmis, blood flow in this area stops and the pink background disappears (no pink sign). The frost then appears solid white.

EPIDERMAL SLIDING

The epidermis is attached to the dermis by means of epidermal projections (rete ridges), corresponding dermal invaginations, and a network of an-

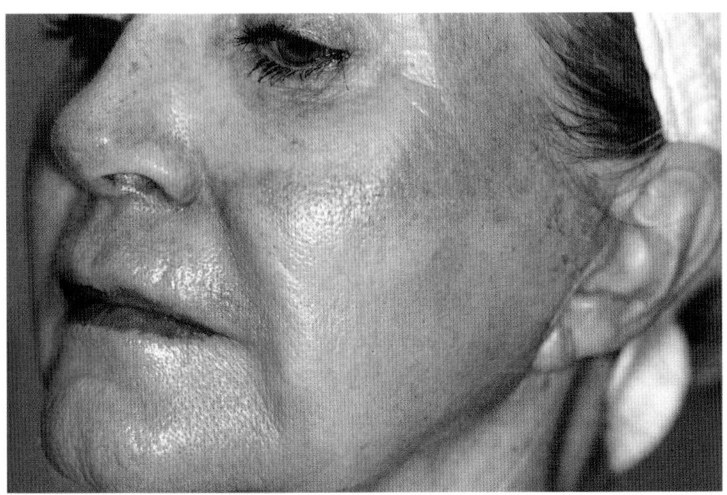

a

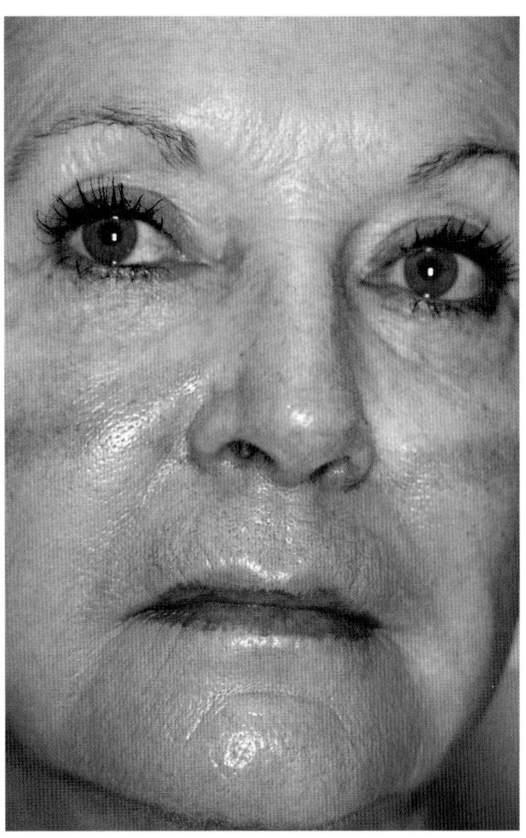

b

FIGURE 8-11. *(a) Another patient showing all levels of frost at the same time (for teaching purposes). This patient's skin shows the difference between 1 coat of the 15% versus 1 coat of the 20% Blue Peel solution. Temples, which received 1 coat of 15% Blue Peel, show light blue color and no frost; ears to jawline to nasolabial folds, which received 1 coat of 20% Blue Peel, show frost with pink; chin, which received 2 coats of 20% Blue Peel, shows frost with less pink; upper lip, which received Design (extra application of 20%), shows frost with no pink. This was a teaching demonstration, and the patient's peel was subsequently evened out. (b) Same patient as in (a), frontal view.*

choring fibrils that extend vertically from the reticular dermis through the papillary dermis and attach themselves to the basement membrane. This attachment is strong in young skin and can be observed clinically by the absence of epidermal movement or wrinkling when the skin is gently pinched (negative "accordion sign"). As skin ages, the rete ridges flatten and the anchoring fibrils are disrupted or lost, allowing the epidermis to wrinkle (slide) upon pinching (positive "accordion sign").

The application of TCA to the skin causes changes, including protein coagulation and precipitation, disruption of the anchoring fibrils, initial vasodilation, and edema, that allow the epidermis to be moved easily if it is pinched or pushed, creating wrinkling effects. This is called the epidermal sliding sign (Figure 8-13), and it indicates that the acid has reached the papillary dermis. (However, the capillary loops and blood flow are still intact, so the frost still shows a pink background.) When the acid has precipitated all of the components of the papillary dermis, the epidermis becomes "fixed" to the dermis as one block and is no longer moveable. The sliding sign disappears when this occurs and indicates that the IRD has been reached. In addition, the frost no longer shows any pink at this stage because the capillary loops in the papillary dermis have been constricted by vasospasm.

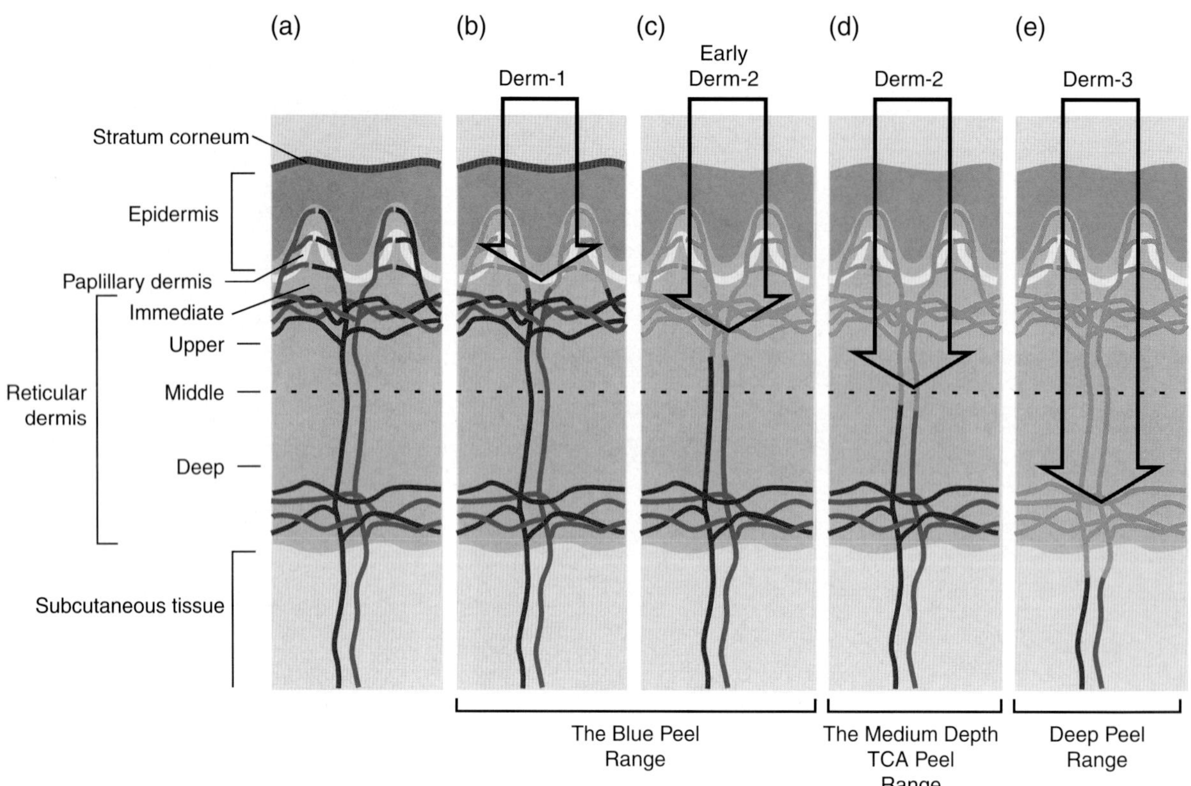

FIGURE 8-12. **Progressive levels of vascular reactions during TCA application.** *(a) Normal vasculature. (b) Derm-1 Peel. TCA penetration to the papillary dermis results in 1) skin frost with pink because blood vessels are intact and 2) epidermal sliding. (c) Early Derm-2 Peel. TCA penetration to the immediate reticular dermis (IRD) leads to 1) skin frost with pink that has just disappeared and 2) loss of epidermal sliding. (d) Derm-2 Peel. TCA penetration to the mid dermis leads to solid white frost. Defrosting takes a minimum of 10 minutes. (e) Derm-3 peel. TCA penetration to below the mid dermis leads to frost that appears gray. Defrosting takes 20 to 30 minutes. Derm-3 rarely utilized (only for very deep scars in extremely thick skin).*

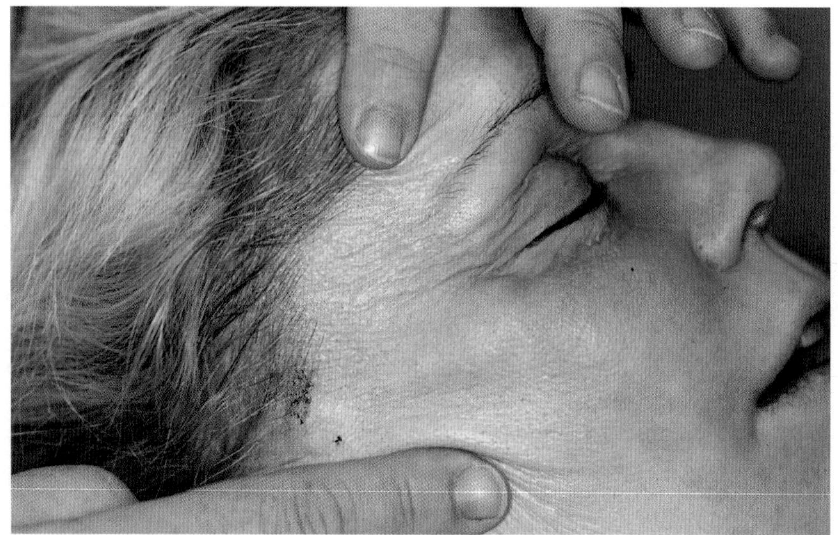

FIGURE 8-13. *The Epidermal sliding sign. Patient showing frost with pink at temples (penetration to papillary dermis) and numerous wrinkles when the skin is pushed together (epidermal sliding). The epidermal sliding sign ends abruptly in the areas where the acid has penetrated to the immediate reticular dermis (where pink sign is absent).*

The epidermal sliding sign is important when peeling dark or Black skin because the pink sign may not be clearly visible. In thick, porous skin, on the other hand, the sliding sign may not be very obvious, and the pink sign has to be used as an endpoint instead. (Table 8-8 summarizes Blue Peel and points at various depth levels.)

PERIOD OF RELATIVE RESISTANCE

The Period of Relative Resistance is a concept that explains the length of time skin resists penetration of TCA. That resistance period can be short or longer, depending on certain factors that affect penetration rate. When an acid is applied to the skin, defenses come into play, the first of which is epidermal protein (keratin), which acts to neutralize and arrest the penetration of the acid. When this epidermal defense has been consumed, application of more acid will allow deeper penetration (to the papillary dermis) where the second line of defense, dermal components (collagen, elastin, glycosaminoglycans, blood vessels, blood, and other proteins) come into play and also act to arrest the penetration of TCA. When these dermal defenses have been consumed, application of more acid will result in penetration deeper to the upper reticular dermis or below.

The ability of skin defenses to neutralize TCA is related to 1) TCA concentration, which determines the speed of penetration, 2) volume of solution applied in relation to the size of the body surface area, and 3) skin thickness. A high concentration of TCA (25% to 40%) will rapidly consume a larger amount of skin protein and thus penetrate faster and deeper than concentrations of 15% to 20%. A large volume of TCA solution also leads to faster consumption of skin protein and faster and deeper penetration, especially if the large volume is applied to a small surface area. Use of plain or augmented

TABLE 8.8

SUMMARY OF BLUE PEEL ENDPOINTS AT DIFFERENT DEPTHS

	Endpoints			
Blue Peel Depth	***Coloring***	***Frosting***	***Pink Background***	***Epidermal Sliding***
Exfoliation to stratum corneum (light exfoliation)	Even blue	Misty or cloudy, no organized frost	Present	Absent
Exfoliation to basal layer (deep exfoliation)	Darker blue	Thin sheet of cloud or fog, no organized frost	Present	Present
Peel to papillary dermis (standard Blue Peel)	Darker blue	Thin transparent, organized sheet	Present	Present
Peel to immediate reticular dermis (IRD) (Designed Blue peel)	Darker blue	Solid organized sheet	Just faded	Just faded

Box 8-8

The Period of Relative Resistance is longer:

- **with 15% than 20% TCA**
- **in Thick Skin vs. Thin Skin**
- **with the Blue Peel solution than equal concentrations of plain TCA**

TCA also leads to faster penetration than occurs with the Blue Peel mixture of the same volume. And because thin skin contains less neutralizing protein than thick skin, penetration is faster in thin skin. With the Blue Peel, the safety margin is higher because there is control of acid concentration and acid volume in relation to skin thickness. Thicker skin has more defenses and requires more solution volume and a longer Period of Relative Resistance.

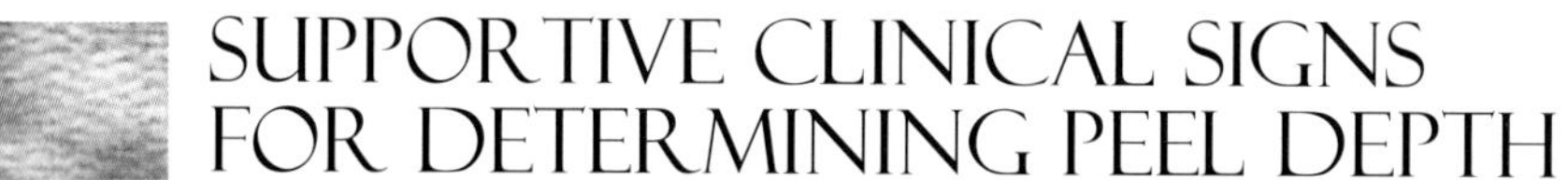

SUPPORTIVE CLINICAL SIGNS FOR DETERMINING PEEL DEPTH

The supportive clinicial signs are 1) defrosting time, 2) skin firmness, and 3) healing time (Table 8-9). While these are not endpoints, they can help in

TABLE 8.9

BLUE PEEL CLINICAL SUPPORTING SIGNS AT DIFFERENT DEPTHS

	Signs			
	Defrosting Time (minutes)			
Blue Peel Depth	***Thin Skin***	***Thick Skin***	***Firmness***	***Healing Time***
Exfoliation to stratum corneum (light exfoliation)	NA	NA	None	3 days
Exfoliation to basal layer (deeper exfoliation)	NA	NA	None	6 days
Peel to papillary dermis (Standard Blue Peel)	5	10	Light	7 to 8 days
Peel to immediate reticular dermis (IRD) (Designed Blue Peel)	10	15	Medium	10 days

determining depth. This applies especially to healing time, which correlates well retrospectively with the depth of skin injury.

DEFROSTING TIME

After frosting has occurred (the coagulation of epidermal and dermal protein), the process of dispersion of the precipitated proteins, called defrosting, begins. With papillary dermal penetration, defrosting time is approximately 10 minutes in thick skin and 5 minutes in thin skin. With IRD penetration, defrosting time is about 15 minutes in thick skin and 10 minutes in thin skin. Persistence of a frost up to 10 minutes before defrosting indicates a good hold on the depth that was reached.

FIRMNESS

The more protein precipitated by the action of TCA, the firmer the skin will feel upon pinching. Thus increased skin firmness is more pronounced with deep peels and in thick skin and is not detectable in exfoliative procedures. The less-experienced peeler may not be able to detect the increased firmness in papillary dermis or IRD peels, but an effort should be made to acquire this ability.

POSTPROCEDURE HEALING TIME

Healing time is the time needed for complete reepithelialization. It can be predicted accurately if the depth guidelines of the Blue Peel are followed, and it correlates well with the depth of skin injury in all skin types. After the procedure, an observation of a patient's healing gives the physician an indication of the depth achieved by the peel, and the time noted should be placed in the patient's record. Expected healing time following chemical peeling is shown in Table 8-10, and the stages of healing after the Blue Peel are shown in Table 8-11.

TABLE 8.10

EXPECTED HEALING TIME

Chemical Peel Depth	*Days for Healing*
Stratum corneum exfoliation	3
Exfoliation above the basal layer	4 to 6
Papillary dermis peel	7 to 8
IRD peel	10
Upper reticular dermis	10 to 14

TABLE 8.11		
THE HEALING STAGES OF THE BLUE PEEL		
The Peel Stage (7–10 Days)	***The Recovery Stage (1–6 weeks)***	***Return to Normal***
■ Procedure completed ■ Home care instructions to be followed ■ The blue color washes away ■ Swelling for 2 to 3 days ■ Skin will appear as a tight, dark mask ■ Skin will start to peel off in 2 to 3 days ■ No pain with normal healing. Pain suggests an infection.	■ Anticipated reaction may appear (erythema, PIH, acne flare-up) ■ Camouflaging with make-up may be necessary ■ Skin reconditioning should be started	■ Results of the procedure can be evaluated at this stage ■ Treatments of any complications to continue ■ Plan for a second Blue Peel, if needed

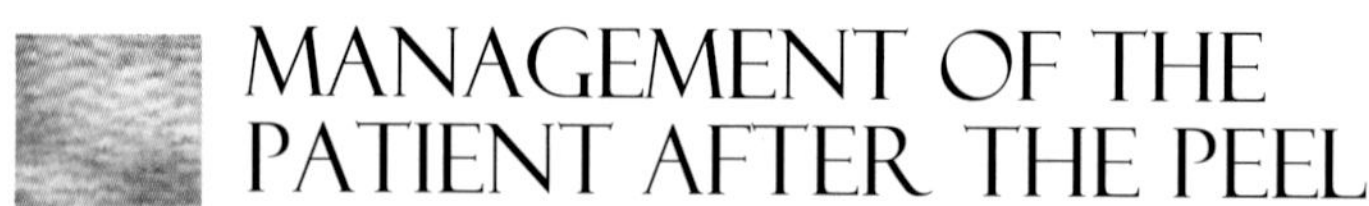

MANAGEMENT OF THE PATIENT AFTER THE PEEL

Healing at home is usually painless. The patient is to follow simple instructions of washing the face twice daily without rubbing off any skin, applying antiseptic compresses, and applying a moisturizer, possibly with 0.5% hydrocortisone, several times daily. If the skin is very tight, a light coat of a heavier lubricant can be applied. The patient should minimize making facial expressions, sleep on his or her back, and avoid being struck on the face with the shower water spray while bathing. Men should shave daily. If Design has been performed with the Blue Peel, the patient may need stronger and more frequent lubrication, such as Aquaphor ointment, petroleum jelly, or Bacitracin or Polysporin ointments, in areas where the skin feels very tight. Figures 8-14 and 8-15 show a patient in the healing stages.

Healing time can be delayed by patient factors (picking, excoriation, facial expressions that lead to cracking of the scabs), postpeel management (excessive dryness or excessive moisture), and minor complications such as infections or irritation. The first stage of healing is complete when the epidermis has been restored (reepithelialization) and the skin can tolerate topical treatment with hydroquinone and tretinoin. In the next stage dermal changes, including collagen production and alignment and neovascularization, take place for 2 to 6 weeks. For that reason, the results of the peel should not be judged until then. After reepithelialization has occurred,

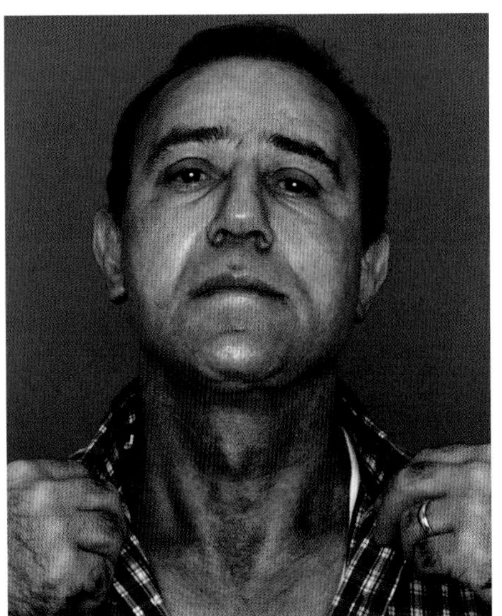

a

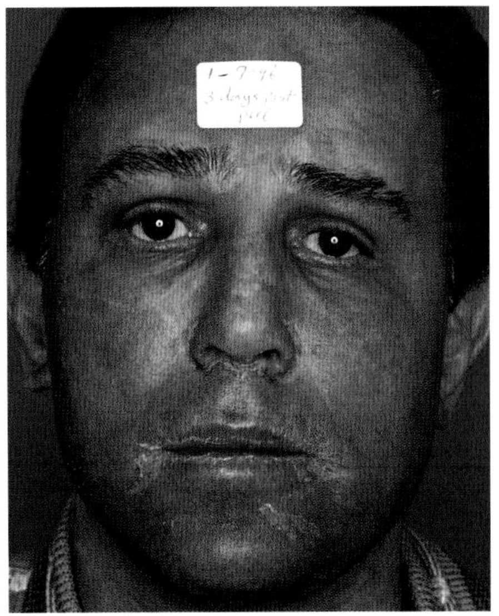

b

FIGURE 8-14. *(a) Patient (the author) underwent a Blue Peel with 2 coats of 20% on the face and 1 coat of 20% on the neck. (b) 3 days after peel shows even healing.*

the patient can resume the Skin Conditioning program, as tolerated, to stabilize skin color, reduce redness, and restore normal skin tolerance. Home care following the Blue Peel is shown in Table 8-12.

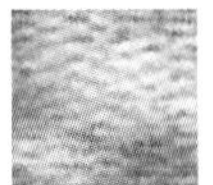

THE DESIGNED BLUE PEEL

The Designed Blue Peel is performed when deeper skin correction or leveling is desired. This involves application of extra Blue Peel solution to selected areas of the face that require penetration up to the immediate retic-

TABLE 8.12

POST-BLUE PEEL HOME CARE

A.M.	*Midmorning*	*Midafternoon*	*Evening*
■ Wash face gently with cleanser; avoid rubbing. ■ Apply the recommended moisturizer alone or mixed with 0.5% hydrocortisone; use an ointment occasionally, if needed.	■ Apply antiseptic compresses for 2 minutes. ■ Following an IRD level peel, perform scab thinning for 2 minutes beginning on day 4 after the peel. ■ Apply the recommended moisturizer mixture, if needed.	■ Apply antiseptic compresses for 2 minutes. ■ Following an IRD-level peel, perform scab thinning as in mid morning. ■ Apply moisturizer mixture, if needed.	■ Wash face. ■ Apply moisturizers as in morning.

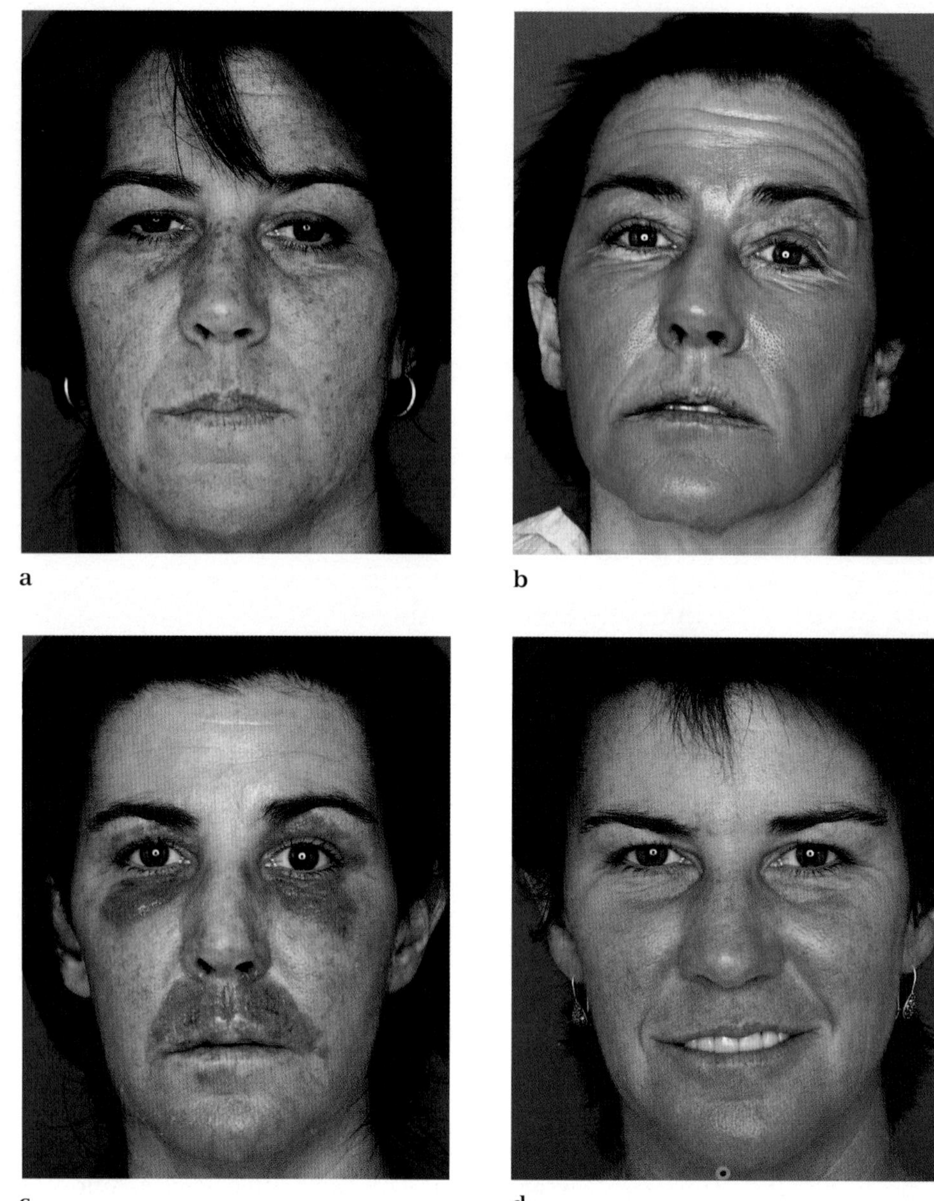

FIGURE 8-15. *(a) Patient (Brunette) with photoaging, uneven pigmentation, perioral and periorbital rhytids, and general laxity. (b) Patient undergoing a Blue Peel with Design with 2 coats of 20% applied on entire face (shows frost with pink) and additional application (Design to upper reticular dermis) periorally and periorbitally (shows frost with less pink). (c) Patient 7 days after the peel. Areas peeled to level of papillary dermis are healed with no erythema or inflammation. Designed areas (immediate reticular dermis) are continuing to heal. (d) Patient 1 year after 2 Blue Peels with Design were performed.*

Box 8-8

The Designed Blue Peel involves application of extra Blue Peel solution to selected areas, such as scars or deep wrinkles, for penetration to the IRD.

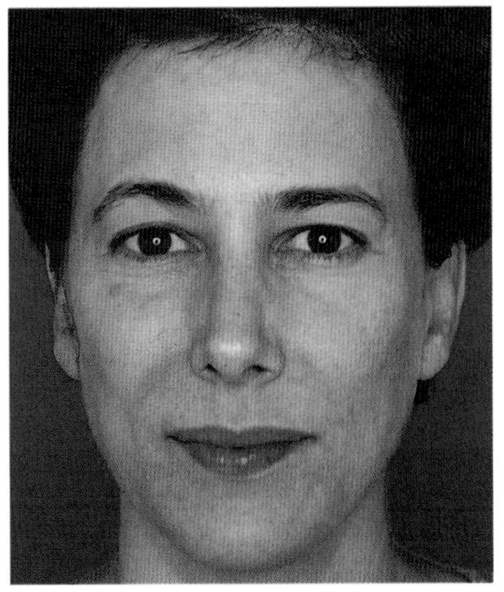
a

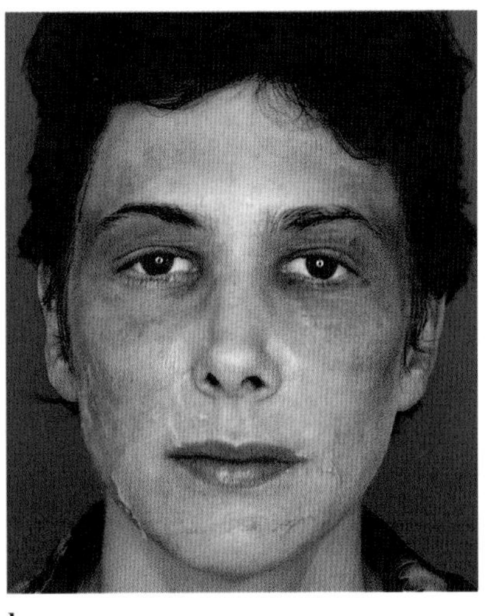
b

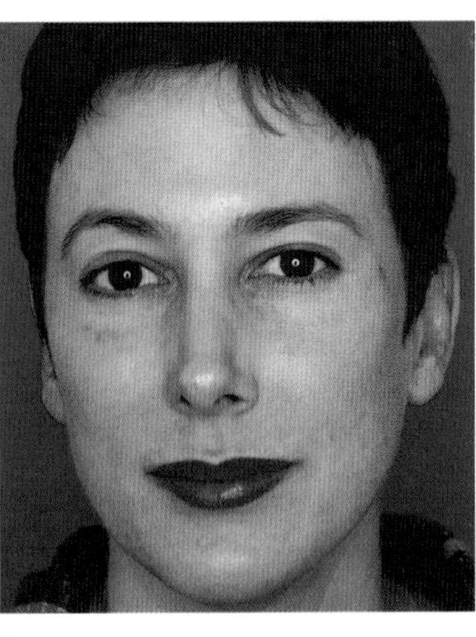
c

FIGURE 8-16. *Before—Patient, White to Brunette, with mild acne scars, uneven pigmentation, and laxity who was treated with Skin Conditioning for correction and stimulation for 5 months. A Blue Peel with Design periorbitally was performed during that period. (She underwent a total of 2 Blue Peel procedures, 2 months apart, with Design.) (b) 5 days after first Blue Peel procedure. Healing occurring at a variable rate. (c) 1 year after second Blue Peel with Design procedure.*

ular dermis. Such deeper penetration is helpful in producing increased leveling for stretchable scars or deep wrinkles or increased tightening for laxity and jowling (Figures 8-16, 8-17). The physician must keep in mind that the depth of the standard Blue Peel is the papillary dermis, and, when Design is added, the maximum recommended depth is the IRD. Also, the Designed Blue Peel is to be used for facial skin only; nonfacial skin is poor in adnexal structures and cannot support this depth of peel.

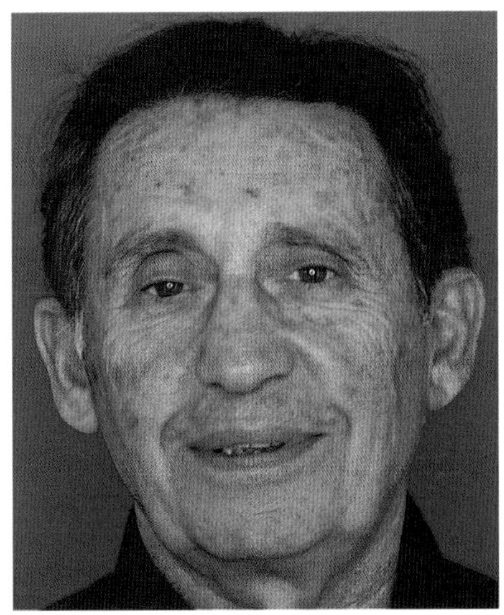
a

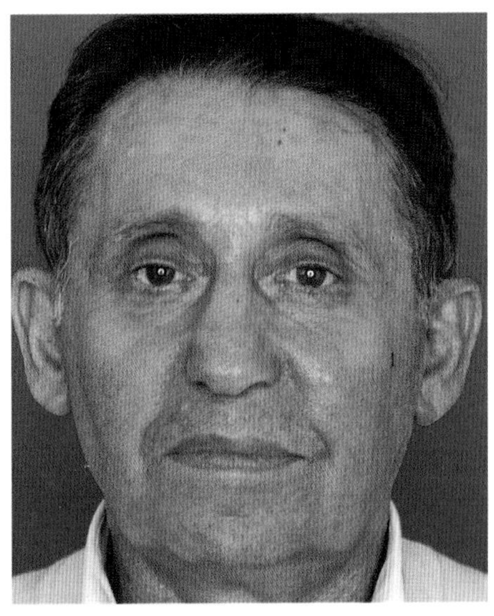
b

FIGURE 8-17. *(a) Before—70-year-old patient, White, with actinic keratoses, history of basal cell carcinomas, photoaging, laxity. (b) 1 year after—Treatment consisted of Skin Conditioning for correction and stimulation for 5 months. A Blue Peel with Design in the periorbital area was performed after 3 months of conditioning.*

To perform the Blue Peel with Design, apply the necessary number of coats to reach the papillary dermis. Then use a cotton swab or sponge to apply additional solution to the chosen areas, and continue solution application until the pink sign begins to disappear in those areas. Feather out the margins to the surrounding areas for a smooth transition between the designed areas and the others. The Blue Peel with Design should be attempted only after the physician has built up sufficient experience in performing the standard Blue Peel penetrating to the papillary dermis and has mastered postpeel management.

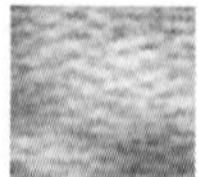

PEELING NONFACIAL SKIN

Facial skin varies in thickness, is rich with sebaceous glands and other adnexal structures, tends to be loose and less bound to underlying muscle with subcutaneous fat present in most areas except the upper lip, and has fairly consistent thickness of the stratum corneum. The skin of nonfacial areas, such as the neck, hands, or arms, on the other hand, tends to be poor in sebaceous units and other adnexal structures and loose in variable degrees, depending on the location. For example, the skin on hands is tight and cannot be pinched in the area of the fingers and is loose on the dorsum (Figures 8-18, 8-19, 8-20). In the neck area, skin is tight in the back and loose in the front because of direct attachment to the underlying muscle with little subcutaneous fat.

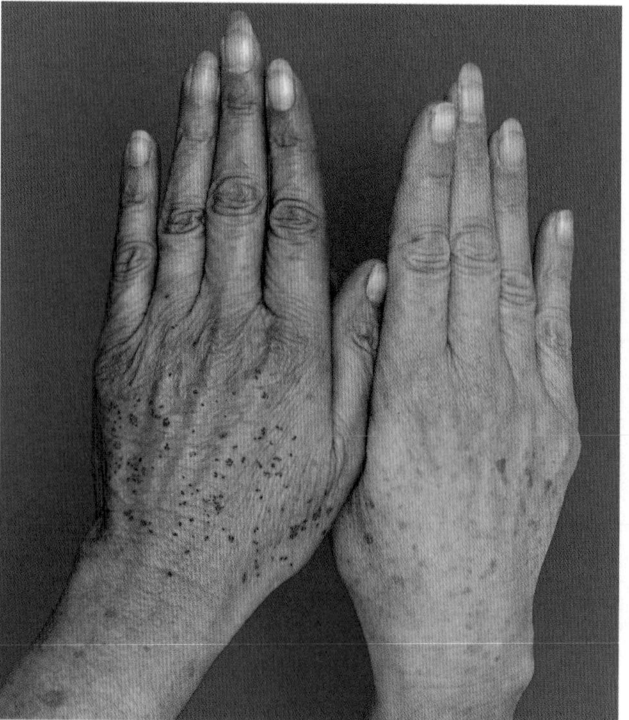

FIGURE 8-18. *Hands with hypertrophic seborrheic and actinic keratoses. Treatment consisted of Q-switched Nd:YAG 532 laser on the lesions followed by 1 coat of 20% Blue Peel. Uneven frosting of hands with peel can be seen.*

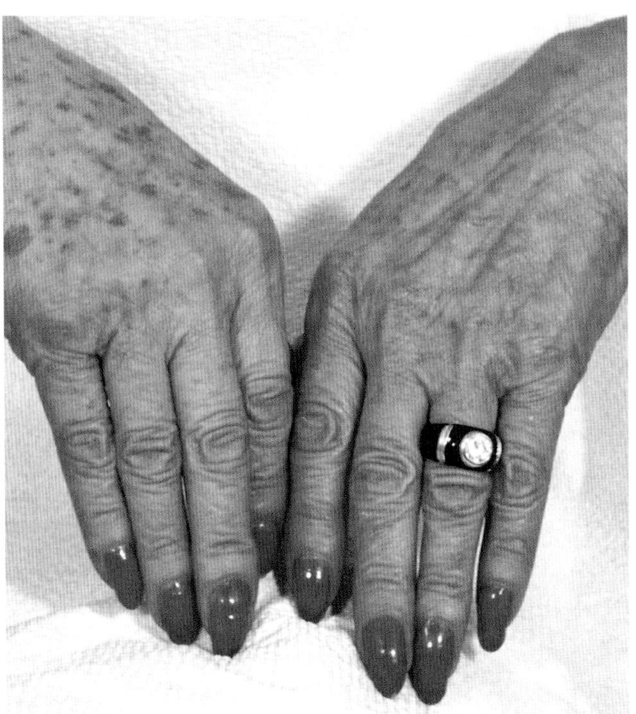

FIGURE 8-19. *Hands with lentigos. Treatment consisted of bleaching and blending, followed by 3 coats of 15% Blue Peel to the papillary dermis level. Left hand, 3 months after treatment.*

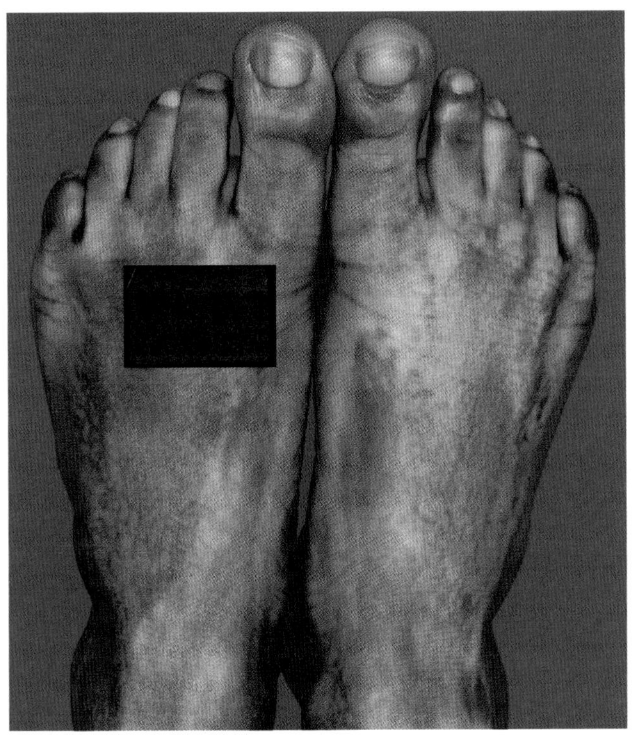

a

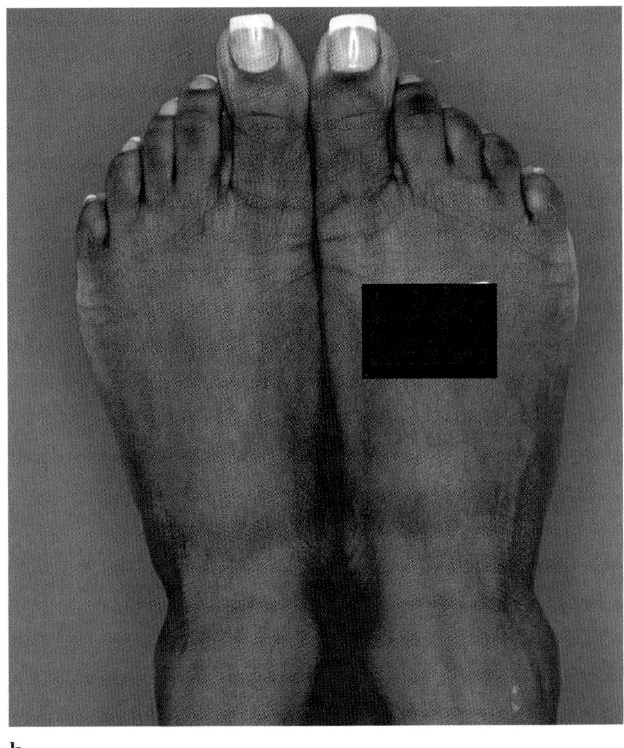

b

FIGURE 8-20. *Feet with pigmentary changes following first- and second-degree burns. Treatment consisted of creams for correction and stimulation with an emphasis on bleaching and blending. A Blue Peel with 1 coat of 20% was performed during that time. Bleaching was performed for 3 months and blending for 5 months.*

Nonfacial skin behaves differently than facial skin during peeling. In areas where the skin is loose (can be pinched) and where the stratum corneum is thin, frost appears faster than in areas where the skin is compact (knuckles, toes) or where the stratum corneum is thick. The latter may show only a cloud of frost or no frost at all, despite equal application of acid solution to both areas. When painting nonfacial skin with a colorless solution, physicians often think that nonfrosted areas have not had solution applied (been skipped) and have a tendency to apply more solution to those areas to induce a frost. This can lead to deep penetration and possible scarring. This does not occur in the Blue Peel due to the blue color guide.

PERFORMING A NONFACIAL PEEL

The 15% Blue Peel coat system should be used when peeling nonfacial skin, and the depth should not exceed the papillary dermis. Skipped areas are made visible by the blue color in the Blue Peel. Select a 5% body surface area and apply the coat in increments, painting the whole area evenly, wait 2 minutes for the acid to be neutralized, then paint again. Maintain an even blue color, similar in intensity, while the frost is slowly progressing. Do not attempt to obtain an even frost. In most cases, 2 coats of the 15% solution will be sufficient for reaching the papillary dermis. The areas that frost should show frost with pink and epidermal sliding.

When peeling an area that is smaller than 5% of the body's surface, such as a spot peel, one of two methods can be followed. In the first method, calculate the amount of solution needed for 1 coat, i.e., if a 5% surface area uses 4 cc, a 2% to 2.5% area will need 2 cc and a 1% area will need 0.75 to 1 cc. Apply the reduced amount to the area to be peeled. In the second method, you are guided by endpoints. Paint the solution evenly, wait 2 minutes, and paint again, maintaining an even blue. Stop applying the peel solution when organized, sheet-like frost with a pink background appears in the areas that have frost, even if other areas are not equally frosted. A little more solution can, however, be applied lightly with a cotton-tipped applicator to feather the margins and reduce demarcation lines.

Box 8-9

PEELING NONFACIAL SKIN

- **Use the 15% coat system.**
- **Select an area that is 5% of the body's surface.**
- **Paint the solution evenly.**
- **For the endpoint, look for an even blue color.**
- **Do not attempt to obtain an even frost.**

REPEATING THE BLUE PEEL

The Blue Peel is a program of gradual correction designed to provide maximal improvement with minimal safety risks. Varying depth levels can be obtained ranging from exfoliation, to a light peel (papillary dermis), to a light-medium (IRD) peel. The recommended waiting periods before repeating a Blue Peel are shown in Table 8-13.

TABLE 8.13

RECOMMENDED WAITING TIME BEFORE REPEATING A BLUE PEEL

Type of Peel Performed	*Depth Reached*	*Minimum Waiting Time Before Repeating Blue Peel*
Light or deep exfoliation	Epidermis	1 to 2 weeks
Standard Blue Peel	Papillary dermis	6 to 8 weeks
Designed Blue Peel	IRD in certain areas	8 to 10 weeks

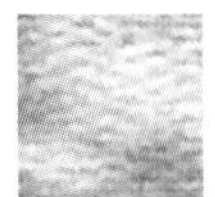

COMBINED PROCEDURES

The incidence of complications following procedures increases with the depth of skin injury: Reticular dermis procedures have more risk than papillary dermis procedures, which have more risk than exfoliating procedures. When a patient has variable levels of epidermal and dermal damage in different areas of the face, different procedures in combination can reduce the depth of skin injury in areas where such depth is not needed. Thus the rationale for performing several procedures on the same surgery date lies in using a less deep procedure where possible, combined with a deeper one only in certain areas. For example, a deeper peel can be used for leveling on unstretchable perioral wrinkles or deep acne scars and solar elastosis on the cheeks, while the standard Blue Peel can be used on the damaged areas for tightening and blending. This spares the normal area from unnecessary penetration depth. It also can reduce skin injury, shorten recovery time, reduce the incidence of complications, and enhance results.

Figures 8-21 and 8-22 are good examples of combined procedures. Figure 8-23 demonstrates the effects of the Blue Peel with Design on the right side of the patient's face, and CO_2 laser resurfacing on the left side of the patient's face (350 milizoul, 2 passes). Notice there is less erythema and more tightness on the Blue Peel side.

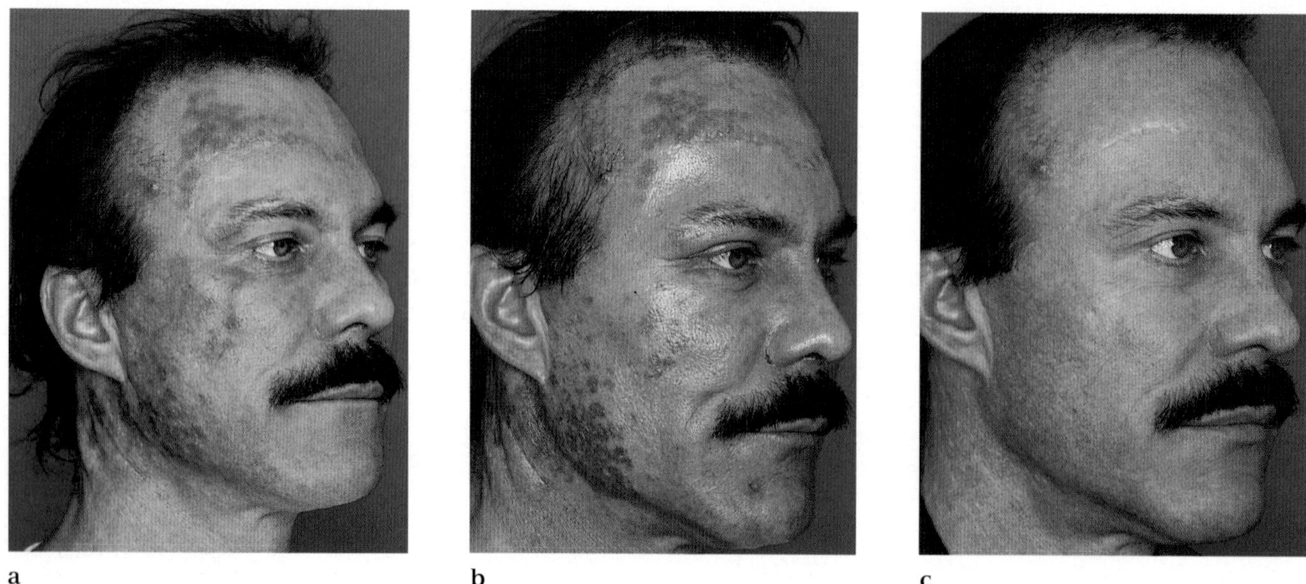

FIGURE 8-21. *(a) Before—Patient with acne scars and sun-induced telangiectasia. (b) Treatment consisted of FLDP laser, 3.7 J/cm^2, along with a Blue Peel with Design on the same day. (c) 1 year after.*

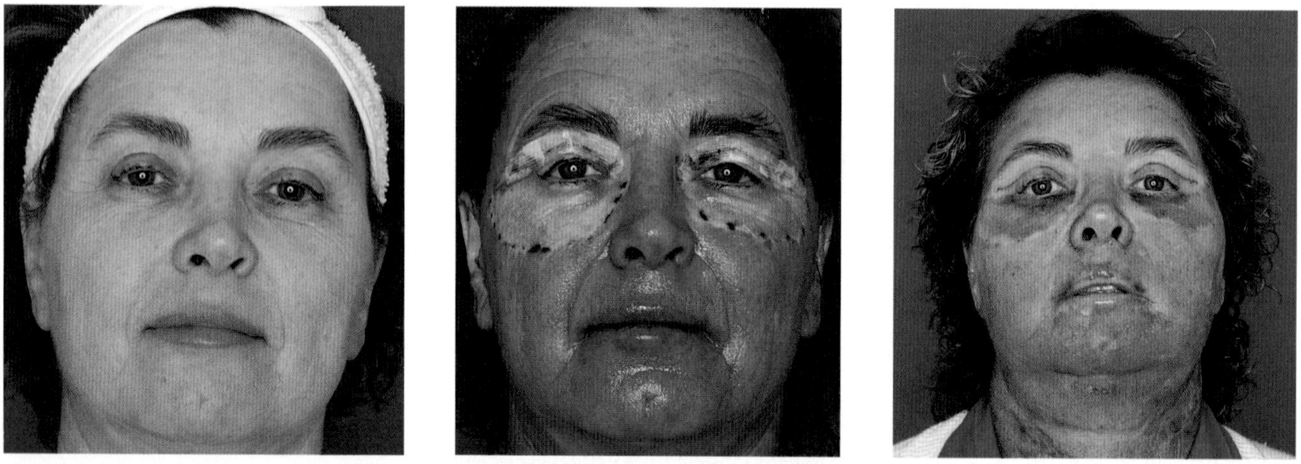

a b c

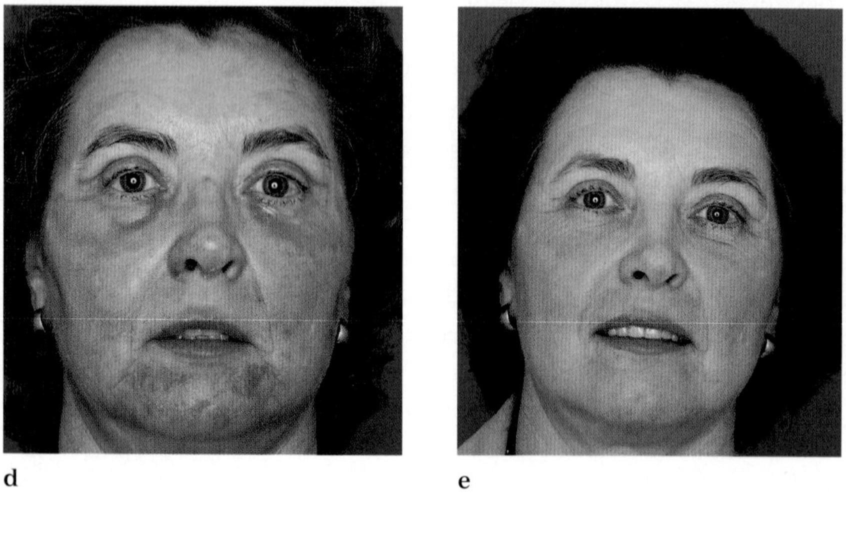

d e

FIGURE 8-22. *(a) Before—51-year-old patient with normal White skin, general laxity following 6 weeks of prepeel correction and stimulation. (b) Treatment consisted of CO_2 laser resurfacing periorbitally, an upper lid blepharoplasty, and 2 coats of 20% Blue Peel on the face and 1 coat of 20% on the neck. (c) 3 days after procedures. (d) 10 days after procedure. (e) 4 months after procedures. Some periorbital redness where CO_2 laser resurfacing was performed is still visible.*

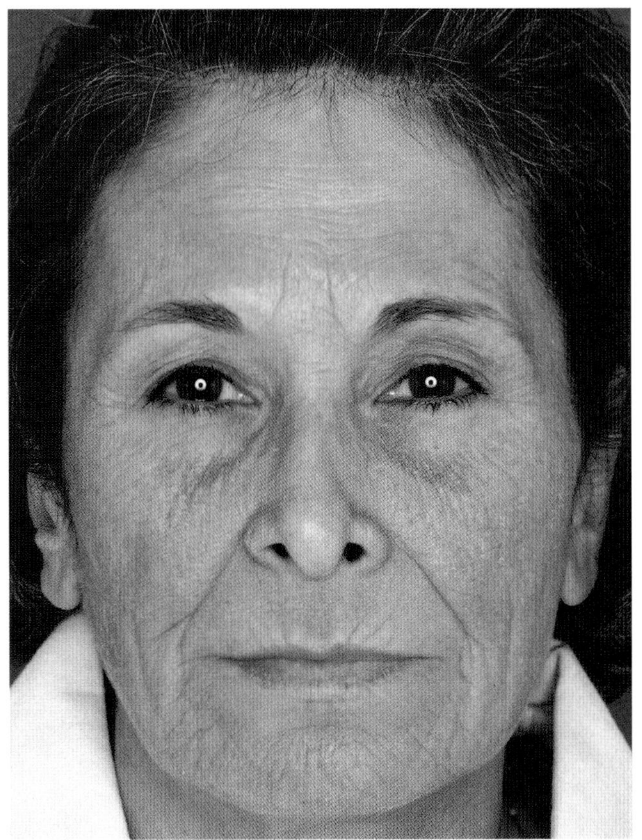

a

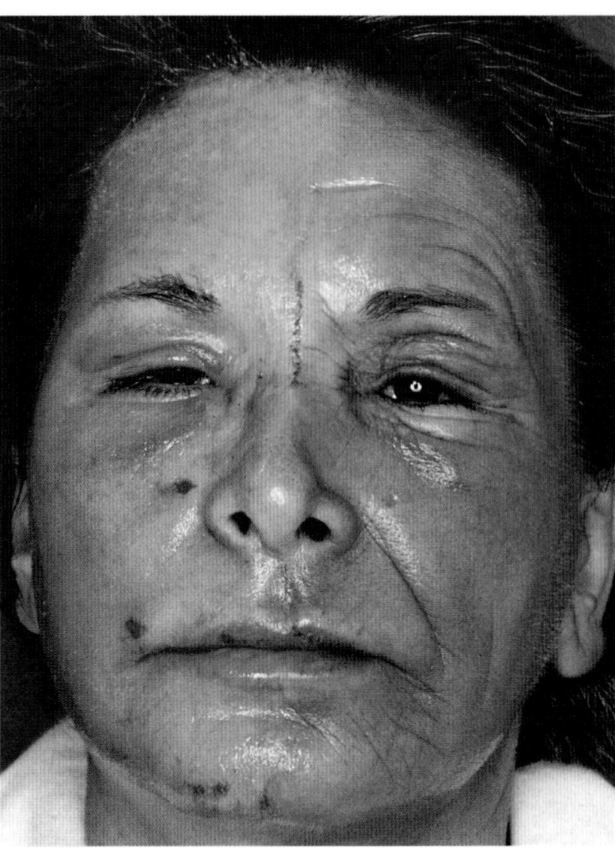

b

FIGURE 8-23. *(a) Before—Patient (White Brunette) with intrinsic aging, thin skin with laxity, following 6 weeks of prepeel correction and stimulation. (b) Right side was treated with CO_2 laser resurfacing. Left side was treated with 20% Blue Peel to papillary dermis level on the eyelids and to the IRD on the other areas.*

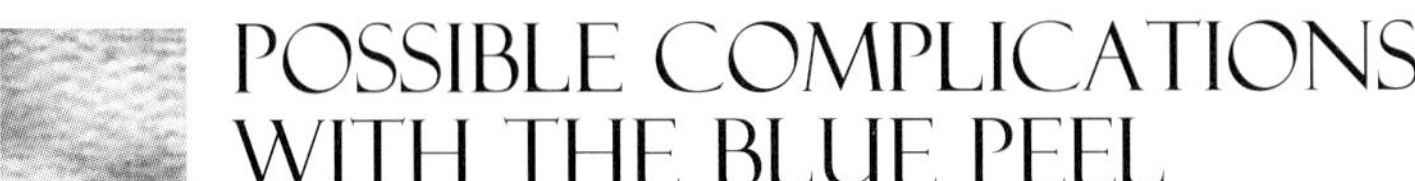

POSSIBLE COMPLICATIONS WITH THE BLUE PEEL

DEPTH ISSUES

All rejuvenation procedures have potential for complications, especially if they are performed improperly, if unsuitable patients are selected, and if patient management is below accepted standards. However, since increased depth is highly associated with an increased incidence of complications, every effort should be taken to avoid the level of depth that may lead to increased risk of scarring. In general, a procedure reaching below the IRD has a higher risk of scarring and permanent hypopigmentation than procedures that stop at the IRD. The phenol peel is a deep peel, dermabrasion is deeper than CO_2 laser resurfacing, and CO_2 laser resurfacing producing chamois yellow changes is deeper and more invasive than the Blue Peel to the papillary dermis or the IRD.

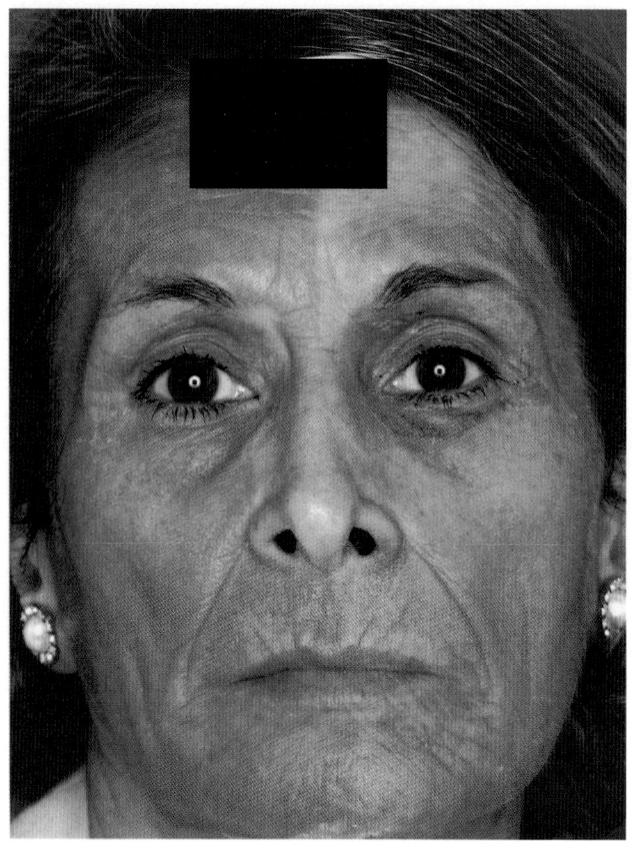

c

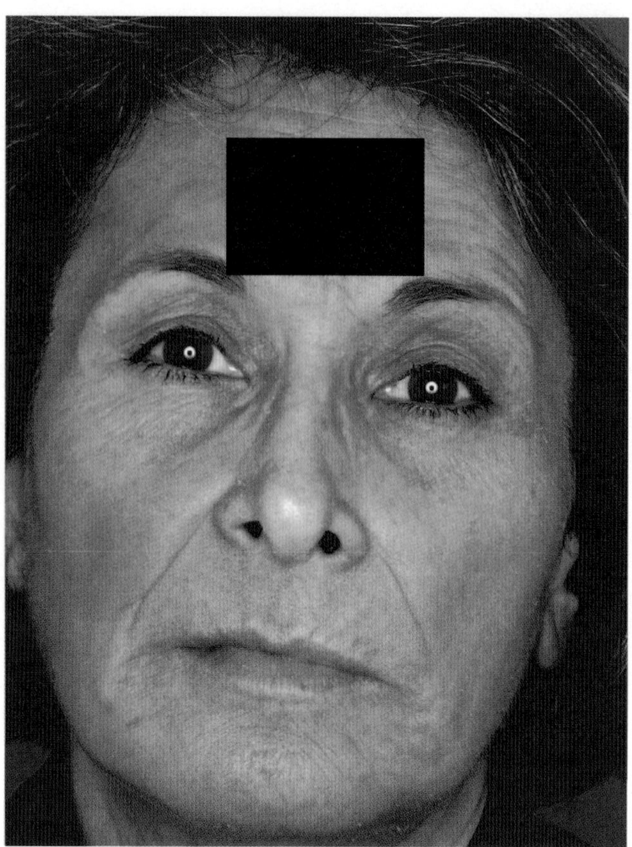

d

(c) 10 days after procedures. Both sides show good healing, but lasered side shows more redness than Blue Peel side. (d) 6 months after procedures. Patient has been treated with skin conditioning consisting of tretinoin and hydroquinone after healing. The Blue peel side (left) shows more tightness, while the lasered side shows more improvement of perioral wrinkles.

While the Blue Peel produces more consistent results and a lower potential for serious complications than conventional TCA peels that have poor depth control, complications can occur. These can be divided into two categories: 1) temporary, usually anticipated, and occurring in the recovery stage, and 2) temporary, occurring in the peeling stage (Table 8-14). Hypertrophic reactions or keloids, however, are possible, are not anticipated, and may not be temporary.

HYPERTROPHIC REACTIONS AND KELOIDS

A hypertrophic reaction is characterized by a well-localized area of red, firm, and thickened skin. The most susceptible areas are the upper lip, cheeks, and lower eyelids, as well as areas with long-standing crusts or cracks that the patient has picked or peeled. Hypertrophic reactions can usually be detected 2 to 3 weeks after healing. Pinching the involved skin reveals texture fuller than that of the surrounding skin. Under a magnifier,

Table 8.14 BLUE PEEL POSSIBLE COMPLICATONS	
Temporary, Anticipated, Occur During Recovery	***Temporary, Occur During Peeling Stage***
■ Erythema—Usually mild, short-lived, often requiring no treatment ■ Postinflammatory hyperpigmentation—Occasionally occurs in type III to VI skin and responds quickly to treatment ■ Acne flare-up—Occurs in acne-prone patients and usually disappears with prompt treatment	■ Infection—Can result from picking or peeling skin, poor hygiene. Responds to antibiotics ■ Herpes simplex infection—Responds to antiviral treatment and can be prevented ■ Irritation—Is caused by excessive moisturization, facial expressions, or skin rubbing

the areas appear as rough, pearly patches with fine, raised threads or papules. Hypertrophic reactions can sometimes resolve slowly without treatment, but resolution can occur faster with use of injected or topical steroids.

A keloid, on the other hand, is an elevated, thickened scar that grows to involve the surrounding skin. Keloids are more likely to form after a procedure below the IRD in the upper lip area, jawline, shoulders, back, and chest, and in individuals with fragile skin. Dr. Obagi has never seen a keloid forming after a papillary dermis or IRD level peel; however, such an occurrence is possible if directions are not followed. Two cases of keloid formation following a Blue Peel have been reported since the peel was introduced 5 years ago, and in both I doubt that the parameters of the Blue Peel were followed.

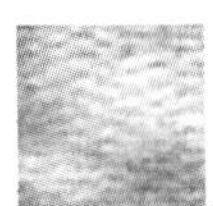

REFERENCES

1. Brody HJ. *Chemical peeling and resurfacing.* 2nd ed. St. Louis, Mo.: CV Mosby; 1997:108–136.
2. Obagi ZE, Sawaf MM, Johnson JB, et al. The controlled depth trichloroacetic acid peel: methodology, outcome, and complication rate. *Int J Aesthetic Restor Surg.* 1996;4:81–94.
3. Johnson JB, Ichinose H, Obagi ZE, Laub DR. Obagi's modified trichloroacetic acid (TCA)-controlled variable depth peel: A study of clinical signs correlating with histological findings. *Annals Plast Surg.* 1996;36:225–237.

CHAPTER

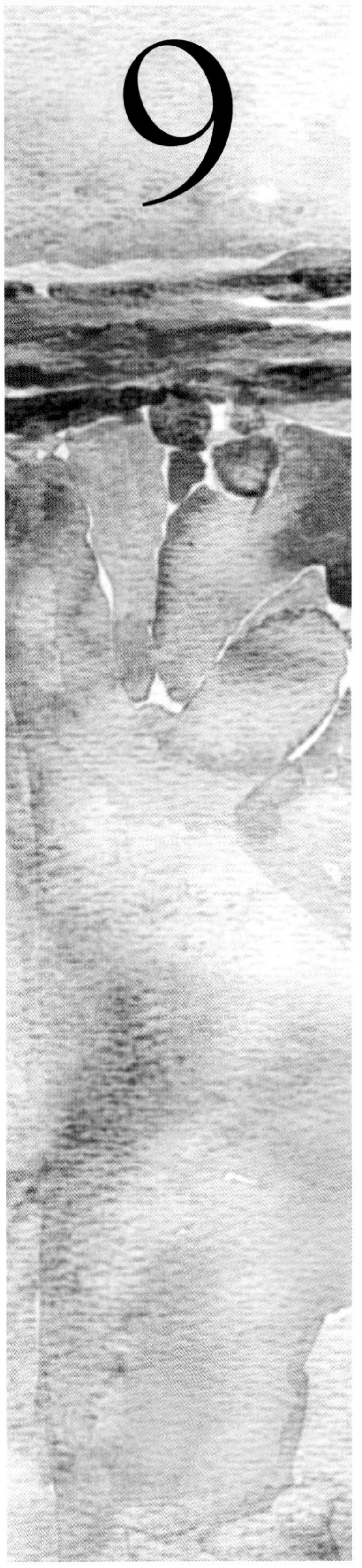

THE OBAGI CONTROLLED MEDIUM-DEPTH PEEL

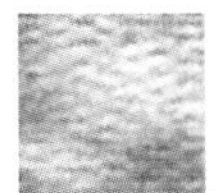

INTRODUCTION

Chapter 8 described the Blue Peel, a highly standardized trichloroacetic acid (TCA)-based procedure that has well-defined endpoints and is recommended as a light or light/medium skin tightening procedure that reaches the papillary dermis and immediate reticular dermis (IRD). This chapter presents a deeper procedure, the Obagi Controlled, Medium-Depth TCA Peel, which reaches the upper reticular dermis to mid and very rarely the lower dermis for correction of deeper wrinkles or scars. This peel is a leveling procedure and uses a higher concentration of TCA than the Blue Peel. Like the Blue Peel, it provides suggested endpoints to determine depth more accurately.[1]

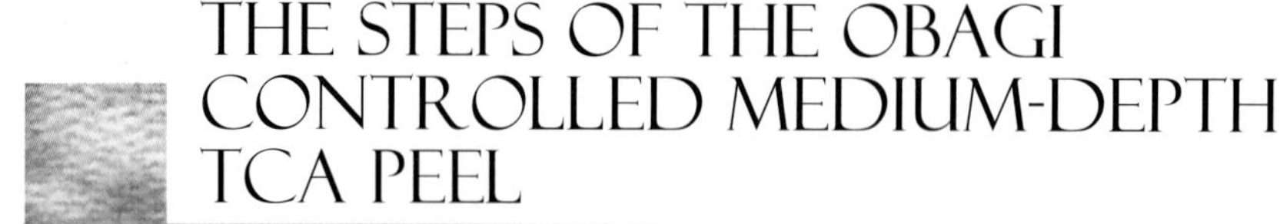

THE STEPS OF THE OBAGI CONTROLLED MEDIUM-DEPTH TCA PEEL

PREOPERATIVE SKIN CLASSIFICATION

Determining a patient's skin type according to the Obagi Skin Classification System was described in detail in Chapter 4, and only a brief overview is presented here. The author has found that the traditional Fitzpatrick skin classification system that categorizes skin in terms of color and reaction to sun exposure is inadequate for selecting a procedure and its depth. The Obagi classification system considers skin color as an important variable but also considers the variables of skin thickness, oiliness, fragility, and laxity, which are not taken into account in other systems (Table 9-1).

Skin Color

In the Obagi classification system, skin color is considered not only from the standpoint of depth of color but also from the standpoint of whether the skin color is Original (not racially or ethnically mixed), Deviated (racially or ethnically mixed), or Complex (present in certain ethnic and racial groups). These distinctions are important because in the Deviated and Com-

TABLE 9.1

OBAGI CLASSIFICATION SYSTEM: SKIN VARIABLES, DEPTH OF PEELS, AND REACTION TO PROCEDURES

Skin Variable	*Recommended Peel Depth**	*Relevance to Procedure*
Color	Light color—all depths Dark color—to the IRD	Hypopigmentation: more common with procedures below the IRD. Hyperpigmentation: more likely with darker or deviated, but can occur with all colors except the very light.
Oiliness	Not a depth determinant by itself	Must be brought to normal before performing peel and controlled afterwards to facilitate the effects of postprocedure Skin Conditioning.
Thickness	Thick—all depths Thin—to the IRD	Thick skin most tolerant of any depth. Safety margin narrow with thin skin.
Laxity	To the IRD	The IRD level is ideal if skin is thin or of normal thickness, but, in thick skin, a medium-depth peel will give better results. For muscle laxity, surgery is needed.
Fragility	Fragile—papillary dermis Nonfragile—all depths	The maximum depth allowed is the papillary dermis.

*Physician must be skilled in light peels before attempting medium or deep peels. Deeper peels have an increased risk of complications.
IRD = immediate reticular dermis.

TABLE 9.2

STABILITY OF OBAGI SKIN COLOR CATEGORIES

Skin Color Category	*Examples*	*Stability**
Original (not racially or ethnically mixed)	Light White Dark Asian (yellow) Dark Black (jet)	Stable
Deviated (racially or ethnically mixed)	Light or Dark Brunette Light or Medium Asian (yellow) Light or Medium Black	Moderately stable
Complex (skin light in some areas and dark in others)	Indian, Pakistani, Bangladeshi, American Indian, Latino Indian, and some persons of mixed racial origin	Extremely unstable

*Following TCA peel or any other rejuvenation procedure.

plex categories, skin has a higher risk of pigmentary changes after any rejuvenation procedure, including a chemical peel, and therefore needs to be conditioned more aggressively pre- and postoperatively (Table 9-2). Most important, there are large differences among the skin color types in their reactions to the depth of a procedure (Table 9-3).

TABLE 9.3

VARIABILITY OF REACTIONS TO INCREASING DEPTH OF PROCEDURES IN DIFFERENT SKIN COLOR TYPES

Skin Color	*Reactions with Increasing Depth*
White: ■ Very Light White ■ Light White ■ Normal White ■ Light Brunette ■ Dark Brunette	All White categories have increased degree and duration of redness. All Brunette categories show longer period of hyperpigmentation and, with increased depth, higher risk of hypopigmentation.
Asian (Yellow): ■ Light Yellow ■ Medium Yellow ■ Dark Yellow	Deviated Asian categories (Light or Medium) show significantly higher incidence of PIH.* Hypopigmentation and keloids possible with deeper procedures.
Black: ■ Light Black ■ Dark Black	Dark Black categories: Shorter duration and less severe PIH, and hypopigmentation with deeper procedures. Deviated Black (light) show prolonged and more severe PIH; hypopigmentation possible with deeper peels.

*PIH = postinflammatory hyperpigmentation

Skin Thickness, Oiliness, Fragility, and Laxity

Skin is classified as thick, normal (medium), or thin based on the amount that can be pinched at the cheek. Thickness is the major determinant of procedure depth because patients with thin skin should not have procedures that exceed the IRD. Thick skin is the best type for deeper procedures such as a chemical peel or dermabrasion, but it is not ideal for CO_2 laser resurfacing. Skin of medium thickness, is suitable for all procedures. Tightening procedures are ideal for thin skin, while leveling procedures carry more risk. Dynamic or expression lines (mistakenly called *wrinkles*) will not be completely corrected and will return to their preprocedure state in thin skin faster than those in thick skin because thin skin folds easily following action of underlying muscles. Thick skin, on the other hand, shows better and long-lasting results with leveling procedures since the muscles cannot fold the skin as easily.

Skin is classified as oily, normal, or dry by visual and tactile examination. Before a procedure, oiliness must be brought down to normal with appropriate topical agents as part of an effective skin conditioning program. After the procedure, when the healing is complete, oiliness should be reduced to facilitate the activity of topical agents that are used to treat PIH or acne flare-up. The author has performed many procedures, especially the Blue Peel, to the level of the papillary dermis in patients who were treated with Accutane before the procedure. For deeper peels, CO_2 laser resurfacing, and dermabrasion, however, Accutane must be discontinued for 6 months before the procedure to decrease the risk of poor wound healing and scarring.

Skin fragility can be assessed by resistance to penetration with a needle or by the feel of the skin during pinching. Fragile skin can be squeezed without resistance. It reacts unpredictably to procedures, heals more slowly, and has a higher potential for scarring. Patients with fragile skin should not have a procedure deeper than the papillary dermis and never below the IRD.

Skin and muscle laxity are assessed by pulling and lifting wrinkles, jowls, nasolabial folds, and eyebrow ptosis. Skin laxity alone responds well to a tightening procedure. Muscle laxity, on the other hand, responds well to incisional surgery.

PREOPERATIVE SKIN CONDITIONING

The standardized protocol for the Obagi Controlled Medium-Depth Peel includes a mandatory preprocedure skin conditioning program for at least 6 weeks. The objectives are to increase skin tolerance; create a soft, compacted stratum corneum; suppress melanocyte activity; increase basal cell mitosis in the adnexal structures for faster postoperative reepithelialization and improve skin hydration. The details of the Obagi Skin Conditioning and Skin Health Restoration programs, including variations in duration and aggressiveness of approach appropriate for different skin types, were discussed in depth in Chapter 5.

Box 9-1

The benefits of skin conditioning before a TCA peel* include:

- **normalization of the stratum corneum for uniform skin uptake of TCA**
- **increase of skin tolerance**
- **improve skin hydration**
- **improved postpeel healing due to faster reepithelialization**
- **prevention or reduction of severity of postprocedure hyperpigmentation**
- **reduced incidence and severity of anticipated early or delayed reactions**

*Skin Conditioning provides the same benefits preceding other procedures, such as CO_2 laser resurfacing and dermabrasion.

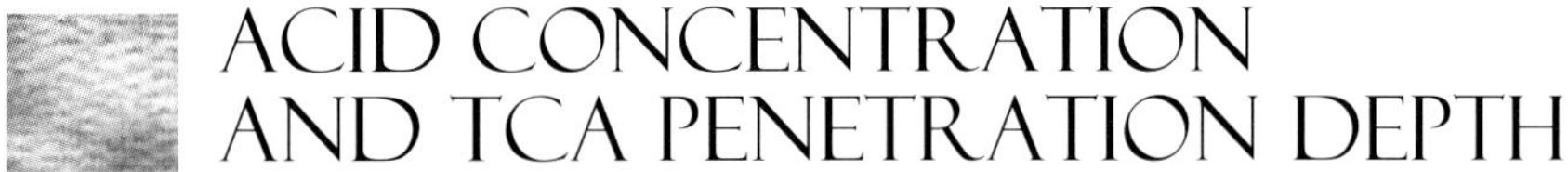

ACID CONCENTRATION AND TCA PENETRATION DEPTH

TCA PENETRATION DEPTH: THE ISSUES

The major determinant of the outcome and safety of a TCA peel procedure is the depth of acid penetration. Penetration to the basal layer generally improves the epidermis and superficial coloration, while penetration to the papillary dermis and the IRD improves texture, increases tightness, eliminates stretchable wrinkles and scars, and helps to improve pigmentation problems. Medium-depth wounding (reaching the upper reticular dermis to mid dermis) generally eliminates or improves deeper, unstretchable wrinkles and scars, treats solar elastosis, softens skin texture, treats deeper discolorations, and increases skin firmness. Deep wounding (mid dermis and lower reticular dermis) to improve deep wrinkles and scars may produce a good outcome in thick, White skin but is not usually suitable for other skin types. Such deep peels penetrate to the mid dermis or below and destroy a large number of adnexal structures and melanocytes, leading to an increased incidence of permanent textural changes and loss of color. Thus, the physician must weigh the benefits of deep chemical peels (TCA or phenol) against the possibility of such changes. Furthermore, since the incidence of complications increases with deeper peels, it is imperative that such procedures be performed 1) by a highly skilled physician, 2) only on patients with the proper skin type, and 3) only if the clinical condition warrants such depth.

Currently the published literature correlates procedure depth (light, medium, or deep) with the concentration of TCA used for the peel. For ex-

Box 9-2

Volume of applied TCA is also important in peel depth. Higher concentrations penetrate the skin faster with less volume used, while lower concentrations can reach the same depth but penetrate more slowly and require a larger volume of solution.

ample, 10% to 20% TCA concentrations are considered more suitable for superficial peels, 35% TCA alone or TCA combined with augmenting agents as suitable for a medium-depth peel, and 50% TCA for deeper peels.[2] The three most common misconceptions of TCA peels are that 1) high concentrations cause scarring, 2) lower concentrations produce superficial peeling, and 3) lower concentrations cannot penetrate deeply and augmentation is needed if a deeper and safer peel is desired.

In contrast, the author has found that *any concentration* of TCA can be made to penetrate to any depth (Table 9-4). The concentration and volume are the important factors, and both of these determine the *speed and depth* of acid penetration.[1,3] Higher concentrations of TCA reach a certain depth faster (with less solution volume needed), while lower concentration can reach the same depth but do so more slowly (with more solution volume needed). Also, it is important to remember that safety is not determined by TCA concentration only, but is affected by patient selection factors, skin type, and peel depth.

TABLE 9.4

RELATIONSHIP OF TCA VOLUME AND CONCENTRATION TO PEEL DEPTH

TCA Concentration (%)	*Volume* for Skin Thickness (cc)*			*Depth Achieved*
	Normal	*Thin*	*Thick*	
15	6	<6	6	Stratum corneum
15	12	<12	12	Basal layer
15	18	<18	>18	Papillary dermis
20	6	6	6	Basal layer
20	12	<12	>12	Papillary dermis
30	6	<6	>6	Papillary dermis
35	6	<6	>6	Immediate reticular dermis (IRD)
40	6	<6	>6	Upper reticular dermis

*Volumes given are estimates only because of skin thickness variations and the absence of end-points when penetration is below the mid dermis.

PENETRATION WITH MODIFIED TCA SOLUTION

TCA for chemical peeling can be used alone or augmented with another agent or device to increase penetration. The Obagi Controlled Medium-Depth TCA Peel uses 25%–35% or 40% TCA, modified with an FDA-approved saponin complex such as Complex 272. The saponin component of this modifier is a plant-derived glycoside with a cyclic penta alpha phenanthrene structure with a steroid nucleus that reduces the surface tension of TCA. The glycerin component is a vehicle that helps to form a TCA/oil/water solution that slows penetration. To reduce variables with this peel, only the 25% or 40% concentrations of TCA are used. The 25% concentration is used to achieve a peel to the papillary dermis or IRD, and the 40% concentration is used to achieve peel depth to the upper reticular or mid dermis.

The modifier solution (Complex 272 and glycerin), has been shown clinically to slow the penetration of TCA into the skin. This approach is in contrast to the approach of augmenting the action of TCA to obtain deeper penetration by pretreating the skin with agents such as solid carbon dioxide, Jessner's solution, or glycolic acid.

The belief that augmentation to increase penetration of lower concentrations of TCA is safer than the use of higher concentrations without augmentation is erroneous. TCA is a powerful, easily penetrating acid at any concentration and does not need to have its penetration enhanced. Use of augmenting agents is detrimental because it increases the number of variables involved in the peel process and may increase the risk of complications. The only benefit from using augmenting agents such as Jessner's solution or glycolic acid before applying TCA is in the more even penetration of TCA after removal of the stratum corneum. Augmentation with certain substances such as solid carbon dioxide can destroy melanocytes and possibly injure the skin from excessively deep penetration of TCA. TCA peels can be better managed and produce better results if TCA is used alone or if its action is slowed and controlled after skin conditioning to regulate the stratum corneum.

THE TIME GAP FOR ACID NEUTRALIZATION

If TCA (an acid soluble in water, ether, or alcohol) is combined with an oily substance such as glycerin, penetration of the acid in skin will be slowed down. However, with its high surface tension, TCA requires the addition of surface-tension reducing agents such as saponins (Complex 272) to mix with glycerin and create a homogenous mixture of acid, glycerin, and water. With such modification, TCA is released into the skin at a slower rate, which leads to more effective neutralization of the acid by skin proteins and slower frost formation.

This results in a shorter *time gap*, a term that describes the time it takes for the penetrating acid to be completely neutralized, as revealed by the rate of frost formation. With a slow-penetrating TCA solution, the time gap is shorter because small amounts of TCA are quickly neutralized, while, with fast-penetrating TCA, the time gap is longer because larger amounts of acid penetrate and neutralization takes longer. The time gap for neutralization

TABLE 9.5	
THE TIME GAP IN SLOW-PENETRATING AND PLAIN OR AUGMENTED TCA	
Obagi Modified TCA (Slow-Penetrating)	***Plain or Augmented TCA***
■ Glycerin competes with the skin for free TCA → slower penetration	■ TCA is free and penetrates rapidly
■ Only a small portion of the applied volume penetrates: any excess can be wiped off	■ All of the applied volume penetrates rapidly; excess cannot be wiped off
■ The smaller volume of penetrating acid is effectively and rapidly neutralized = short time gap	■ The larger volume of penetrating acid needs more time for neutralization = longer time gap
■ Slow penetration = slower frost formation = more time to observe depth signs	■ Faster penetration = rapid appearance of frost = less time to observe depth signs
■ Slow penetration → fewer acid pockets in the skin = even penetration, more uniform results, less irritation, less pain	■ Fast penetration leads to formation of acid pockets = uneven penetration, less even results, more irritation, more pain

of modified TCA is 1 to 2 minutes, compared with approximately 2 to 4 minutes for unmodified TCA (Table 9-5). This leads to one of the main advantages of slower-penetrating TCA: more time for the physician to recognize the clinical depth signs and stop applying TCA if the signs show that the desired depth has been reached. In addition, the presence of glycerin in the modified solution reduces irritation and duration of the burning sensation and allows for more even application of the peel solution.

The modifier used for 25% to 40% TCA solution is designed to work at these higher TCA concentrations. After modification, these concentrations can be used to reach any depth of the skin, from exfoliation to a deep peel. Lower TCA concentrations, however, are not useful for deeper peels because the cumulative time gap is too long, depth signs cannot be accurately observed, and the large volume of solution needed can macerate the skin and increase the chances of irritation and necrosis.

The time gap should not be confused with the Period of Relative Resistance (discussed in relation to the Blue Peel), which describes the time

Box 9-3

With slow-penetrating TCA, the smaller volume of acid that penetrates is rapidly neutralized, resulting in a short time gap.

Box 9-4

The time gap (time for each application of TCA to complete its action and be neutralized) is 1 to 2 minutes with the modified TCA solution. It is longer and variable with plain TCA solution and unknown with augmented TCA peels.

needed to reach a specific depth. The Period of Relative Resistance is much longer with slow-penetrating TCA solution than with plain or augmented TCA and is usually related to TCA concentration, volume, and skin thickness. The time gap, on the other hand, is mostly related to the amount of TCA penetrating the skin with each application and is not related to depth or skin thickness.

SAFETY OF MEDIUM-DEPTH PEELS

Although conventional (unmodified) TCA has been used in concentrations of 25% to 50% to perform light, medium, and deep peels for treating a variety of dermatological conditions, light peels are most often performed. Deeper peels are not performed because of the fear of uncontrolled penetration and subsequent complications. Such fears are unfounded and may be based on a statistical misperception. The *absolute number* of TCA complications may be notable because more TCA peels are performed worldwide each year than any other rejuvenation procedure. However, when the *incidence* (number of cases per 100 procedures) of complications is examined, TCA peels are no more likely to result in complications than any other type of rejuvenation procedure *that reaches the same depth*. With a standardized approach and use of the modified, slow-penetrating TCA solution, penetration is more controlled, giving more time to observe the depth signs and to stop application when the desired depth has been reached. With proper patient selection and peel management, TCA peels are no less safe than laser resurfacing, dermabrasion, or other modalities. The safety of a procedure is affected by many factors, including patient selection, physician training and skill, and proper prepeel and postpeel management.

Box 9-5

Medium-deep and deeper peels can be performed with greater safety if penetration of TCA is slowed down, patients are selected properly, and the physician performing the peel is properly trained and skilled.

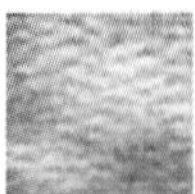

PREPEEL CONSIDERATIONS

After the patient has had skin typed (see the Obagi Skin Classification System, Chapter 4) and the diagnosis and depth of the problem have been determined at a consultation visit, the physician can determine the most suitable type and depth of procedure for that patient (Table 9-6, Figure 9-1). The patient should start a prepeel conditioning program, as previously described (see Chapter 5), continuing up to 4 or 5 days before the day of the peel. Discuss the options for anesthesia or sedation with all patients, regardless of the depth of peel planned. Topical anesthetics such as EMLA are not recommended because they can cause uneven epidermal hydration, which can lead to an uneven peel.

TABLE 9.6

PENETRATION LEVELS OF OBAGI CONTROLLED-DEPTH TCA PEELS

Peel Description (per Obagi Classification)	*Level and Peel Terminology*	*Skin Layer Reached*	*Volume and Costs According to Skin Thickness*		
			Normal	*Thin*	*Thick*
Light exfoliation	Blue Peel (Epi-1)	Stratum corneum Stratum granulosum	1 coat of 15%	1 coat of 15%	1 coat of 15%
Medium exfoliation	Blue Peel (Epi-2)	Above the basal layer	2 coats of 15%	1 coat of 15%	2 coats of 15%
Deep exfoliation	Blue Peel (Epi-3)	Basal layer	3 coats of 15% or 1 coat of 20%	2 coats of 15% or 1 coat of 20%	3 coats of 15% or 1 coat of 20%
Light peel	Standard Blue Peel (Derm-1)	Papillary dermis	4 coats of 15% or 2 coats of 20%	2 to 3 coats of 15% or 1 coat of 20%	4 coats of 15% or 2 coats of 20%
Light/medium peel	Designed Blue Peel (Early Derm-2)	IRD	After Blue Peel coats, extra coat of 15% or 20%	After Blue Peel coats, extra coat of 15%	After Blue Peel coats, extra coat of 20%
Medium peel	Controlled Medium-Depth Peel (Derm-2)	Upper reticular dermis	6 cc of 40% modified TCA	<6 cc of 40% modified TCA	>6 cc of 40% modified TCA
Deep peel	Controlled Medium-Depth Peel (Derm-3)	Mid dermis or below	>6 cc of 40% modified TCA	Not recommended	>6 cc of 40% modified TCA

Schedule a prepeel office visit between 2 days and 1 week before the procedure. At that visit, tell the patient about the extent of expected correction with the peel, describe the anticipated postpeel reactions, and inform her or him of the time needed for recovery. Present alternative treatments to the peel, describe in detail any possible complications, and give instructions for postpeel home care, such as a home-care information kit. Be sure patients understand the possible risks of the procedure when they sign the consent forms, preferably 1 week before the peel.

Patients who have a history of Herpes simplex infection should be treated prophylactically with oral medication such as 400 mg of acyclovir (Zovirax) four times daily or valcyclovir (Valtrex) 500 mg twice daily beginning the day before the peel and continuing for 7 to 10 days after the peel, with a longer duration for a deeper peel.

Ask the patient to arrive without facial make-up or jewelry and dressed in a blouse or shirt that is easily removable. Position the patient comfortably in a chair and place a roll under the neck to extend the neck position. A room lit by daylight fluorescent lamps is best for color observation. A spot or multiple-beam surgical light is not ideal. Have a syringe of normal

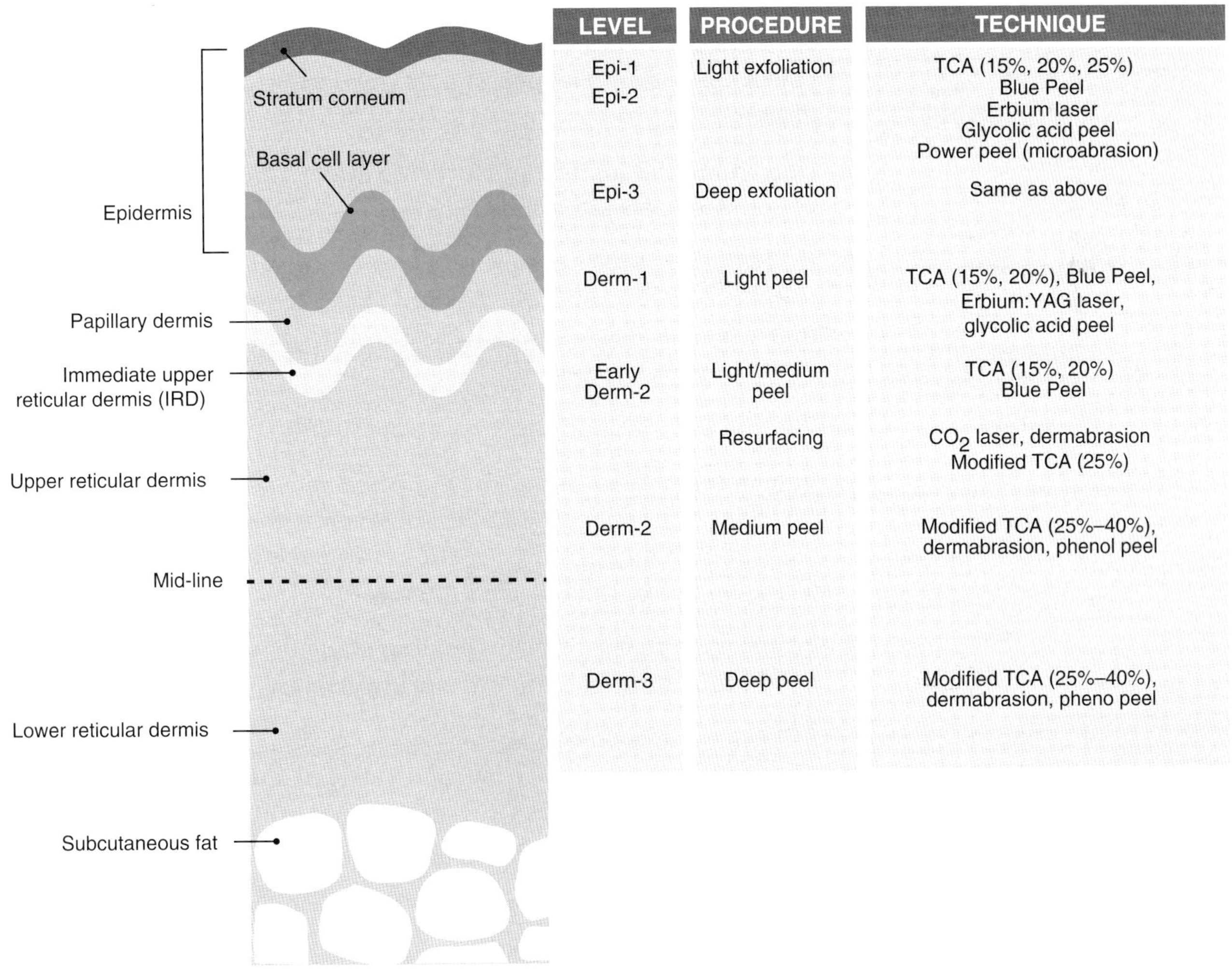

LEVEL	PROCEDURE	TECHNIQUE
Epi-1 Epi-2	Light exfoliation	TCA (15%, 20%, 25%) Blue Peel Erbium laser Glycolic acid peel Power peel (microabrasion)
Epi-3	Deep exfoliation	Same as above
Derm-1	Light peel	TCA (15%, 20%), Blue Peel, Erbium:YAG laser, glycolic acid peel
Early Derm-2	Light/medium peel	TCA (15%, 20%) Blue Peel
	Resurfacing	CO_2 laser, dermabrasion Modified TCA (25%)
Derm-2	Medium peel	Modified TCA (25%–40%), dermabrasion, phenol peel
Derm-3	Deep peel	Modified TCA (25%–40%), dermabrasion, pheno peel

FIGURE 9-1. *Spectrum of depth with various procedures.*

Box 9-5a

PATIENT PREPARATION FOR THE PEEL

- Plan to perform a peel only if a patient follows the skin conditioning program, has realistic expectations, and is dependable and cooperative.
- Do not perform a peel (or CO_2 laser resurfacing or other invasive procedure) on a pregnant patient.
- Have all patients follow the skin conditioning program for 6 weeks before the procedure or until tolerance has been restored. Patients who complain that skin is sensitive should not have the procedure until sensitivity has been eliminated (tolerance restored).
- Give detailed informed consent forms. Let the patient take the forms home to read at least 1 week before the procedure. If appropriate, tell the patient that more than 1 peel may be needed for optimal results.
- Treat and control all inflammatory conditions (acne, folliculitis, infection, Herpes simplex eruption) before the peel date.
- Determine the history of Herpes simplex infection and start prophylactic treatment.
- Discuss the sedation modality and the need for the patient to be escorted home on the day of the procedure. The author uses the services of an anesthesiologist for sedating patients during the peel.
- Photograph the patient for documentation.
- Inform the patient about the expected recovery time, the anticipated reactions (PIH, milia, acne, etc.), the potential complications (hypertrophic reactions, keloids, etc.), and the alternative modalities of treatment.
- Prepare the patient for the healing stage by showing a video or photographs of patients during various stages of healing.
- Give the patient instructions and supplies for postpeel home care. Instruct the patient to purchase certain other needed items (antiseptic solution, etc.).
- Have your staff arrange the postpeel schedule of follow-up visits with the patient.

saline available for flushing the eyes if acid accidentally gets into the eyes, but do not place shields in the patient's eyes. Have cotton swabs available for application of solution to the eyelids and ice-pick scars.

Prior to application of the peel solution, degrease the patient's face with gauze dipped in alcohol or acetone and dry the skin with facial tissue. Wear 2 pairs of surgical gloves to protect your hands when applying the TCA. For a peel that is below the papillary dermis, have the patient lightly sedated by an anesthesiologist.

Patients usually feel fine after even deep TCA peel procedures, but most do not return to work or social activities for 7 to 16 days, depending on the depth of the peel. Normal activities do not need to be curtailed, but strenuous exercise and the perspiration it induces should be avoided during the peeling stage. Initially, prolonged sun exposure should be avoided; limited exposure is permitted in 2 to 3 weeks when sunscreens are tolerated.

PEEL MATERIALS

Have your pharmacist prepare TCA in 30% and 50% concentrations or purchase it already prepared (Delasco, Council Bluffs, Iowa) (Figure 9-2). If stored in a sealed bottle, at room temperature, away from light, pure TCA can be stored for more than 1 year. Add the proper amount of modifier to the 30% and 50% TCA to obtain a 25% or 40% concentration of modified TCA (Table 9-7). Add a few drops of methylene blue dye to the 25% solution and a few more drops to the 40% solution to make it easier to distinguish the two concentrations visually (the 40% solution will be darker blue), and label the solutions. The modified TCA should be used immediately after being mixed with the modifier. Be sure to always prepare a known vol-

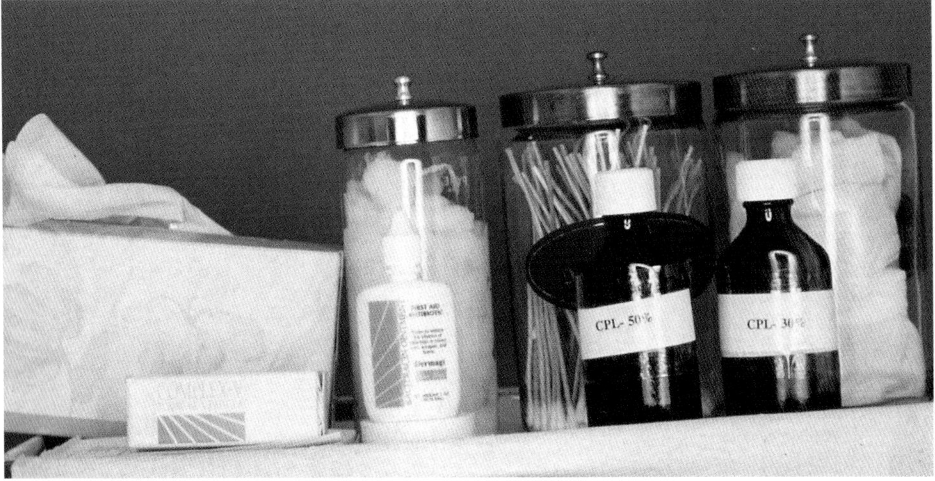

FIGURE 9-2. *50% and 30% TCA solutions for the Controlled Medium-Depth Peel before modification to 40% and 25%, respectively. Other materials for the peel include the Complex V modifier, cotton-tipped applicators, 2-in by 2-in gauze, Bacitracin or other ointment, and facial tissues.*

TABLE 9.7

PREPARATION OF 25% AND 35% TCA SOLUTIONS FOR A CONTROLLED MEDIUM-DEPTH TCA PEEL

Amount of Pure TCA Solution	*Amount of Complex V*	*Amount of Methylene Blue Coloring*	*Final Concentration of TCA*
5 cc of 50% TCA**	2 cc	4 drops (0.2 cc)	34.7% = 35%*
5 cc of 30% TCA	1 cc	2 drops	24.59% = 25%*

*The 35% and 25% concentrations differ markedly in their action during a Controlled Medium-Depth Peel.
**5cc TCA and 1cc modifier yield 40% concentration; 35% and 40% concentrations act almost the same.

ume of modified TCA, such as 4 cc or 6 cc, and record the volume in the patient's chart. Also, prepare 4 cc of a modified 25% solution along with the 40% solution to use at the end for saturation and feathering.

Box 9-6

MATERIALS FOR THE CONTROLLED MEDIUM-DEPTH PEEL

2 pairs surgical gloves
30% and 50% TCA solution
Complex V modifier
2-in by 2-in gauze
Cotton balls soaked in alcohol
Small cotton swabs
Box of facial tissue
5-cc syringe of normal saline
Bacitracin or Aquaphor ointments
Methylene blue dye (optional)

PERFORMING THE CONTROLLED MEDIUM-DEPTH PEEL

PEEL DEPTH

In performing the Controlled Medium-Depth peel, select the desired depth and proceed from one level to another. For example, peel the entire face to the Derm-1 (papillary dermis) level, then proceed to the Derm-2 (upper reticular dermis) level, and then to the Derm-3 (mid reticular dermis), and so forth. If still greater depth is desired, more solution can be applied very cautiously, because there is no clear endpoint for the lower dermis (below mid dermis).

HANDLING THE GAUZE

Dip 2 squares of the gauze into the modified TCA solution until one corner is moderately saturated, but not dripping. Paint the skin without pressure, using most of the wet gauze surface. Avoid dripping on or overwetting the skin surface. Do not apply pressure with the gauze, for that may lead to increased acid release and subsequently uneven TCA penetration. Keep the gauze square, and do not crumble it. Do not leave any loose hanging "tags" of gauze that can unintentionally add more solution to already painted areas. Rotate the gauze to use all of its edges and surfaces. When the gauze begins to feel dry, dip one corner into the modified TCA solution, but do not oversaturate. To prevent oversaturation, even out the solution in the gauze with your fingers before applying it again to the skin. Your objective is to use the least amount of solution to perform the peel.

SOLUTION APPLICATION

Begin by applying the solution until the depth of the papillary dermis is reached. Observe the depth signs, such as frost with pink and epidermal sliding. If you need to stop the peel at the papillary dermis level for any reason, the frost on the skin should be even. Proceed deeper if required for a particular case. Always follow the depth limits for specific areas, such as the Derm-1 level for the eyelids, Early Derm-2 for the upper lips and the jawline, Derm-2 or Derm-3 for the cheeks (depending on skin thickness), and Derm-1 for nonfacial skin. Before returning to paint the same area again, you must wait 2 minutes to allow complete neutralization of the applied acid (time gap) and permit the clinical depth signs to develop.

You can proceed clockwise or counterclockwise in applying the solution (painting). Paint the solution in light, short, gentle, and rapid strokes, which tend to have a more even pressure and deliver more equal amounts of solution than long strokes. Do not use the tips of your fingers to support the gauze; instead, use the length of your thumb, index finger, or middle and index fingers. When you reach the jawline, use your thumb to support the gauze for feathering.

Work at a steady rhythm, not too slowly and not too fast. Apply 2 to 3 strokes to an area and then move to the next area. You must work fast enough to maintain the ability to use the depth signs (i.e., epidermal sliding lasts approximately 5 minutes). Speed also helps keep the pressure uniform and the amount of solution delivered equal. Complete your run on the entire face in 2 minutes, then repeat while observing frost quality and related depth signs. Coat the hairline, earlobes, and postauricular areas,

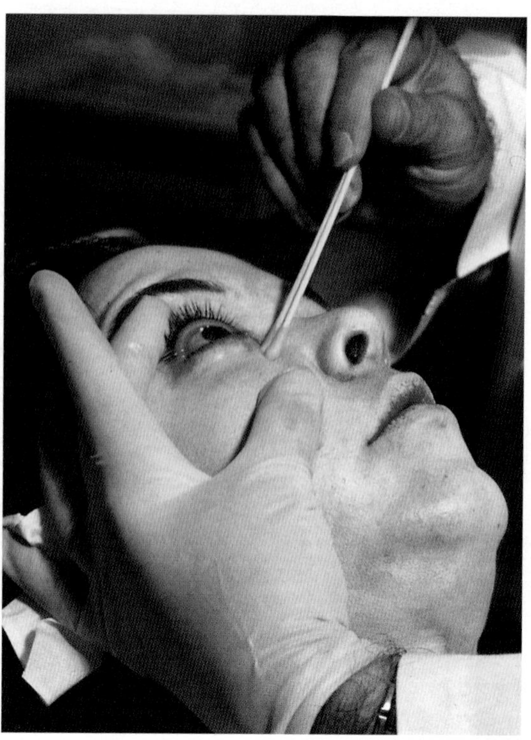

FIGURE 9-3. *Application of peel solution to eyelids. The upper lid is painted in the lateral direction. The lower lid is painted in a similar manner with the eye open, and the upper lid is fixed open with one finger.*

but keep at least 1 inch away from the jawline, for you will need that much space to extend downward toward the neck when feathering out any demarcation lines. Peel the upper and lower eyelids last, either at the same time or at the end of the peel, using a cotton-tipped applicator.

To change the direction of your strokes, move your wrist or move your body around the patient's head. It takes 2 minutes for the modified TCA solution to complete its activity and be neutralized (the time gap). Thus, you must respect the time gap and wait at least that amount of time before applying more solution to the same area. If frosting of facial skin is not even, continue the application to even out the frost before trying to reach deeper levels in the dermis. Nonfacial skin should be peeled only to the level of the papillary dermis.

Peeling of the eyelids helps to eliminate wrinkles and tighten the lids for better cosmetic results (Figure 9-3). Coat the eyelids with solution as you coat the rest of the face. Keep the patient's eyes open while coating the lower lids by lifting and holding the upper lid against the eyebrow bone with your thumb. This can also be done by your assistant. Apply the solution to the lower lid by stroking sideways. Extend the application beyond the lateral canthi, inward toward the nasal canthus, upward toward the eylashes, and downward to the infraorbital rim. Coat the upper eyelids with the patient's eyes closed and apply the solution downward and sideways to prevent opening the eye. Do not allow the solution to drip or run onto the skin. To prevent solution from getting into the patient's eyes, you must apply the solution without any pressure on the gauze. Refine the eyelids at the end of the procedure with a cotton swab dipped in the solution. The maximum depth for the eyelids is the papillary dermis.

Paint the upper and lower lip areas down to the chin in the usual fashion to the depth of the papillary dermis. Avoid greater depth because the dermis here is thin and lies on the muscles with almost no subcutaneous fat. Scarring can easily occur in these areas at the Derm-2 level, especially in thin skin.

When the desired depth has been achieved with the 40% solution, apply a modifed 25% TCA solution to blend the deeper peeled areas with the more lightly peeled areas and quickly create a uniform frost. This essential step is called the *saturation process*. Feather out at the jawline with the same solution. Then apply a thin coat of an ointment such as Bacitracin, Aquaphor, or another.

The entire peel process usually takes 20 to 30 minutes. On the average, a physician must properly perform at least 30 peels to the Derm-1 level before attempting to perform deeper peels. Workshop attendance and performance of deeper peels under the supervision of a skilled physician are highly recommended.

FEATHERING

Feathering is performed to prevent abrupt termination of the peel at the edges, which can leave sharp demarcation lines. It should gradually achieve a decreasing peel depth, moving from the deepest penetration at the peeled area to progressively less deep penetration and ending with a light exfoliation 1 to 2 inches away from the peeled area. Feathering can be accomplished by two methods (Figure 9-4).

Progressively Lighter Pressure Method: Touch the acid-filled gauze to the skin with light pressure at the peeled areas, as usual. Then, moving away from the jawline toward the neck, lighten the pressure with the gauze so that it barely touches the skin at the end. Dry the area where the feathering will end with tissue. The application maneuver could be compared to an airplane take-off with a 1- to 2-in runway. If the upper reticular dermis is reached at the jawline, the depth in the feathered areas should decrease from the upper reticular dermis to the papillary dermis, to the basal layer, and end with a stratum corneum exfoliation, all in the space of 1 to 2 in. Wait 1 to 2 minutes between each application. Be sure to use the modified 25% TCA solution for saturation (see below) and for feathering.

Limited Time of Contact Method: Feathering can also be accomplished by progressively shortening the time the acid is left in contact with the skin as the physician moves away from the edge of the peeled area. As described before, TCA penetrates deeper when all of the applied solution is allowed to penetrate. Thus, wiping the applied solution off with a tissue after short contact with the skin decreases the penetration depth because less volume is allowed to penetrate. To perform this technique for feathering, apply the modified 25% TCA solution in the direction away from the frosted peeled area. Allow 5 seconds to pass, then wipe off firmly with a tissue. Repeat after 2 minutes, this time counting to 4, then next time to 3, etc. In other words, wipe the first application after 5 seconds, the second application (2 minutes later) after 4 seconds, then after 3, etc.

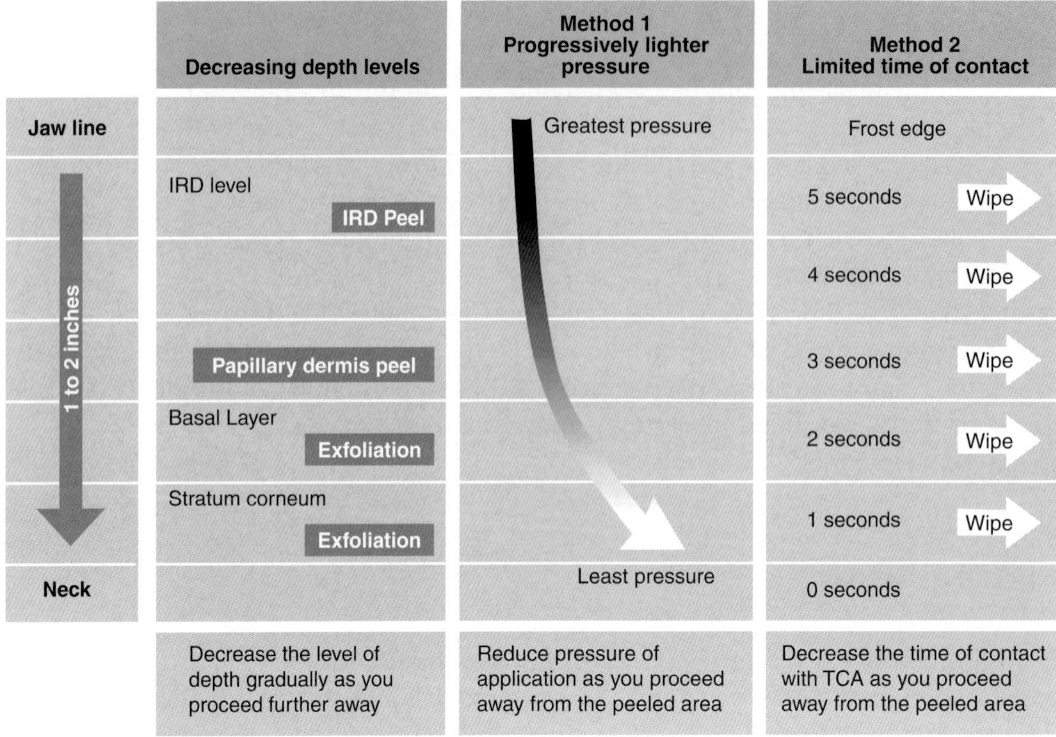

FIGURE 9-4. **Feathering methods.** Method 1: *Apply 25% modified TCA solution 1 to 2 in beyond the peeled areas using progressively lighter pressure while moving from the jawline to the neck. Wipe with tissue after each application. Repeat every 2 minutes until desired levels have been reached.* Method 2: *Apply 25% modified TCA solution 1 to 2 in beyond the peeled areas using progressively shorter time of acid contact with the skin by wiping up the solution with a tissue after 5, 4, 3, 2, 1, and 0 seconds, progressing from the jawline to the neck. Contact time is longer near the peeled area and shorter near the neck. Repeat every 2 minutes until desired levels have been reached.*

Both feathering methods help to create a smooth transition between peeled and unpeeled skin areas and prevent demarcation lines.

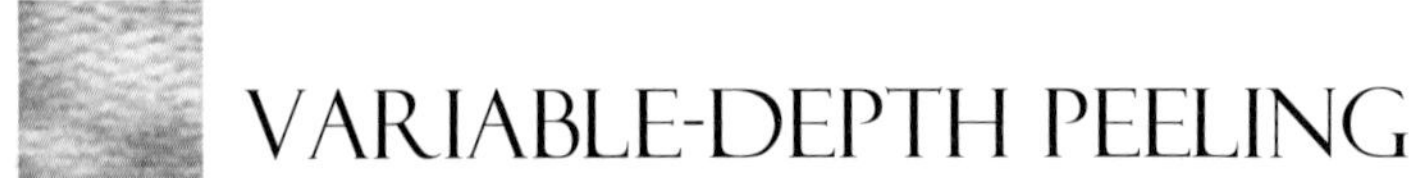

VARIABLE-DEPTH PEELING

Variable-depth peeling is a technique that customizes the peel depth to the different thicknesses found on the face, such as the thinner skin on the eyelids, medium on the forehead, and thicker on the cheeks. Variable-depth peeling should be used to correct skin with variable depths of damage. For example, an early Derm-2 peel (IRD) can be performed for the periocular area, a Derm-2 peel for deeper wrinkles or scars on the cheeks, and a Derm-1 (papillary dermis) peel on the eyelids and the neck. To perform the peel accurately, safely, and evenly, the depths shown in Table 9-8 are recommended.

TABLE 9.8

RECOMMENDED PEEL DEPTHS FOR DIFFERENT SKIN AREAS

Facial Area	*Recommended Depth*
Eyelids	Papillary dermis (Derm-1 = Standard Blue Peel)
Jawline	Papillary dermis or IRD (Derm-1, Early Derm-2)
Normal areas of cheeks	IRD (Early Derm-2)
Deep scars or wrinkles on cheeks	Upper reticular dermis (Derm-2); or, if needed for thick skin with proper color, Derm-3
Upper lip	Papillary dermis, IRD (Derm-1 or Early Derm-2); or, in thick skin, upper reticular dermis (Derm-2)
Crow's-feet and temples	IRD (Early Derm-2); or, in thick skin, upper reticular dermis (Derm-2)
Forehead	Papillary dermis, IRD (Derm-1 or Early Derm-2); or,in thick skin upper reticular dermis (Derm-2 or Derm-3)
Nonfacial skin (neck, chest, hands, arms)	Papillary dermis (Derm-1)

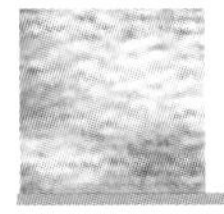

SATURATION

Saturation is performed after completion of a variable-depth peel to prevent demarcation lines and obtain an even skin surface after healing. The method is similar to performing a rapid light peel over the 40% variable-depth peel. To perform saturation, apply some or all of the 4 cc of a modified 25% solution (prepared before starting the peel) evenly and all over the face, with emphasis on the edges of the variable-depth frost. This creates a gradual transition between the different depths, which prevents demarcation lines.

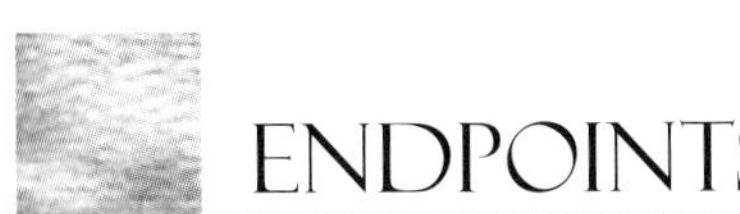

ENDPOINTS

SKIN REACTIONS TO TCA APPLICATION

When TCA is applied to the skin, body defenses in the form of epidermal protein (keratin) act to neutralize the acid and arrest its penetration. With more acid application, epidermal keratin is eventually denatured through the coagulation process. Clinically, this phenomenon is recognized as a frost. If additional acid is applied, penetration extends to the papillary der-

Box 9-7

The variables responsible for inconsistent results after chemical peels are:

- **TCA concentration**
- **TCA volume**
- **Skin thickness**

Box 9-8

Recognition of peel depth signs is very important in performing a safe, effective, Controlled Medium-Depth TCA Peel.

mis where more efficient defenses (collagen, elastin, glycosamninoglycans, blood vessels, blood, and other proteins) are available to prevent further penetration. When these defenses have been consumed, the acid penetrates deeper into the IRD, then into the upper reticular dermis, and then deeper into the dermis.

The ability of body defenses to successfully oppose the acid is related to 1) acid concentration, 2) volume of solution applied, and 3) skin thickness. When the concentration is low, the solution volume is small, or the skin is thick, there are sufficient defenses to counteract and neutralize the acid. However, when the acid concentration is high, the volume is large, or the skin is thin, the defenses are easily consumed and the acid is able to penetrate faster and deeper into the dermis.

In the author's experience, 6 cc to 7 cc (depending on skin thickness) of the 40% solution and 8 cc to 10 cc of the 25% solution are needed for each concentration to reach the IRD. However, for peels deeper than the IRD, the exact volume of solution needed to reach a specific depth cannot be determined, and recognition of endpoints is especially important in performing such peels safely. While a higher level of physician skill is required to perform deeper peels, the author believes that such peels can be performed effectively and safely if the associated variables (Box 9-7) are controlled.

SIGNIFICANCE OF ENDPOINTS

Endpoints are clinical depth signs demonstrating skin changes that correlate with a specific depth reached by the acid. When physicians see certain endpoints, they can determine whether they should stop acid application because the desired depth has been reached or continue to apply more acid to reach the desired depth. In the Obagi Controlled Medium-Depth TCA Peel, the following endpoints should be monitored: 1) degree and color of frost, 2) presence or absence of a pink background, and 3) presence or absence of epidermal sliding (Table 9-9). In addition, 3 supportive signs are used, with the latter 2 helpful only retrospectively: 1) skin firmness, 2) defrosting time, and 3) healing time (Table 9-10). Conventional peels using plain or augmented TCA cannot clearly and reliably produce such endpoints because the TCA penetrates rapidly. Control is poor with these peels, and penetration can be too deep in certain areas, increasing the risk of complications.

FROSTING AND PINK BACKGROUND

When TCA encounters protein present in the epidermis or dermis, it coagulates and precipitates the protein and forms a frost. Frosting will occur more quickly in areas where the stratum corneum is thin or absent and in skin that has been conditioned with tretinoin. Application of more TCA to areas that frost more slowly in an attempt to create an equal frost can inadvertently result in deeper than desired penetration. This should be avoided in nonfacial skin, such as skin on the hands (Figure 9-5).

TABLE 9.9

ENDPOINTS AT DIFFERENT DEPTHS OF THE CONTROLLED-DEPTH TCA PEEL

Obagi Controlled-Depth Peel Classification	*Obagi Peel Depth Terminology*	*Skin Level Reached*	*Frosting*	*Pink Background*	*Epidermal Sliding*
Epi-1	Light exfoliation	Stratum corneum	Light mist or cloud; no organized frost	Present	Absent
Epi-2	Medium exfoliation	Above basal layer	Dense cloud or fog; no organized frost	Present	Absent
Epi-3	Deep exfoliation	Basal layer	Thin sheet of cloud or fog, no organized frost	Present	Starts to appear
Derm-1	Light peel	Papillary dermis	Thin, transparent, organized sheet of frost	Present	Present
Early Derm-2	Light/medium peel	Immediate reticular dermis (IRD)	Solid, organized, white frost	Fading or just faded	Absent
Derm-2	Medium-depth peel	Upper reticular to mid dermis	Solid, thick, organized white frost	Absent	Absent
Derm-3	Deep peel	Mid to lower reticular dermis	Thick, gray sheet of frost	Absent	Absent

Table 9.10			
SUPPORTIVE CLINICAL SIGNS AT DIFFERENT DEPTHS OF THE CONTROLLED-DEPTH TCA PEEL			
Obagi Controlled-Depth TCA Peel Classification	***Skin Firmness***	***Average Defrosting Time***	***Healing Time (Days)***
Epi-1	Not firm	<3 min	2 to 3
Epi-2	Not firm	<3 min	3 to 4
Epi-3	May feel firm	<3 min	5 to 6
Derm-1	Begins to be firm	Thin skin—5 min Thick skin—10 min	7 to 8
Early Derm-2	Firmness felt	Thin skin—10 min Thick skin—15 min	8 to 10
Derm-2	Solidly firm	Thin skin—15 min Thick skin—20 min	10 to 12
Derm-3	Very solid	Thin skin—20 min Thick skin—30 min	12 to 14

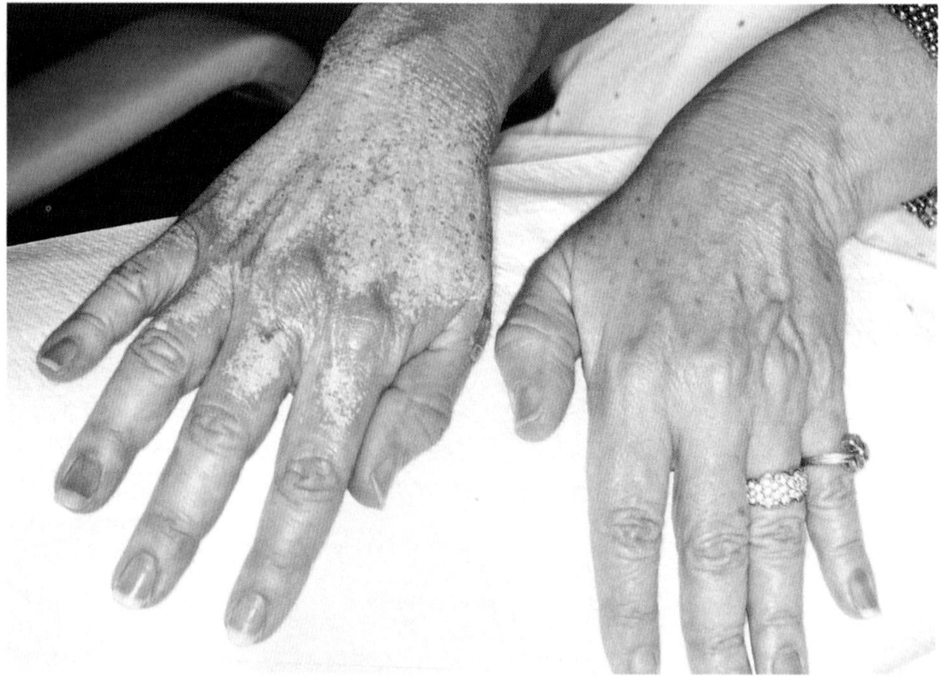

Figure 9-5. **Peeling of hands.** *The right hand, which had a colorless solution of TCA applied equally from the wrist to the nails, shows the uneven development of frost that is characteristic of nonfacial skin. Frost with pink is present on the dorsum of the hand and the proximal phalanges, but no frost appears on the knuckles or the distal phalanges. When colorless solutions are used for peeling, unfrosted areas appear untreated. The Blue Peel can reduce the uncertainty because the physician looks for development of an even blue color as an endpoint for nonfacial skin.*

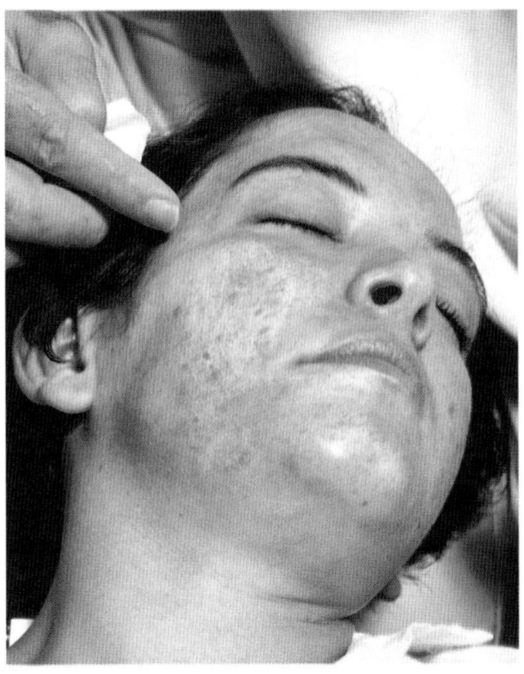

FIGURE 9-6. *Patient in early stages of frosting. A nonorganized cloud is present, but not a solid frost. This indicates exfoliation.*

Frosting is not a permanent event. The precipitated protein disperses with time, and the frost disappears. If the penetration is limited to the epidermal layer (Epi-1 and Epi-2 levels), the skin shows either no frost or a nonorganized, white, cloudy, or foggy appearance that quickly disappears (Figure 9-6). Following the application of more solution and deeper penetration of the acid, the nonorganized fog or cloud starts to organize and appears as a sheet. This will appear earlier in thin skin. When the papillary dermis has been reached (Derm-1), the frost will look like a thin, transparent, organized sheet with a pink background (Figure 9-7). Frosting of the papillary dermis should last for 5 minutes in thin skin and 10 minutes in thick skin before defrosting. When the IRD has been reached (Early Derm-2), the frost will show less pink background or the pink background will have just disappeared (Figure 9-8). If penetration continues to the mid dermis, the frost starts to appear "grayish," and defrosting will take 15 to 20 minutes. The progression of frost formation is summarized in Figure 9-9.

Pink Background

The pink background to the frost is called the "pink sign." When TCA begins to penetrate the papillary dermis, the frost has a pink background due to the intact blood vessels and continuous blood flow in the capillary loops of the papillary dermis (Epi-1, Epi-2, Derm-1 peel levels). When the IRD level is reached (Early Derm-2 level), TCA induces vasospasm, resulting in occluded blood vessels and cessation of normal blood flow. The pink background disappears, and the frost becomes white. The pink background does not return until defrosting is complete. The loss of the pink sign indicates a light/medium peel, known as an early Derm-2 or IRD-level peel.

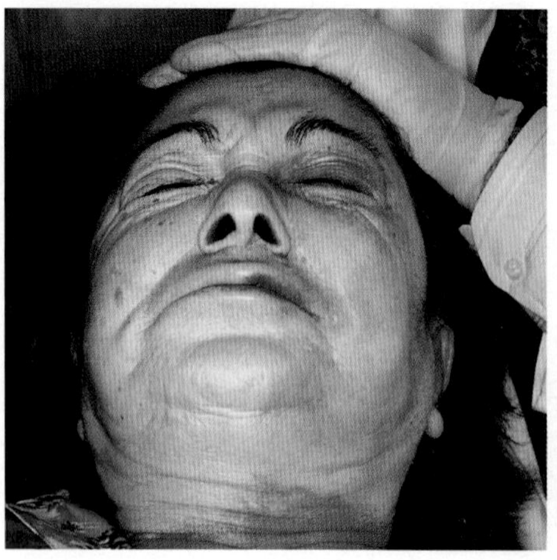

FIGURE 9-7. *Left side of patient's face shows an organized frost with pink background (papillary dermis level), while the right side shows an organized frost with the pink background just disappeared (IRD level).*

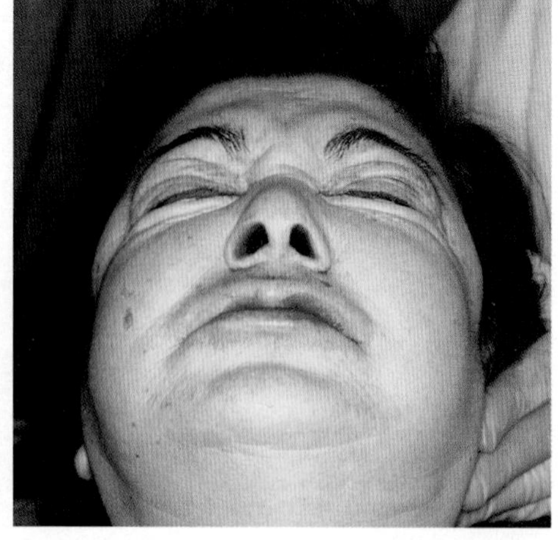

FIGURE 9-8. *Both sides of patient's face show a solid, organized frost with no pink, indicating IRD-level penetration, while the upper eyelids and neck show frost with pink, indicating papillary dermis-level penetration.*

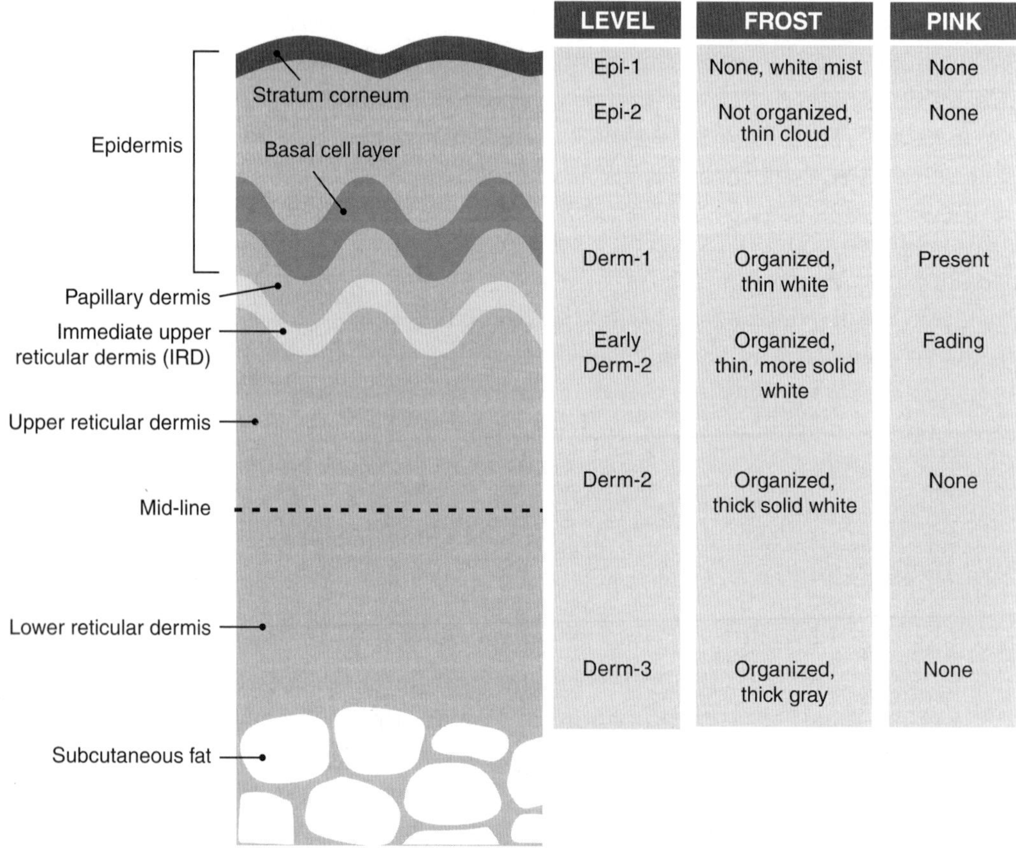

LEVEL	FROST	PINK
Epi-1	None, white mist	None
Epi-2	Not organized, thin cloud	None
Derm-1	Organized, thin white	Present
Early Derm-2	Organized, thin, more solid white	Fading
Derm-2	Organized, thick solid white	None
Derm-3	Organized, thick gray	None

FIGURE 9-9. *Level of skin penetrated and frost description for Obagi Controlled Medium-Depth TCA Peels.*

Box 9-9

The pink sign disappears when TCA-induced vasospasm stops blood flow in the papillary dermis.

Upon reaching the papillary dermis, the pink color may disappear and then quickly reappear through the frost; in other words, defrosting was not maintained for 10 to 15 minutes. This indicates that the peel did not sufficiently involve the blood vessels in the papillary dermis and that the IRD was not reached. Additional solution has to be applied to frost the area for the proper amount of time.

EPIDERMAL SLIDING

The epidermis is attached to the dermis by means of epidermal projections (rete ridges), corresponding dermal invaginations, and a network of anchoring fibrils that extend vertically from the reticular dermis through the papillary dermis and attach themselves to the basement membrane. When TCA is applied to the skin, the epidermal/dermal junction is altered, the anchoring fibers are disrupted, and edema fluid accumulates between the epidermis and the papillary dermis. This allows the epidermis to slide over the firmer, nonmovable dermis and allows exaggerated wrinkles to appear when the skin is tugged; this is called the "epidermal sliding sign" (Figure 9-10). The epidermal sliding sign disappears when the peel reaches the IRD because all of the protein in the epidermis and papillary dermis has precipitated as one block.

The epidermal sliding sign and the pink sign go hand in hand. Both indicate that the peel is not deeper than the papillary dermis. When peeling

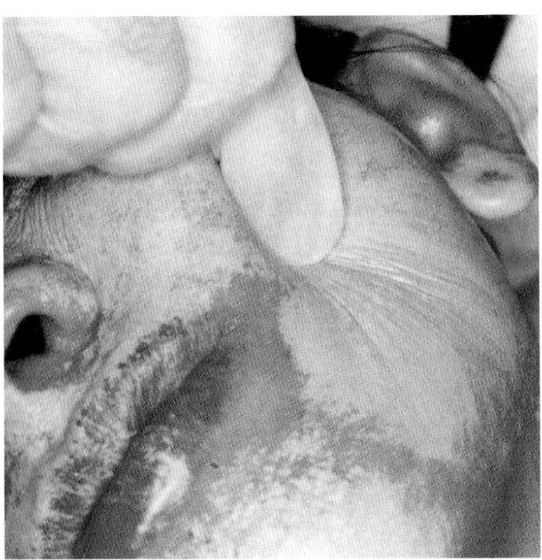

FIGURE **9-10.** *Penetration of the TCA solution to the depth of the papillary dermis allows the epidermis to slide over the dermis when the skin is pinched, producing the epidermal sliding sign. The pink sign will also be observed at this level.*

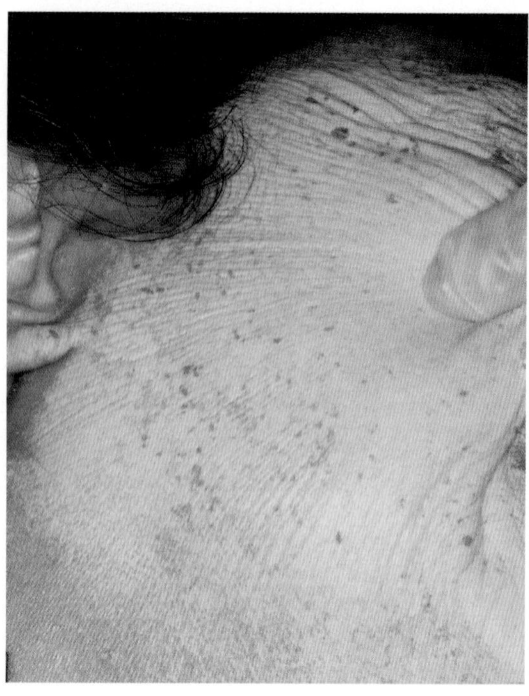

FIGURE 9-11. *A patient during a Controlled Medium-Depth Peel showing frosting with and without pink. Epidermal sliding appears upon tugging of the skin where penetration was to papillary dermis and shows frost with pink (above jawline), but does not appear in the immediate area of the physician's finger, where acid penetration was deeper and shows frost with no pink. Proper feathering on the neck is also shown.*

dark or Black skin, the pink sign may not be clearly visible, so the epidermal sliding sign may be the only indicator of the papillary dermis level. In very thick or porous skin, on the other hand, the sliding sign may not be very obvious, and the pink sign has to be used as an endpoint instead. A patient during a Controlled Medium-Depth Peel showing frosting with and without pink, epidermal sliding, and proper feathering on the neck is shown in Figure 9-11.

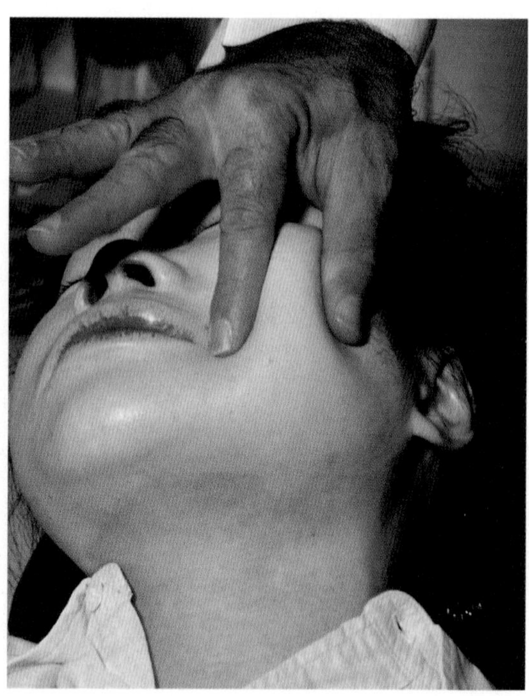

FIGURE 9-12. *Feeling skin firmess with pinching. Patient's skin shows a solid frost with no pink. Note also the absence of demarcation lines on the chin and neck following proper feathering.*

FIRMNESS

The more protein precipitated by the action of TCA, the firmer the skin will feel upon grasping (Figure 9-12). Thus the "firmness sign" can be used as a supportive sign by a skilled peeler. The sign is more pronounced with deeper peels and in thick skin and may not be detectable in exfoliative procedures and light peels. The less-experienced peeler may not be able to detect skin firmness in papillary dermis or upper dermis peels, but an effort should be made to acquire this ability.

DEFROSTING TIME

While defrosting and healing times are not endpoints, they are helpful retrospectively for determining the peel depth that was achieved. After epidermal and dermal proteins have been coagulated to form a frost, the process of dispersion of the precipitated proteins, called *defrosting*, begins. As the precipitated proteins are dispersed by cellular and edema fluids, the frost gradually disappears, and the skin changes back to being pink and edematous. The time for defrosting to take place correlates well with peel depth (longer in deeper peels) and skin thickness (longer in thick skin) (Figure 9-13). Typical defrosting times for different peel depths were shown in Table 9-10. In an early Derm-2 peel, persistence of a frost for 10 to 15 minutes (depending on skin thickness) before disappearance (defrosting) indicates a good hold on the depth that was reached.

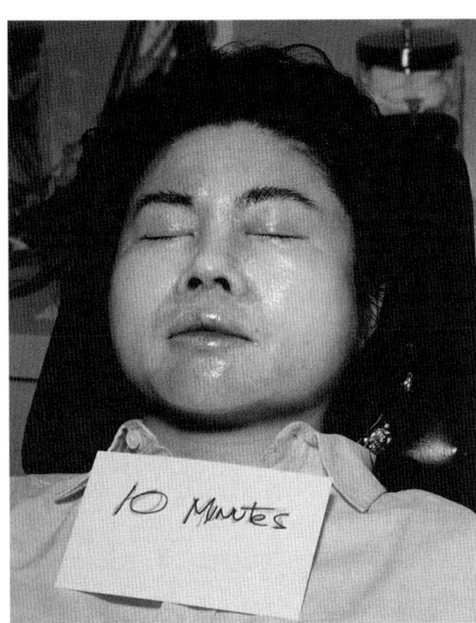

a

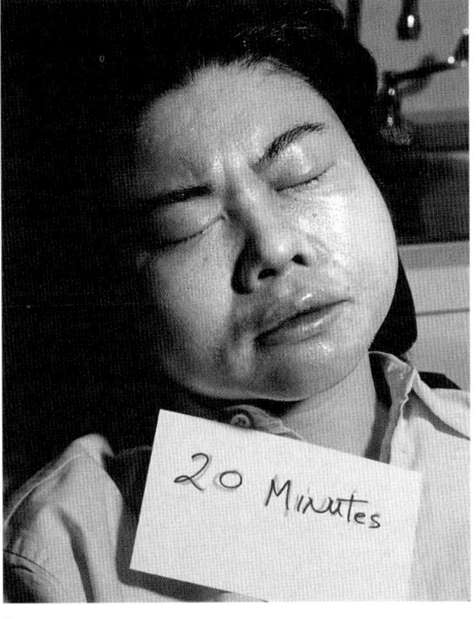

b

FIGURES **9-13.** *Defrosting. (a) After 10 minutes, pink has returned to the chin, upper lip, upper lids, and forehead, where the papillary dermis was reached. Pink has not returned to the cheeks, indicating greater depth of penetration (upper reticular dermis). (b) After 20 minutes, there has been total defrosting in the areas peeled to the papillary dermis, while frost remains on cheeks.*

TABLE 9.11

POSTPEEL TOPICAL CARE

Morning	*Mid-morning*	*Mid-afternoon*	*Evening*
■ Wash face ■ Apply the recommended moisturizer or ointment, with or without 0.5% hydrocortisone	■ Apply compresses for 2 min ■ Perform scab thinning for 2 min beginning on day 1 if scabs are present ■ Apply the recommended moisturizer or ointment, if needed. Keep skin somewhat dry (not too moist, not too dry)	■ Apply compresses for 2 min ■ Perform scab thinning for 2 min on thick scabs ■ Apply moisturizers or ointment, if needed	■ Wash face ■ Apply moisturizers

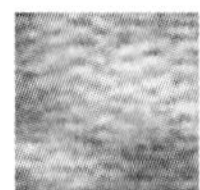

POSTPROCEDURE HEALING

HEALING TIME CONCEPTS

As can be seen in Table 9-10 and Figure 9-14, postprocedure healing time correlates well with the depth of skin injury. In other words, the deeper

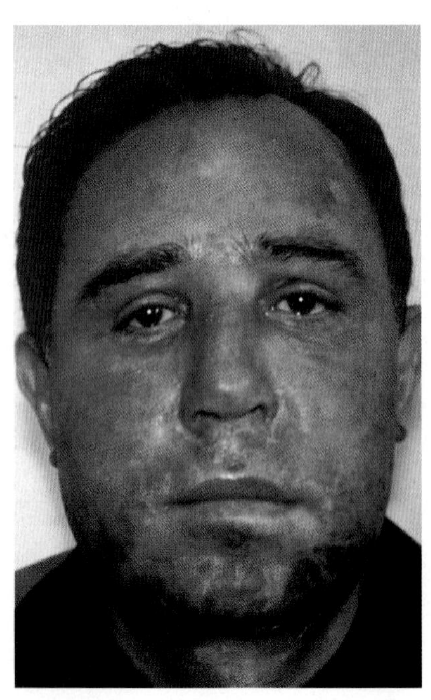

a

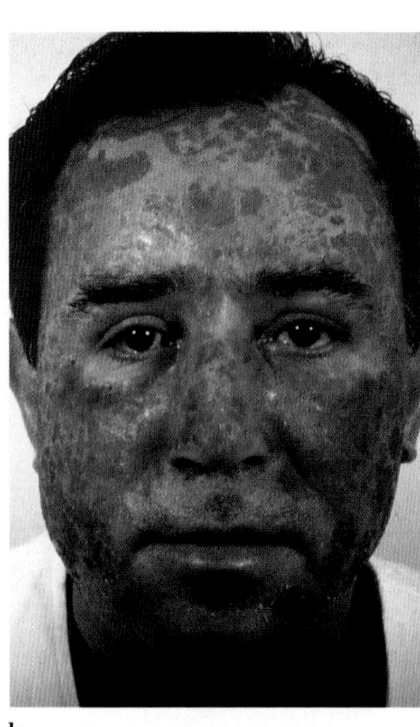

b

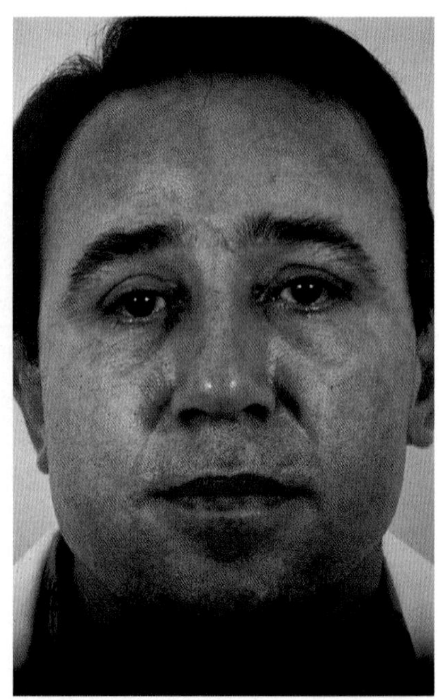

c

FIGURE 9-14. *Patient during healing. (a) Patient (the author) on the fourth day after a Controlled Medium-Depth TCA Peel to the upper reticular dermis. (b) Same patient on day 7. Areas of penetration to the papillary dermis (lower eyelids) show complete healing. The rest of the face, where penetration was to the upper reticular dermis, is still healing. (c) Same patient 1 year after a Controlled Medium-Depth TCA Peel to the upper reticular dermis.*

the procedure, the longer it takes for the skin to heal. Healing time correlates well with achieved depth, regardless of the type of procedure (laser resurfacing, chemical peeling) that was performed. Variations in healing time are related to the exact depth that was achieved, whether skin conditioning had been performed, and whether complications occurred.

THE STAGES OF HEALING

The healing of skin after any procedure can be divided into three stages: 1) the injury and initial healing, 2) extended healing, and 3) the return to normal (Table 9-12). The patient should be made aware of these stages before undergoing a procedure.

The first stage of healing is complete when the epidermis has been restored (reepithelialization) and the patient can tolerate normal activities and topical treatments with tretinoin and hydroquinone. Dermal healing or extended healing, on the other hand, involves collagen and elastin production

TABLE 9.12
THE STAGES OF HEALING

	Procedure Stage	*Recovery Stage*	*Normal Stage*
Duration	■ 7 to 14 days of initial healing, depending on depth of procedure	■ 1 to 6 weeks	NA
Expected Reactions	■ After deeper procedures: more swelling, oozing, thicker scabbing, and a longer time to heal, in general	■ After deeper procedures: Anticipated reactions include erythema, inflammatory hyperpigmentation, milia, acne flareup, larger pores, tight skin, rough skin, "marblized" appearance Unanticipated reactions include delayed healing from unintended excess depth; severe, patchy erythema with skin thickening or itching that can be precursors of keloids or hypertrophic reactions	■ Residual, unanticipated reactions: hypopigmentation, demarcation lines, large pores, persistent erythema, keloid or hypertrophic reaction
Pain	■ Painless healing is the norm with the Blue Peel and the Controlled, Medium-Depth Peel (pain is common after CO_2 and erbium laser resurfacing) ■ The presence of pain after chemical peels indicate infection		
Care	■ Home-care instruction to be followed	■ Home care instruction to be followed	

Box 9-9

After procedures that remove the epidermis, keratinocytes and melanocytes migrate from the epithelium of adenexal structures to reepithelialize the skin. Thus, remaining adnexal structures and fibroblasts play a significant role in postprocedure healing.

and neovascularization, which continues for 2 to 6 weeks after a procedure to the IRD level and 3 to 4 months after a Derm-2 or Derm-3 peel. Proper healing depends on the remaining integrity of the dermis and adnexal structures, which are needed to form new epidermis, melanocytes, and other cells.

Being able to estimate healing time is very desirable because patients want to schedule the necessary amount of time away from work or social activities after their procedure. Healing time also provides a retrospective indication of the peel depth. For example, if the physician performed a Derm-2 peel (upper reticular dermis), the patient's expected healing time is 10 to 12 days. If, however, the patient's skin healed in 7 to 8 days, the intended depth was not attained and a papillary dermis peel was performed instead.

HEALING TIME AND SKIN APPEARANCE

Exfoliations

After exfoliative procedures (Epi-1, Epi-2), skin appears erythematous and may become darker and start to exfoliate rapidly without pain or crust formation. Healing time is short, completed in 3 to 5 days.

Papillary Dermis Peels

In peels that involve the papillary dermis (Derm-1), the skin is initially erythematous, and there may be mild or no edema. The skin darkens and begins to peel on the second or third day and is healed in 7 to 8 days. Scab formation is minimal. There is no pain, but the skin feels tight and occasionally there is itching or burning. The neck and chest tend to be more sensitive than the face.

IRD and Medium Depth Peels

Following peels below the papillary dermis (early Derm-2 or deeper), edema is present for 3 to 4 days, but the overall healing stage is painless. The skin becomes darker, feels tight like a mask, and crusts and scabs form. Peeling begins on the third or fourth day. Recovery after a light/medium peel (early Derm-2) is 8 to 10 days, and after a medium-depth peel, 10 to 12 days. Crusting may be uneven, and some areas may heal faster than others due to variable depth.

In acne-prone patients or those with oily skin, acne may be activated with the appearance of comedones and cysts during the healing stage or after healing has been completed. These conditions should be treated promptly to prevent scarring and discolorations. Pores may appear larger in patients with thick or oily skin, especially after procedures that reach the upper reticular dermis. Pores usually return to normal gradually over a few months following an aggressive skin conditioning program with tretinoin. Newly produced elastin (3 to 4 weeks after the procedure) in the papillary dermis helps to tighten the pores.

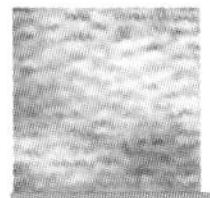

POSTPEEL HOME CARE

The physician can use his or her preferred methods for home care. The author's home care instructions include topical treatment and systemic treatment.

TOPICAL TREATMENT

Washing: The face should be washed gently, twice daily, with no rubbing, using a gentle cleanser and warm or cold water. Then the face should be rinsed and patted dry with a soft cloth. Showers are permitted as long as the water and shampoo are kept away from the face.

Lubrication: After a papillary dermis peel, such as the Blue Peel, a non-oil-based moisturizer can be used alone or mixed with 0.05% hydrocortisone cream and applied 2 to 4 times daily, as shown in Table 9-11. After an IRD-level peel, such as the Blue Peel with Design, the same moisturizer, alone or with an ointment such as Aquaphor, petroleum jelly, A&D ointment, or antibiotic ointment is preferable for more deeply peeled areas to release tightness and prevent cracking of scabs. The skin should be kept comfortable, not too dry, to avoid cracking, and not too moist, to avoid maceration of scabs and premature skin separation.

Antiseptic Compresses: Acetic acid, 2% to 5% with water (Domebro or other) is used to prevent both bacterial and fungal infections. Apply the solution with gauze to the skin with gentle pressure. This is to be done twice daily for 2 minutes each time. This antiseptic solution can also to be used to wipe away any fluid oozing from the skin.

Scab Thinning: Thick crusts and thick scabs should be prevented by keeping scabs as thin as possible. The scabs should not be rubbed hard or forced off. To keep scabs thin, gauze saturated with antiseptic solution or Cetaphil lotion cleanser can be applied with a *gentle* brushing motion for 1 to 2 minutes up to 2 times daily. This process should start when the scabs become thicker or approximately 4 days after a medium-depth peel. Thin scabs on the eyelids, neck, and jawline should not be thinned, to avoid premature separation. Scab thinning should increase in frequency and duration on about the seventh day following a medium-depth peel to ensure that no scabs remain on the face by day 10.

Patients should avoid making facial expressions, such as smiling or opening the mouth wide, for these may cause cracks and fissures. Loose skin can be trimmed with small scissors. Patients should sleep on their backs and avoid being struck on the face with the shower water spray while bathing. Men should shave daily since facial hair tends to have associated thick crusts that heal slowly and can lead to complications. A summary of postpeel topical care is shown in Table 9-11.

SYSTEMIC POSTPEEL TREATMENT

Following a medium-depth peel, a 7-day tapering regimen of oral prednisone (60 mg, 50 mg, 40 mg, 30 mg, 20 mg, 10 mg, none) or Medrol dose pack can make healing more comfortable and possibly reduce the swelling. Antihistamines, such as Atarax or Benadryl, can be taken if needed for itching and to provide sedation for sleeping. Some patients may need systemic antibiotics and prophylactic Herpes simplex medication. Sleeping pills or sedative medications may also be helpful for some patients.

RECOMMENDED TREATMENT DURING RECOVERY STAGES

If the patient's skin feels sensitive, with itching, burning, or dryness after a papillary dermis or IRD-level procedure, use a mild moisturizer, with or without topical steroid, 2 times daily for 1 week during the first week after the peel. Usually the steroid can be discontinued by the end of the first week. Begin the conditioning program (cleaning, correction, bleaching, blending, stimulation), as tolerated, as soon as possible, especially if PIH is anticipated.

After all scabs are off the face following an upper reticular or mid dermis level procedure (10 days), a potent steroid such as clobetasol propionate (Temovate) should be applied liberally and massaged into the skin 2 times daily for 1 week. One 30 g tube should be used up in 1 week. This helps to reduce skin sensitivity and irritation, increases smoothness, and may help to suppress or prevent the formation of keloids or hypertrophic reactions in susceptible individuals. On the third day of steroid use, the bleaching and blending steps of the skin conditioning program should be started. Discontinue the use of topical steroids after 1 week and continue with the conditioning program alone. If CO_2 laser resurfacing has been performed, bleaching and blending are essential after healing to prevent PIH and shorten the erythema phase. Reconditioning should continue for 4 to 6 weeks.

PROPER HEALING

Healing after any skin rejuvenation procedure can be classified as proper, average, poor, or abnormal. Proper skin healing is characterized by retention of normal color and the presence of normal texture, tolerance, and function. It is also free of anticipated and unanticipated reactions or complications. With average healing, skin has normal texture, tolerance, and function. However, the peeled area may remain lighter than the nonpeeled areas, but there are no demarcation lines. Healing is considered poor when 1 or more skin abnormalities, such as change in color or texture, demarcation lines, or minor uneveness from resolved scars or keloids, are present. With abnormal healing, there are serious sequelae, such as depigmentation, significant textural changes, and deformity from scars or keloids. Postpeel complications are discussed in depth in Chapter 10.

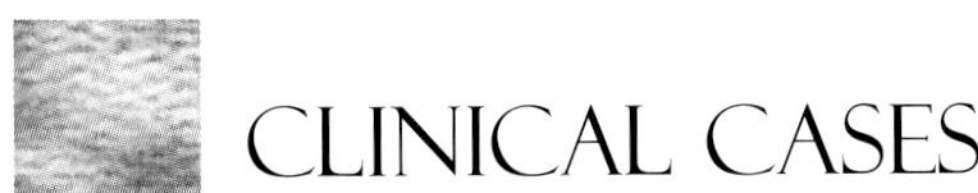

CLINICAL CASES

The case histories of patients who underwent a Controlled Medium-Depth TCA Peel are shown in Figures 9-15 to 9-21. Laxity was scored on a scale of 0 to +5, with 5 indicating the highest severity.

FIGURE 9-15

Skin Classification:

Color—Deviated (Medium Black)

Thickness—Thick (the fold at the cheek is 2 cm)

Oiliness—Oily

Laxity—+2

Fragility—None

Diagnosis: Acne scars, dilated pores, sebaceous gland hyperplasia, hamartomatous changes, excessive oilinees, and discoloration.

Treatment Plan:

1. Skin Conditioning for at least 6 weeks, preferably longer, to soften the scars and control the acne.

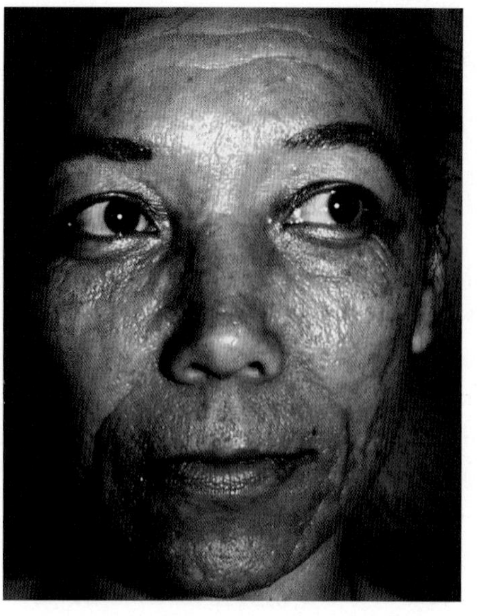

a

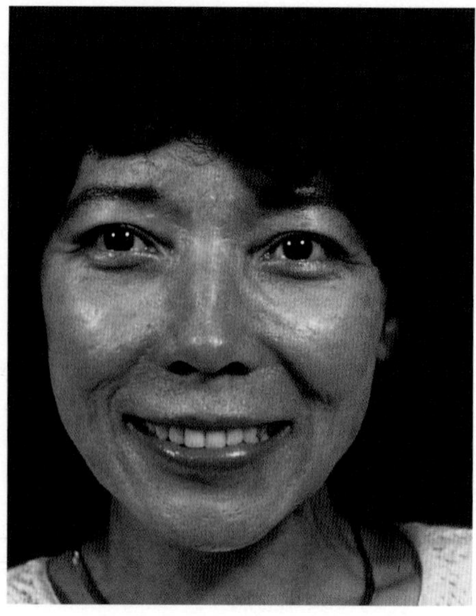

b

FIGURE 9-15. *(a) Before treatment. (b) After—1 year.*

2. A medium-depth peel with modified TCA was performed after 3 months of Skin Conditioning. A Derm-2 level was obtained. The potential for hypopigmentation and other complications was explained to the patient before the procedure.

   Treatment possibilities that were rejected were dermabrasion, CO_2 laser resurfacing, erbium laser resurfacing, and a Blue Peel with Design. The patient had already had a dermabrasion with unsatisfactory results. Furthermore, dermabrasion is a high-risk procedure for this patient's skin type. CO_2 laser resurfacing is also high risk, with the potential for permanent texture and color changes. Erbium laser resurfacing would not be effective since the mid dermis needs to be reached to correct this patient's skin. The Blue Peel with Design may give some improvement, but possibly not enough.

3. Three weeks after the procedure, Skin Conditioning was reinstituted. Thereafter, the patient could follow a maintenance program, if desired. Accutane (isotretinoin) 20 mg/day was started 3 weeks after the procedure and administered for 5 months.

Results: One year after—The photograph 1 year after the procedure shows soft, firm, and uniformly colored skin with normal tolerance.

FIGURE 9-16

Skin Classification:

Color—Normal White

Thickness—Thick

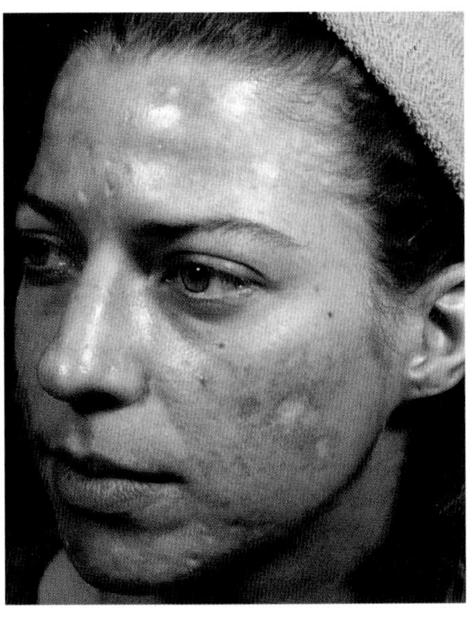

a

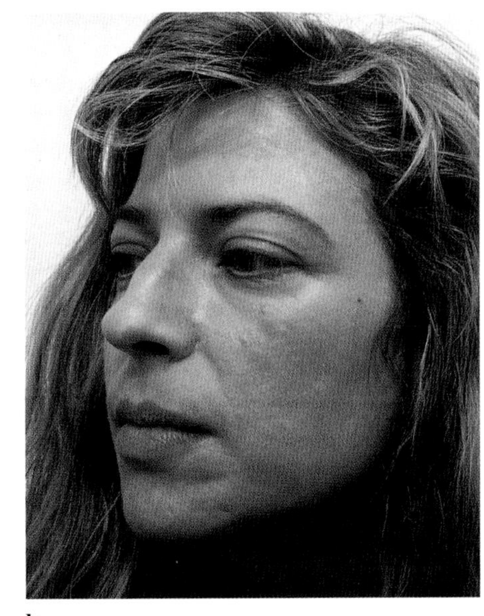

b

FIGURE 9-16. *(a) Before treatment. (b) After—1 year.*

Oiliness—Normal

Laxity—0

Fragility—None

Diagnosis: Acne scars, ice-pick scars, excoriation scars, discoloration.

Treatment Plan:

1. Skin Conditioning for 3 months.
2. Six weeks before the peel procedure, the base of the large, depressed scars was lifted with a 22-gauge needle and punch grafts were performed on the ice-pick scars that did not respond to base lifting. A Derm-2-level peel was performed with modified TCA.

   The patient responded well to the base lifting and punch grafts, which reduced the need for a very deep procedure and allowed a medium-depth procedure to be performed. The benefits of the medium-depth peel were skin leveling and tightening.

   Other treatment possibilities for this patient were CO_2 laser resurfacing or dermabrasion. Collagen injections could also have improved the deeper scars.
3. After the skin was healed, skin conditioning was reinstituted and continued for 2 months. Thereafter, the patient could follow a maintenance program, if desired.

Results: One year after—The photograph 1 year after the procedure shows that the criteria for healthy skin have been met. Skin is smooth, firm, and evenly colored and has normal tolerance.

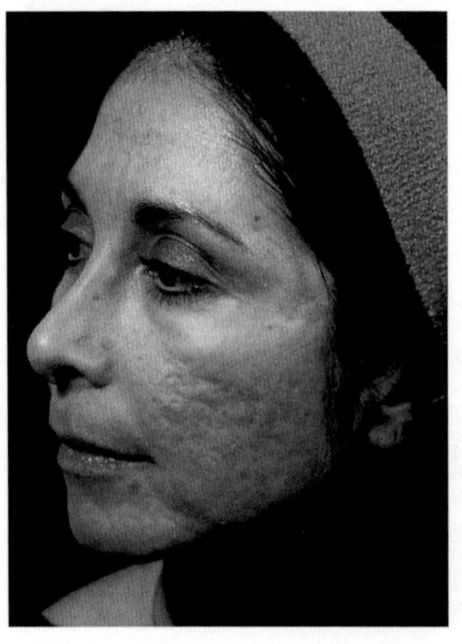

a

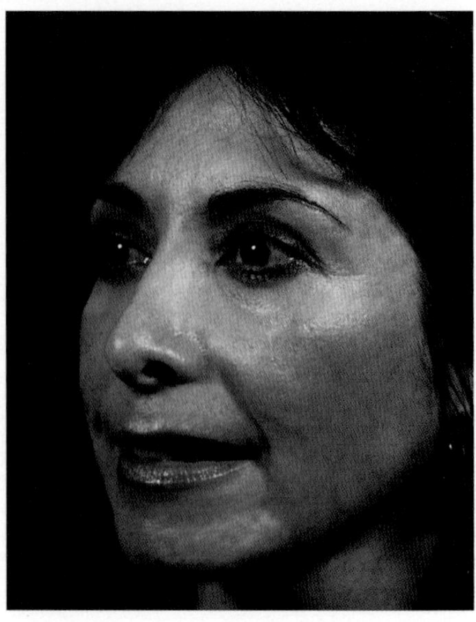

b

FIGURE 9-17. *(a) Before treatment. (b) After—1 year.*

FIGURE 9-17

Skin Classification:

Color—Deviated White (Brunette)

Thickness—Thick

Oiliness—Oily

Laxity—+1

Fragility—None

Diagnosis: Active cystic acne and acne scars.

Treatment Plan:

1. Skin Conditioning for 6 weeks.
2. The scars were stretchable except for those in the central cheek area. Thus, since both leveling and tightening were required, 2 depth levels of peel were chosen to reduce the overall depth of skin injury.

   A modified Controlled Medium-Depth TCA Peel was peformed for a Derm-2 level for the cheeks and a Derm-1 level for the rest of the face. Feathering was performed between the 2 levels and at the jawline.
3. After the skin was healed, Skin Conditioning was reinstituted and continued for 3 months. Thereafter, the patient could follow a maintenance program, if desired. Accutane (isotretinoin) 20 mg/day was started 3 weeks after the procedure.

Results: One year after—The photograph 1 year after the procedure shows that the criteria for healthy skin have been met. Skin is smooth, firm, and evenly colored and has normal tolerance.

FIGURE 9-18

Skin Classification:

Color—Deviated (Medium Asian)

Thickness—Thick

Oiliness—Oily

Laxity—0

Fragility—None

Diagnosis: Fibrotic and depressed scars from chicken pox infection.

Treatment Plan:

1. Skin Conditioning for 8 weeks.
2. The scars did not disappear or improve with stretching. Scar base lifting was performed and improved the uppermost scars.

   A modified Controlled Medium-Depth TCA Peel was peformed to the Derm-2 level for a leveling effect on the scarred area. The rest of the face was treated with a standard Blue Peel for tightening. Feathering was performed to blend the 2 areas.

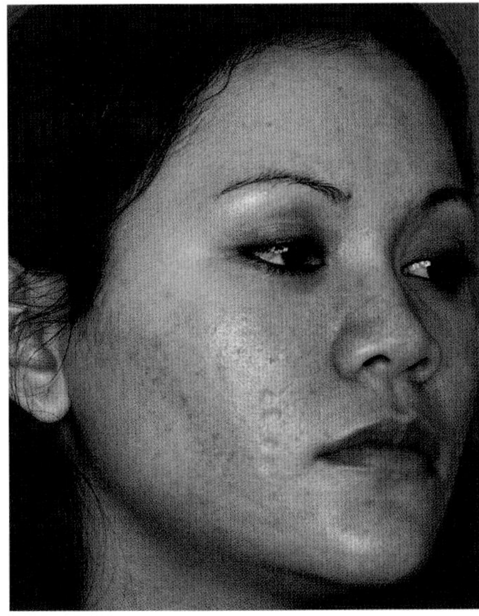

a

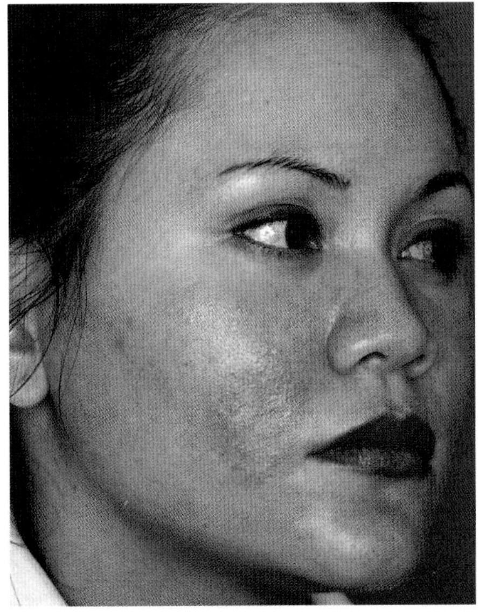

b

FIGURE **9-18.** *(a) Before treatment. (b) After—3 months.*

3. After the skin was healed, Skin Conditioning was reinstituted and continued for 3 months. Thereafter, the patient could follow a maintenance program, if desired.

Results: 3 months after—The photograph 3 months after the procedure shows that the criteria for healthy skin have been met. Skin is smooth, firm, and evenly colored and has normal tolerance.

FIGURE 9-19

Skin Classification:

Color—Deviated White (Brunette)

Thickness—Normal (1.5 cm fold on the cheek)

Oiliness—Dry

Laxity—+3

Fragility—None

Diagnosis: Photoaging, solar elastosis, wrinkles, discoloration.

Treatment Plan:

1. Skin Conditioning for 8 months.
2. After 2 months of conditioning, a variable-depth TCA peel procedure was performed to achieve tightening and leveling. The procedure con-

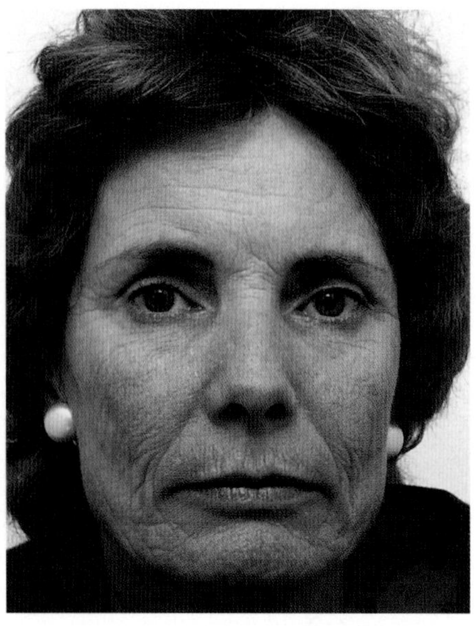

a

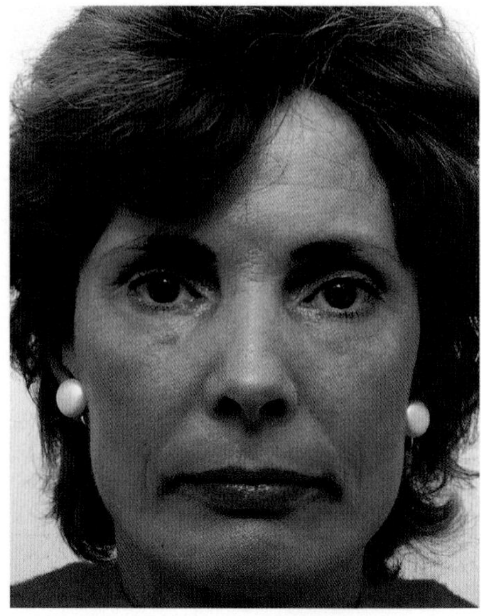

b

FIGURE **9-19.** *(a) Before treatment. (b) After—1 year.*

sisted of an early Derm-2 peel on the upper lip, cheeks, and forehead and a Derm-1 peel on the eyelids.

Three months later, a Blue Peel with Design was performed, with the IRD level reached on the upper lip. Saturation and feathering were performed to blend the areas.

3. After the skin was healed, Skin Conditioning was reinstituted and continued for 2 months. Thereafter, the patient could follow a maintenance program, if desired.

Results: One year after—The photograph 1 year after the procedure shows that the criteria for healthy skin have been met. Skin is smooth, firm, and evenly colored and has normal tolerance.

FIGURE 9-20

Skin Classification:

Color—Normal White

Thickness—Very thick (3 cm fold on the cheek)

Oiliness—Normal

Laxity—+5

Fragility—None

Diagnosis: Actinic keratoses, solar lentigos, rosacea, very weak snap test in both lower eyelids.

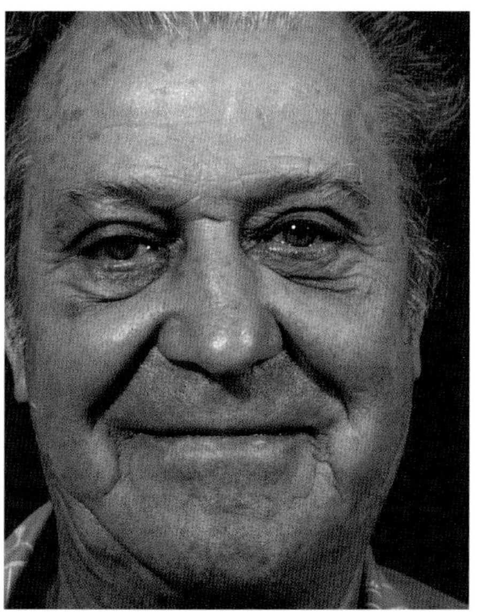

a

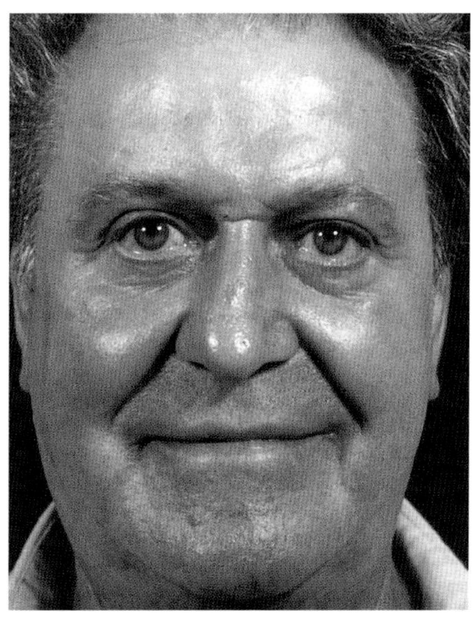

b

FIGURE 9-20. *(a) Before treatment. (b) After—1 year.*

Treatment Plan:

1. Skin Conditioning for 8 weeks.
2. This patient could benefit from a variety of procedures, including a facelift, liposuction of the neck, laser resurfacing, and blepharoplasty. Lower eyelid fat had been previously removed (see scars), but lower lid blepharoplasty had not been performed, and excessive skin laxity and wrinkles remained in this area.

   The patient underwent a variable-depth peel with modified TCA to achieve both leveling and tightening. The Derm-1 level was reached on the eyelids, Derm-2 on the cheeks and forehead, and Derm-2+ in the preauricular areas, lateral canthi, and temples. Saturation and feathering were performed.
3. After the skin was healed, Skin Conditioning was reinstituted and continued for 2 months. Thereafter, the patient could follow a maintenance program, if desired.

Results: One year after—The photograph 1 year after the procedure shows that the criteria for healthy skin have been met. Skin is smooth, firm, evenly colored and has normal tolerance.

FIGURE 9-21

Skin Classification:

Color—Deviated White (Brunette)

Thickness—Normal

Oiliness—normal

Laxity—+3

Fragility—None

Diagnosis: Lentigos, actinic keratoses, solar elastosis, wrinkles.

Treatment Plan:

1. Skin Conditioning for 2 months.
2. In contrast with the patient shown in Figure 9-20, this patient would not benefit from a facelift, which had been performed 3 months earlier. CO_2 or erbium laser resurfacing may give good results, but dermabrasion would not be useful because the eyelids need improvement. The Blue Peel with Design would not eliminate the perioral and lateral canthi wrinkles. A glycolic acid peel would not be effective. A program of Skin Health Restoration would improve skin quality but not the wrinkles.

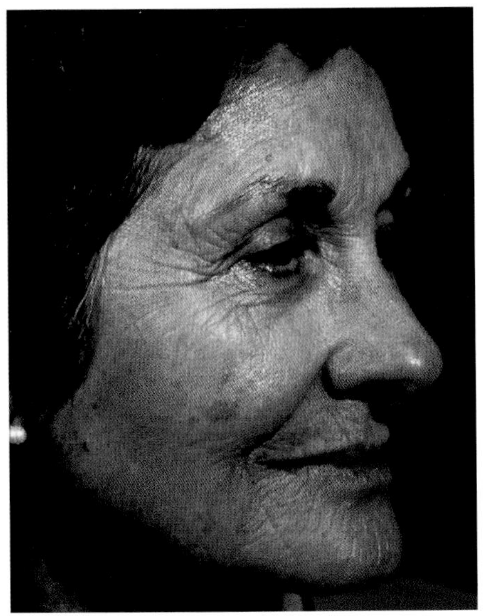
a

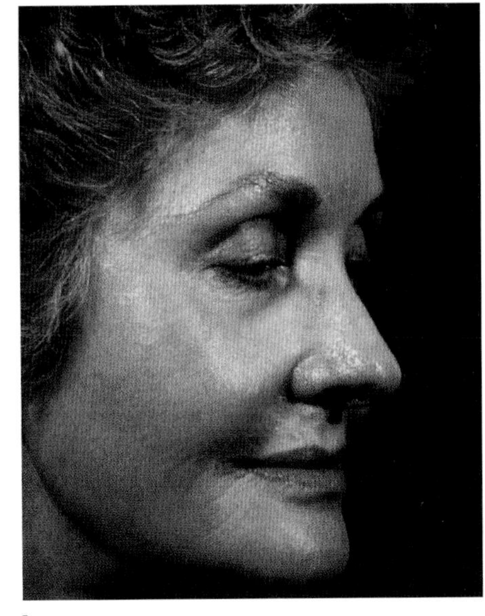
b

FIGURE 9-21. *(a) Before treatment. (b) After—1 year.*

The patient underwent a variable-depth peel with modified TCA. A Derm-2 peel was performed on all of the face except the eyelids, which were treated with a Derm-1 peel on the lids proper and an early Derm-2 peel at the junction of the lids proper and the surrounding skin. Saturation and feathering were performed.

3. After the skin was healed, Skin Conditioning was reinstituted and continued for 2 months. Thereafter, the patient could follow a maintenance program, if desired.

Results: One year after—The photograph 1 year after the procedure shows that the criteria for healthy skin have been met. Skin is smooth, firm, and evenly colored, and has normal tolerance.

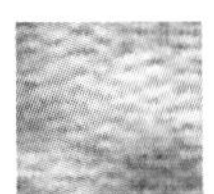

REFERENCES

1. Obagi ZO, Mazen M, Sawaf MM, Johnson JB, Laub DR, Stevens MB. The Controlled, Medium-Depth trichloroacetic acid peel: methodology, outcome, and complication rate. *Int J Aesthetic Restor Surg.* 1996;4:81–94.
2. Brody HJ. Chemical peeling wounding spectrum. In: *Chemical Peeling and Resurfacing.* 2nd ed. St Louis, Mo.: CV Mosby; 1997: inside cover.
3. Johnson JB, Ichinose H, Obagi ZE, Laub DR. Obagi's modified trichloroacetic acid (TCA)-controlled variable depth peel: a study of clinical signs correlating with histological findings. *Ann Plast Surg.* 1996; 36:225–237.

CHAPTER

10

IDENTIFYING AND TREATING ANTICIPATED REACTIONS AND COMPLICATIONS AFTER CHEMICAL PEELS AND OTHER RESURFACING PROCEDURES

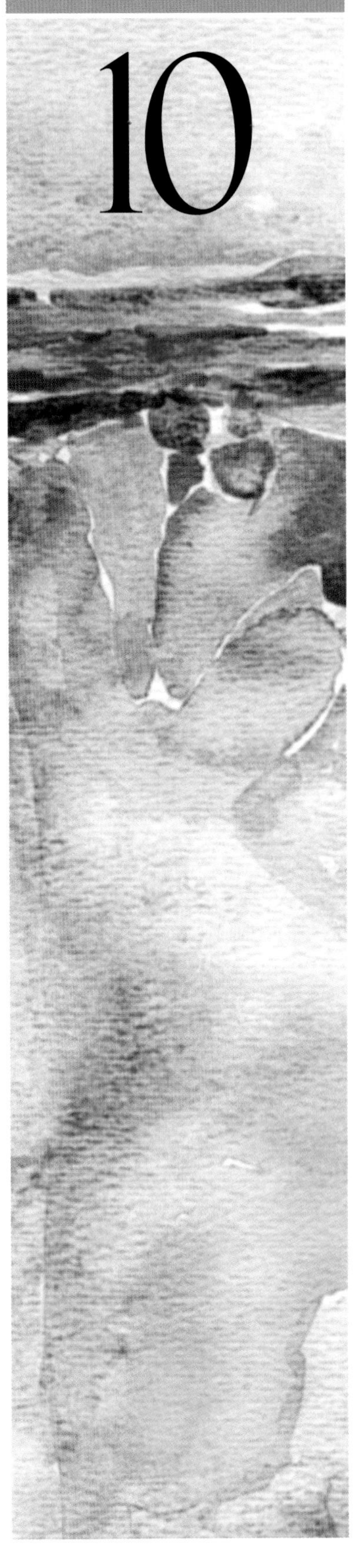

Reactions occuring after a skin rejuvenation procedure can be divided into 3 types: 1) immediate reactions (1 to 14 days after the procedure), which are further subdivided into a) immediate anticipated reactions and b) immediate unanticipated reactions; 2) reactions during recovery (2 to 6 weeks after the procedure); and 3) reactions remaining after recovery (3 to 10 weeks after the procedure) (Table 10-1).

Table 10.1

POSSIBLE REACTIONS FOLLOWING REJUVENATION PROCEDURES AND THE STAGE OF OCCURRENCE

Immediate (1–14 days after procedure)		*Recovery (2–6 weeks after procedure)*	*Delayed (3–10 weeks after procedure)*
Anticipated Reactions	***Unanticipated Reactions***	***Anticipated Reactions***	***Unanticipated Reactions/Complications***
Edema	Herpes simplex eruption	Erythema	Hypertrophic reactions/keloids
Erythema	Infection	Postinflammatory hyperpigmentation (PIH)	Scars
Darkening	Allergic reactions	Acne flare-up	Hypopigmentation/ depigmentation sharp demarcation lines
Oozing	Irritation	Milia	Ectropion
Scabbing	Premature skin separation	Demarcation lines	
		Large pores	
		Marbleization	
		Persistent skin sensitivity	

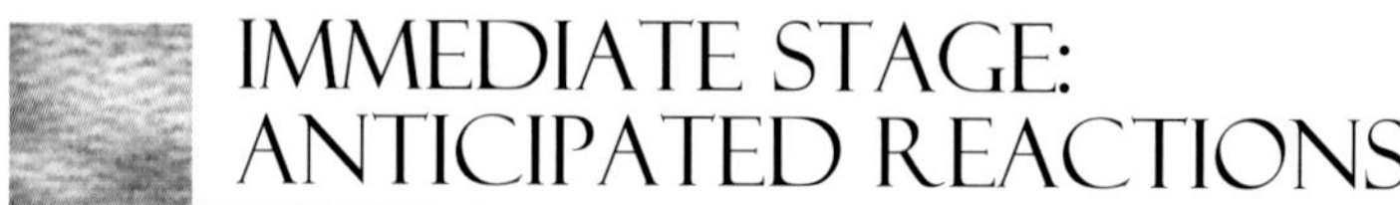

IMMEDIATE STAGE: ANTICIPATED REACTIONS

EDEMA

Edema is mild following procedures that reach the papillary dermis and stronger after procedures reaching the reticular dermis. It appears within 24 hours, peaks by the third day, and disapppears by the fifth day. The extent of edema varies with each patient. Generally it is more extensive in thin and lax skin and after deeper procedures. In rare cases, it can extend to the neck and upper chest, and the patient's eyes may seal shut. The edema generally does not cause laryngeal symptoms or any other systemic reaction or cause pain.

Edema does not have to be treated. If the physician desires, 10 mg of Decadron can be administered intravenously during the procedure followed by a Medrol dose-pack for 5 days on a tapering schedule (6 mg orally first day, 5 mg the next day, etc.) following the procedure to minimize edema. Alternatively, oral prednisone can be used for 7 days, starting with 60 mg the morning after the procedure, tapered daily to 50 mg, 40 mg, 30 mg, 20 mg, 10 mg, and ending with 5 mg. Edema cannot be prevented, even with oral steroids, but the swelling can be reduced and the patient made more comfortable. Cold, dry compresses, started early and applied gently over the eyes, may help reduce eyelid swelling.

REDNESS

CO_2 laser resurfacing, erbium laser resurfacing, and dermabrasion remove surface layers of the skin and expose the dermis. This produces intense redness immediately after the procedure that disappears in 7 to 10 days but is followed by less intense erythema that may last a few months. Chemically peeled skin, on the other hand, may appear slightly red for only 3 to 4 days because the dermis was not exposed as after laser or dermabrasion treatments. After healing, the erythema phase may last a few weeks following a light peel or 1 to 2 months following a deep peel.

DARKENING OF THE SKIN SURFACE

In contrast with CO_2 laser resurfacing and dermabrasion, which leave exposed pink dermis, TCA peels leave treated skin on the face as a natural dressing that gradually separates and peels off. After chemical peeling with TCA or glycolic acid, the treated surface layers of the skin become darker (after a TCA peel it may appear like a dark mask), and later separate and begin to peel away. Separation and peeling begin by the third day, accelerate by the fifth or sixth day, and are completed in 7 to 14 days, revealing pinkish and smooth skin.

OOZING

Serum fluid exudate will immediately begin to ooze from the skin after a procedure that reached the IRD or below into the reticular dermis and will last 3 to 4 days. To prevent infection and the formation of thick scabs and crusts, oozing fluid must be removed through gentle washing or patting with antiseptic solution, such as Domebro. Scabs consist of oozing fluid and dead surface skin and can appear thin and translucent like cellophane after exfoliation and papillary dermis procedures or be quite thick after deeper procedures.

SCABBING

Scab thinning should be performed after chemical peel or dermabrasion procedures to decrease the chances of infection. The scab surface is to be brushed gently with gauze saturated with antiseptic solution or Cetaphil lotion cleanser, 2 to 3 times daily, until healing has occurred. Gentle brushing should be encouraged, and the scabs should not be forced off. The skin surface should be free of scabs 10 days after the procedure. Scab thinning, however, is not permitted after laser resurfacing; heavy lubrication and washing are done instead.

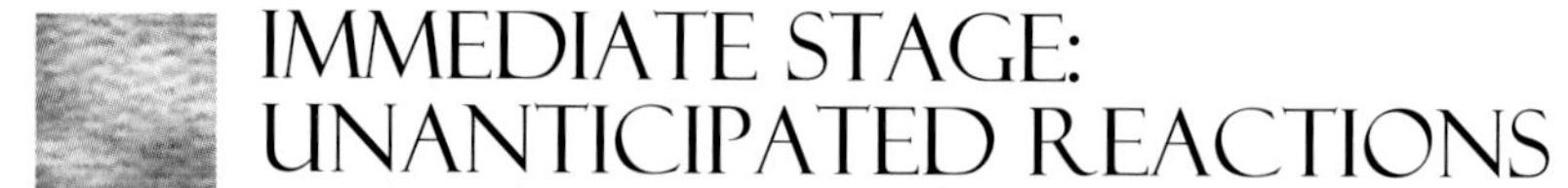

IMMEDIATE STAGE: UNANTICIPATED REACTIONS

HERPES SIMPLEX INFECTION

In patients with a positive history of Herpes simplex labialis or even genital Herpes, every precaution needs to be taken to prevent the activation of the Herpes virus and its appearance on the treated skin area after a procedure. Prophylactic treatment should start before any rejuvenation procedure and before fat or collagen injections in labial areas.

Herpes simplex virus spreads rapidly on deepithelialized, wet skin, especially during the first 7 days after a procedure. Patients can often predict the onset approximately 24 hours before the actual eruption with prodromal symptoms that include itching, slight tenderness, or ache in an area of previous eruption. This is followed by the formation of vesicles that contain infectious virus. The vesicles turn crusty and heal in approximately 7 to 10 days. The labial eruption is usually only slightly painful and, unless it is a primary eruption of the virus, does not cause systemic symptoms. However, a disseminated infection in which vesicular lesions erupt over the entire peeled area is painful, can happen very quickly, and has the potential for leaving scars. Patients must be instructed to notify the physician immediately and return to the office for examination if prodromal symptoms signaling the onset of an outbreak occur or if they experience any unusual pain 3 to 4 days after the peel. The author's treatment plans are shown in Tables 10-2 and 10-3. Figure 10-1 is an example of Herpes simplex labialis after a peel. Figure 10-2 is an example of disseminated Herpes simplex after laser resurfacing.

BACTERIAL INFECTION

Bacterial infections after procedures are rare if the patient follows the home-care instructions. However, patients with poor hygiene, diabetes,

TABLE 10.2

HERPES SIMPLEX PROPHYLAXIS TAILORED TO PATIENT HISTORY

	Low-Risk Patients	*Medium-Risk Patients*	*High-Risk Patients*
Number of occurrences/year	1 or less per year	2 to 3 per year	>3 per year
Prophylaxis	Famvir (famciclovir), 500 mg bid or Zovirax (acyclovir), 400 mg tid or Valtrex (valacyclovir), 400 mg bid started day before procedure and continued for 10 days	Same agents as for low-risk group but started 1 week before the procedure	Same agents as for low-risk group but started 3 months before the procedure. Perform procedure while patient is on the treatment

Table 10.3

TREATMENT OF HERPES SIMPLEX INFECTION

General	Allow skin to dry. Avoid ointments and moisturizers.
Compresses	2% to 5% acetic acid applied with change of gauze after each contact with skin
Antiviral ointment	5% Zovirax ointment or 1% Denavir (penciclovir) cream applied 4–5 times daily to lesions only. Discontinue after all lesions have cleared
Severe cases	May require hospitalization for intravenous antiviral administration

a depressed immune system, and those who are poorly compliant are at risk for infection. Pain is the hallmark. The infected areas have tender, macerated patches with a purulent exudate. Systemic symptoms of fever and chills may develop. Obtain a culture and start a broad-spectrum antibiotic, such as Cipro, Duracef, or Keflex. Allow the infected area to dry up by avoiding lubrication, and immediately start application of antiseptic compresses 3 or 4 times daily. Also have the patient apply topical antibiotic cream (not ointment), such as Bactroban. Bacterial infections usually respond quickly to treatment. Fungal and yeast infections are rare but can occur, especially in women with a previous history of yeast infection. Treat these with Fluconazole tablets 200 mg daily on the first day

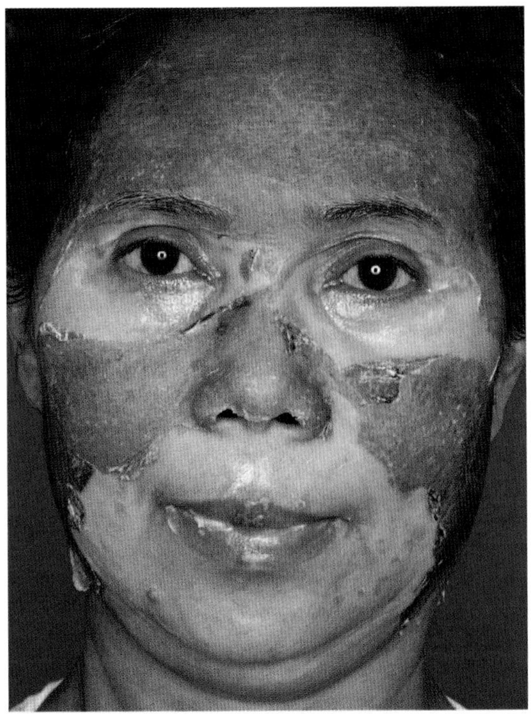

Figure 10-1. *Herpes simplex infection 5 days after a peel procedure.*

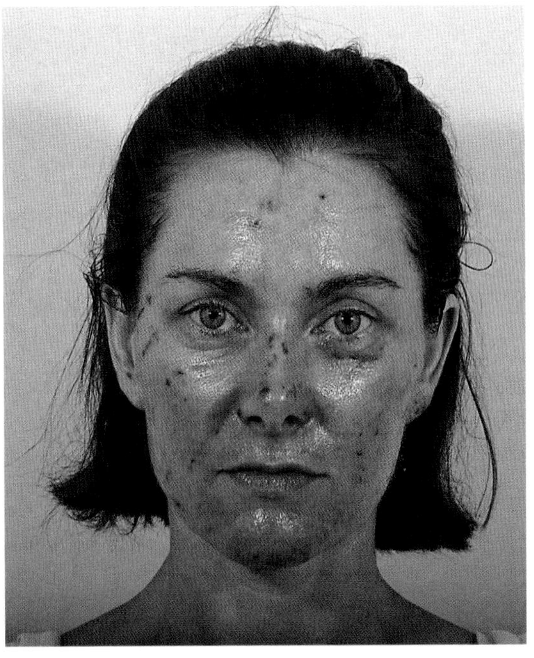

Figure 10-2. *Disseminated Herpes simplex following a peel procedure.*

followed by 100 mg daily for the next 2 weeks. Compresses, as described above, are also advised. After the infection has cleared, lubrication can be resumed. Figure 10-3 is a good example of a case of bacterial infection after laser resurfacing with permanent depigmentation and transient postinflammatory hyperpigmentation.

ALLERGIC REACTIONS

Allergic reactions are rare during the initial healing stage and can be resolved quickly with proper treatment. These reactions are signaled by the appearance of swelling, itching, and erythema in the treated areas and the surrounding skin. The simplest topical agents not containing an antimicrobial agent, such as Aquaphor, petroleum jelly, and K-Y jelly, are preferred since some topical antibiotics are highly allergenic. Treatment of allergic reactions can include use of Medrol dose pack or another form of systemic steroid, oral antihistamines, and allowing the skin to dry up for 24 hours. Once the reaction has cleared, lubrication with a bland ointment can be resumed.

IRRITATION

Irritation of the skin surface after a procedure is common and is usually caused by excessive skin manipulation, such as rubbing, overzealous washing, or scratching before the skin has reepithelialized (the first 7 days). Af-

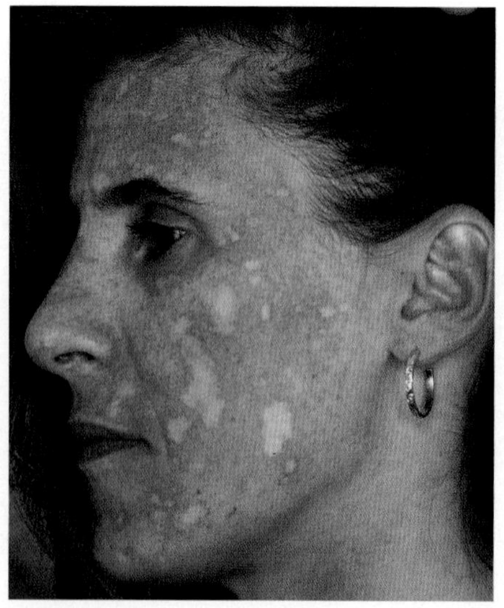
a

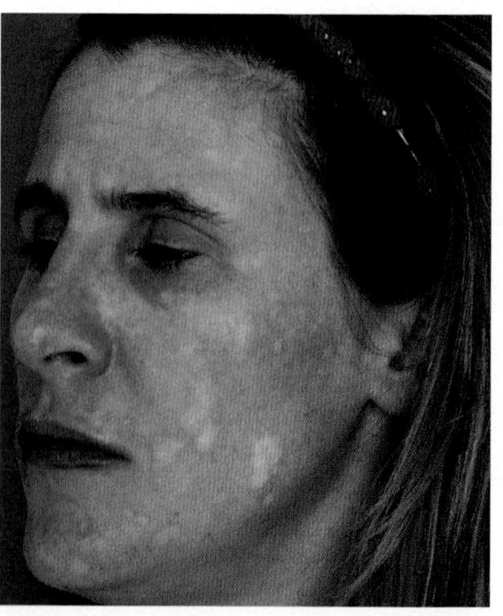
b

FIGURE 10-3. *(a) Postinflammatory hyperpigmentation and depigmentation, complicated by bacterial infection, following CO_2 laser resurfacing. (b) Improvement in same patient after 2 months of treatment with Skin Conditioning for correction and stimulation followed by a Blue Peel.*

ter a chemical peel, irritation can also be caused by excessive moisturization, scab maceration, and early skin separation. Irritation involves only the treated area and, unlike allergic reactions, does not affect the surrounding skin. Symptoms consist of burning, redness, and discomfort. Treatment involves more gentle handling of skin, use of antiseptic compresses, and keeping the skin dry for 24 hours. Home care, including keeping the skin not too dry and not too moist, can then be resumed.

PREMATURE SKIN SEPARATION

Premature skin separation can occur only after a chemical peel because the peeled surface areas remain and separate slowly and progressively as skin is reepithelializing. The gradual skin separation is advantageous in that old, peeled skin acts as a natural dressing, providing comfort and allowing reepithelialization to proceed smoothly. However, if the old skin is lifted off before reepithelialization is complete, a raw, unepithelialized, sensitive surface becomes exposed. This can follow excessively vigorous washing of highly moisturized skin or by the patient's allowing water to run on the skin for a long time during showering. Premature skin separation is associated with significant pain and extreme tightness, but it is not harmful to the skin and does not affect the outcome. However, the patient may be frightened by the occurrence. Immediate treatment consists of a heavy application of a bland ointment and a prescription for oral pain medication.

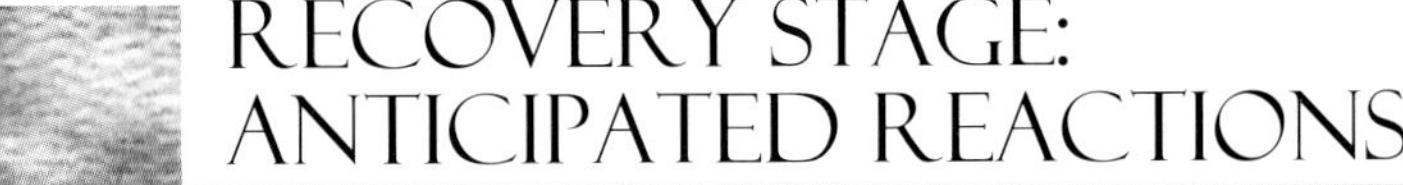

RECOVERY STAGE: ANTICIPATED REACTIONS

ERYTHEMA

Erythema (redness) after healing can be uniform, so that the skin is smooth and has normal texture, or it can be uneven (blotchy), with the redder areas usually indicating deeper penetration. Erythema is stronger and of longer duration in procedures deeper than the immediate reticular dermis (IRD), especially in light-colored skin and after CO_2 laser resurfacing. Localized areas of intense erythema with roughness or gradually increasing thickness could signify keloid formation. Uniform erythema is common, especially in White and Deviated Dark skin types, and is not a complication. Erythema is usually mild and disappears after 1 week after a Blue Peel to the IRD, is rare after a papillary dermis Blue Peel, and may last 4 to 6 weeks after a medium-depth Blue Peel. Following a deep peel or CO_2 laser resurfacing in Very Light White or Light White skin, erythema may last up to 6 months. The duration and intensity of redness ranked according to occurrence after certain procedures are as follows: CO_2 laser resurfacing > dermabrasion > phenol peel > medium-depth TCA peel > Blue Peel > glycolic acid peel.

Some patients may find that the redness increases upon bending, exercise, or drinking wine. This is usually a vascular phenomenon that diminishes with time without treatment. Use of AHA products in concentrations higher than 4% should be avoided for 3 weeks after deeper procedures or CO_2 laser resurfacing since these agents strip the stratum corneum and may worsen and prolong the erythema.

Uneven redness (blotchy color) is more likely to occur after combined procedures since these achieve a variable depth. Erythema may be longer lasting in fair or thin skin and in individuals who previously have had CO_2 laser resurfacing, phenol peel, or dermabrasion. Fissuring, cracking, picking, or rubbing of scabs after a procedure can produce more intense, localized erythema. Patients with severe solar elastosis may exhibit intense, blotchy erythema mingled with less erythematous or normal-appearing areas, which the author calls *marbleization*. This is due to uneven penetration or an uneven response to the procedure.

Treatment of Erythema

When the severity of erythema is mild, it can be left untreated, or 0.5% to 1.0% nonfluorinated hydrocortisone can be used for 1 week and then repeated 2 to 3 times in an off-and-on cycle. Stimulation with topical tretinoin cream is preferred, which can increase the intensity of erythema initially but should shorten the duration. Sunscreen should be used as well as moisturizer if there is dryness. For severe erythema and significant, uneven redness, treatment with a florinated topical steroid (e.g., Temovate) for 1 week, stopping for 1 week, and repeating the off-on schedule 2 to 3 times may help while the patient is using tretinoin. Occasionally, in patients who have severely photodamaged skin and irregular redness (marbleization) that is not responding to the above-mentioned topical creams, it may be necessary to perform a Blue Peel with Design to even out the blotchiness. Do not repeat CO_2 laser resurfacing in hopes of treating irregular erythema because the skin may not tolerate the effects of additional thermal damage. In severe cases, topical vitamin C, oral beta carotene, and oral ginko biloba tablets can be helpful.

Box 10-1

Postprocedure erythema may be prolonged in certain cases, but it eventually disappears and is never permanent.

Uneven pigmentation and postinflammatory hyperpigmentation (PIH) are the result of temporary melanocytic hyperactivity following skin injury from any procedure that reaches the papillary dermis or below. PIH is usually limited to the epidermis, but the dermis may be involved on rare occasions. Occurrence increases with deeper procedures and in patients with Deviated skin color. Sun exposure without sunscreen protection soon after the procedure worsens the condition. PIH can also result from complications, such as irritation, allergic reaction, or infection during the healing stage.

PIH can last 2 to 3 weeks after light procedures and 4 to 6 months after deeper procedures, but with vigorous early treatment (bleaching and blending), it can resolve completely in 2 to 6 weeks. Use of the Obagi Skin Conditioning principles before and after the procedure also helps to reduce both the incidence and severity of PIH. Repeated standard Blue Peels to blend skin color and any demarcation lines can be performed if topical treatment does not restore an even skin tone. Excessive skin oiliness can reduce the effectiveness of topical agents used for Skin Conditioning. In difficult cases, reduction of sebum, possibly with the use of isotretinoin (Accutane) for 2 to 3 weeks, may be necessary. Figure 10-4 shows PIH after a facelift. Figure 10-5 shows PIH after laser resurfacing.

ACNE FLARE-UP

Patients with oily or thick skin and those who are acne prone may have a flare-up of cystic or comedogenic acne, usually 2 to 4 weeks after healing, but, in rare cases, it may begin as early as 4 to 5 days after the procedure.

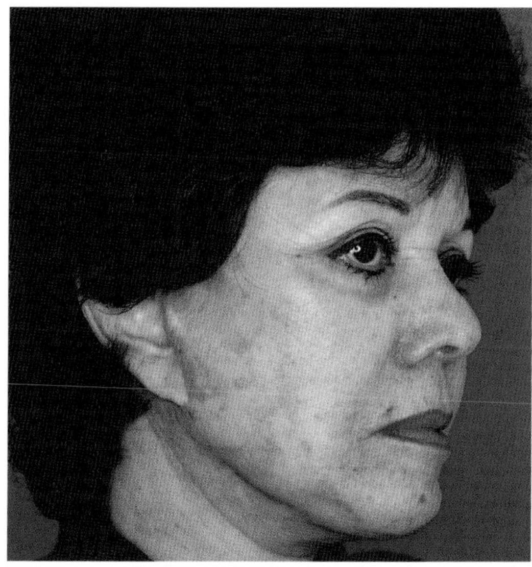

FIGURE 10-4. *Postinflammatory hyperpigmentation following a facelift.*

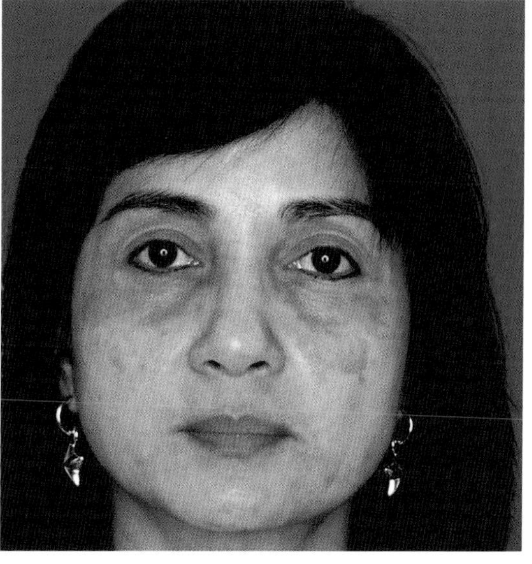

FIGURE 10-5. *Postinflammatory hyperpigmentation following CO_2 laser resurfacing.*

Large, inflamed cysts should be injected with 2 mg/cc of Kenalog. Topical ointment or moisturizer may be applied lightly when needed for comfort, but the skin should be kept somewhat dry in the healing stage. Acne flare-ups can be minimized or prevented by conditioning the skin before and immediately after healing and, if necessary, by using topical and systemic antibiotics in acne-prone individuals. Patients with a history of active acne can be given a 7- to 10-day course of oral antibiotics, such as Dynacin 50 mg twice daily, erythromycin, Keflex, or Cipro, before the procedure and continued until the acne is no longer active. If necessary, a 4- to 5-month course of isotretinoin (Accutane) can be prescribed for patients who are to have a peel not exceeding the papillary dermis. If the acne is severe, Accutane can also be started 3 weeks after the procedure. The author has performed many peels, even to the IRD level, in patients taking Accutane prior to the procedure without any ill effects. However, for procedures penetrating below the IRD, Accutane should be discontinued for 6 to 8 months.

MILIA

The author believes that milia are caused by excessive reepithelialization that leads to pore closure and accumulation of sebum and keratin or by the excessive oil produced by some patients with oily skin. Milia are more common in procedures reaching below the IRD. If not treated, milia can persist 3 to 4 months or longer and be quite problematic. Treatment consists of mechanical removal with a number 11 blade or comedone extractor, light hypercation with an epilating needle, and the use of tretinoin.

DEMARCATION LINES

Demarcation lines are the result of no feathering or improper feathering between treated and untreated areas during a procedure, especially in procedures that reach below the IRD. They can be prevented by learning proper feathering technique. One combination treatment that prevents demarcation is to perform a CO_2 laser procedure for resurfacing the face combined with the Blue Peel for resurfacing the neck. Demarcation lines can be treated by performing a second procedure (exfoliation or a light procedure) to even out abrupt changes in treated and untreated areas. One or more Blue Peels to the papillary dermis may be needed for correction. During these peels, special attention should be given to the process of feathering. The peel should reach the IRD on the dark edge of the demarcation line, and progressively lighter depth proceeding away from the line, ending with an exfoliation 3 to 4 inches away from the line. Demarcation lines can also be treated by aggressive skin conditioning with aggressive bleaching, blending, and stimulation extending beyond the treated areas. Figure 10-6 is a good example of the demarcation lines.

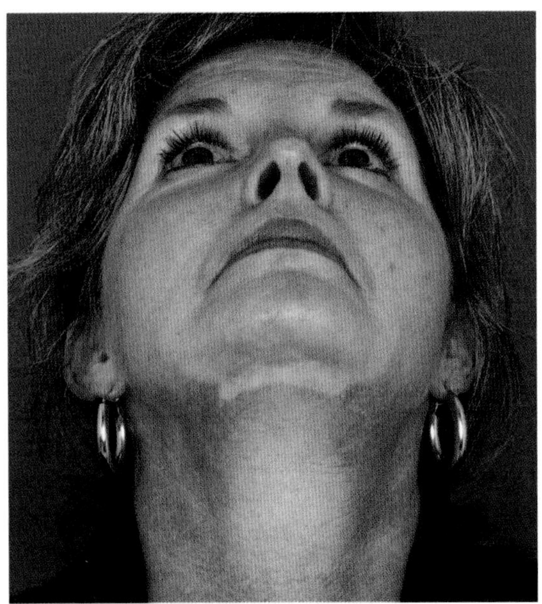

FIGURE 10-6. *Demarcation lines after CO_2 laser resurfacing.*

LARGE PORES

In individuals with thick skin, enlarged pores, sebaceous gland hyperplasia, acne vulgaris, or excessive oiliness, pores may appear larger 3 or 4 weeks after healing following a procedure reaching below the IRD. The pores will return to normal size in 6 to 10 weeks after elastin and collagen are newly formed. However, after certain procedures, such as a phenol peel, dermabrasion, CO_2 laser resurfacing or a medium-depth peel, a mild degree of fibrosis surrounding the hair follicle in the vicinity of the papillary dermis can prevent the restoration of elastic tissue in that area and lead to the appearance of enlarged pores. Loss of elastin in the papillary and upper reticular dermis, as seen in aging, is also responsible for the appearance of enlarged pores. No available treatment is completely effective, but a few cycles of Skin Conditioning with aggressive stimulation may increase the production of elastin in the papillary dermis and soften the fibrotic tissue to induce the desired pore tightening. A Blue Peel to the papillary dermis level can be helpful, repeated 2 to 3 times every 4 to 6 weeks, if needed. For large pores that are a result of sebaceous gland hyperplasia and excessive skin oiliness, 3 to 5 months of isotretinoin (Accutane) treatment added to the Skin Conditioning or Skin Health Restoration programs is quite beneficial.

MARBLEIZATION

Marbleization, a term coined by the author to describe the uneven response of skin to an evenly performed procedure, may be seen following a medium-depth peel, dermabrasion, or CO_2 laser resurfacing of severely photodamaged skin with severe solar elastosis or skin with deep, fibrotic scars. Certain areas of damaged skin do not frost equally after a TCA peel or evaporate properly even after extra passes with the CO_2 laser. After healing, certain areas that appear as if they were not peeled or lasered may be mingled with areas that responded well to treatment and and appear red and smooth. The poorly responding areas may represent very dense, damaged elastin or severely fibrotic tissue that did not react with the acid or the laser treatment. Further peeling or lasering may be needed. In most cases, aggressive use of tretinoin for stimulation tends to reduce the differences in appearance within 3 to 4 months. The occurrence of marbleization can be minimized by a longer and more aggressive Skin Conditioning program prior to the procedure. Figure 10-7 is a good example of marbleization.

PERSISTENT SKIN SENSITIVITY

After a procedure reaching the upper reticular or mid dermis in persons with thin, dry, fragile skin or skin poor in adnexal structures, skin may become intolerant to external factors and topical treatments. This state of extreme sensitivity can last from weeks to months and is often accompanied by severe erythema. Multiple factors are probably at fault, including poor skin circulation, defective keratinization, an excessively deep procedure in a thin skin, inadequate adnexal structures, or a defective skin barrier function. The author has had success in treating such patients by gradually building skin tolerance and improving the skin's barrier function through a program of stimulation with tretinoin (see Chapter 5) that usually takes 2 to 3 months. Topical steroids should generally not be used in these cases for they thin the epidermis, increase skin fragility, and further weaken the barrier function. However, they can be used occasionally to reduce the reaction to tretinoin.

PERSISTENT ERYTHEMA

Erythema is quite common after deeper procedures reaching below the IRD or mid dermis. It is more severe and prolonged in patients with thin, dry, or severely sun-damaged skin. Persistent erythema is that which lasts for 6 months to 1 year. The cause is not known, but the author believes a defect in keratinization that leads to a weak barrier function (as discussed in the previous section) is at fault. Persistent erythema is difficult to treat, and long-term steroid treatment should be avoided. The author has been successful in certain situations by correcting the keratinization defect and building up skin tolerance gradually using the principles of correction and stimulation.

The treatment can be compared to "treating fire with fire." Tretinoin is used in gradually increasing concentration, amount, and frequency of application to which the patient's skin initially responds with more severe erythema and sensitivity. Occasional use of a mild steroid and mois-

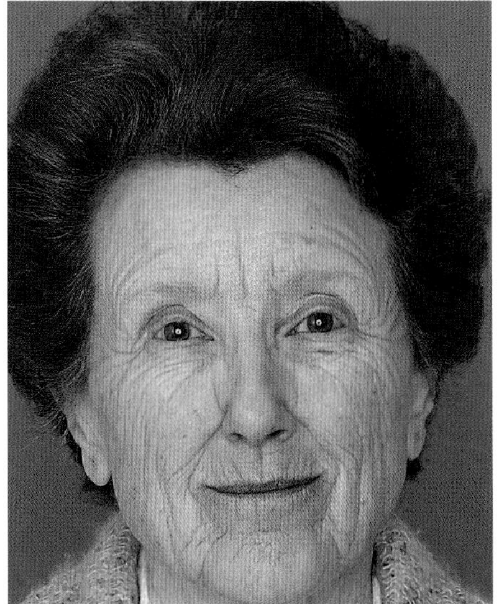

a

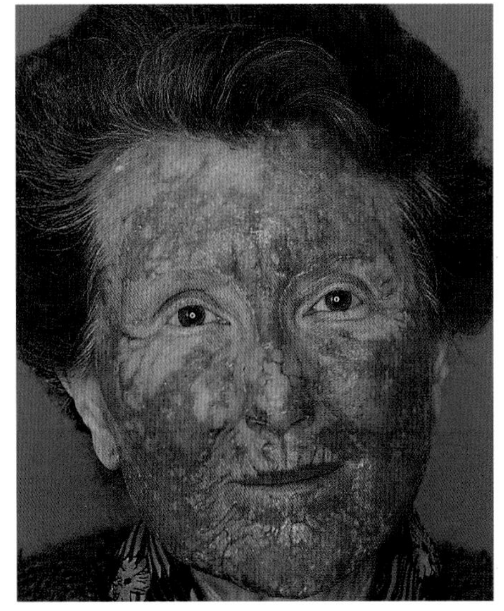

b

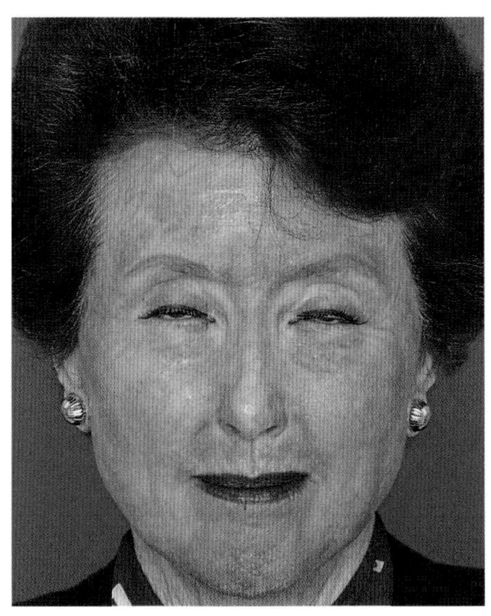

c

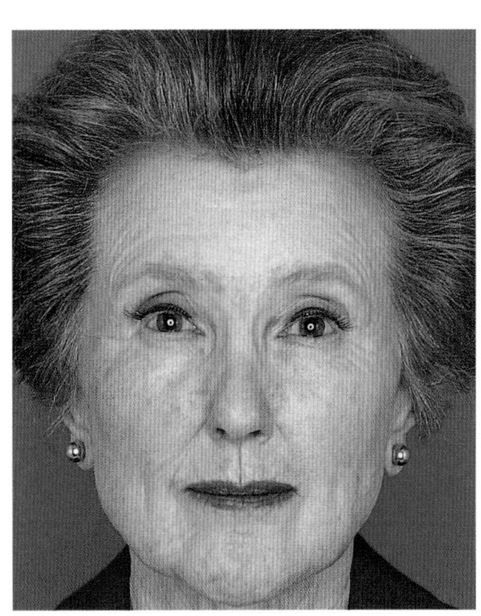

d

FIGURE 10-7. *Marbleization. (a) Before—Patient with White skin, solar elastosis, and laxity. (b) Marbleization phenomenon 10 days after a medium Controlled-Depth TCA Peel. Damaged elastic tissue led to uneven uptake of TCA; deeper red areas indicate proper depth level. Periorbital area where penetration was to papillary dermis level shows good healing. (c) Gradual resolution of marbleization 4 weeks after the Controlled-Depth Peel. Treatment consisted of correction and stimulation with creams. (d) Marbleization was completely resolved by 6 months. Photo shows patient at 1 year.*

turizers for 1 to 2 days is allowed with decreasing frequency. This should continue until natural skin tolerance has been restored, which may take 5 to 6 months. Short-lived hypersensitivity, on the other hand, is common in all skin types after a procedure. It is characterized by poor tolerance of skin products, sun exposure, or changing temperature for 1 to 2 weeks. This may occur with or without erythema and is treated in the same manner.

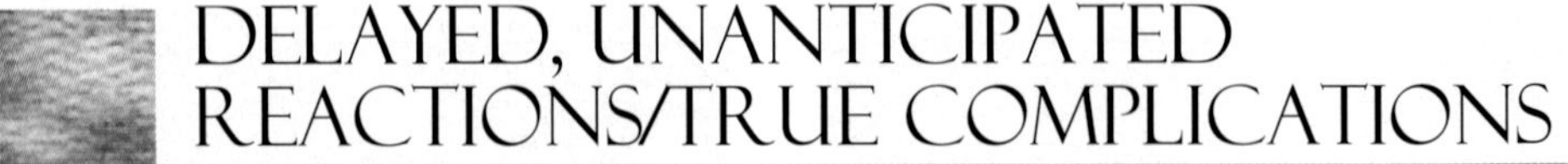

DELAYED, UNANTICIPATED REACTIONS/TRUE COMPLICATIONS

Unlike the immediate, anticipated reactions that appear early, are temporary, and resolve spontaneously, delayed, unanticipated reactions are true complications that appear later and may be permanent. The more common complications in this category are hypertrophic reactions, keloids, hypopigmentation/depigmentation, and ectropion.

HYPERTROPHIC REACTIONS AND KELOIDS

Hypertrophic Reactions

Hypertrophic reactions are distinct from hypertrophic scars or keloids. They are erythematous, firm areas of thickened skin that can be flat or raised; appear in patches, streaks, or cobblestones; and may be pruritic. Hypertrophic areas are usually well demarcated, do not expand to adjacent normal skin, and have limited growth. The most susceptible areas are the upper lip, cheeks, and lower eyelids, especially in areas peeled or resurfaced below the IRD. Areas with long-standing crusts or cracks, areas that the patient has picked or peeled, and previously infected areas are also at risk. Hypertrophic reactions can usually be detected 2 to 3 weeks after healing. The area may or may not appear erythematous. Pinching the involved skin reveals texture fuller than that of the surrounding skin. Under a magnifier, the areas appear as rough, pearly patches with fine, raised threads or papules.

Hypertrophic reactions can sometimes resolve slowly without treatment, but resolution can occur faster with use of injected or topical steroids. A potent steroid cream, such as Temovate (clobetasol, Glaxo-Wellcome, Inc.), should be liberally applied twice daily with massage as soon as the reaction has been identified. Fluradrenolide (Cordran, Oclassen Pharmaceuticals) transparent tape, applied at bedtime, releases a steady dose of steroid that can help in rapid resolution. Intralesional injection of steroid (Kenalog, 10 mg/cc) into the stroma of the thickened areas is helpful, but an effort should be made to avoid injecting into normal skin and causing atrophy. FLPD laser treatment combined with topical steroid may also be

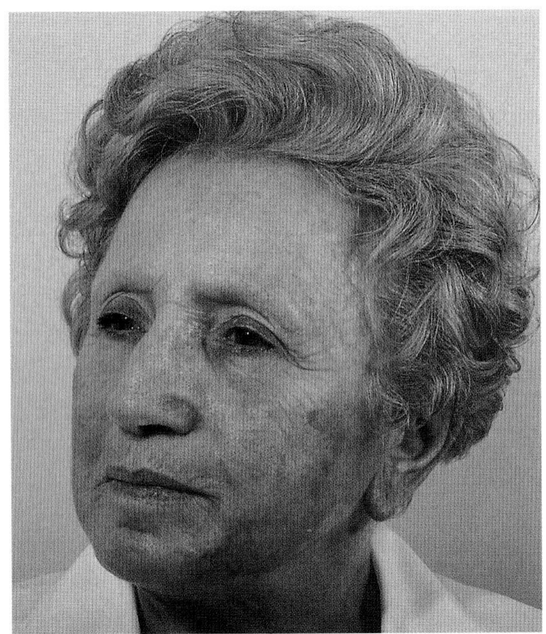

FIGURE 10-8. *Hypertrophic reaction on the chin after a medium Controlled-Depth TCA Peel.*

effective. The laser treatment should be performed 2 weeks apart from the steroid injection because the heat of the laser inactivates the steroid. With proper treatment, hypertrophic reactions usually disappear quickly without residual scarring (Figure 10-8).

Keloids

Keloids (hypertrophic scars) should be suspected in areas showing localized thickening and persistent erythema after a procedure. The affected areas thicken quickly to produce a tumor-like growth that extends to normal skin. Deformity and retraction of surrounding skin are often seen, and symptoms of redness, itching, and pain are common. Keloids are more likely to form after a medium-deep to deep procedure in the upper lip area, jawline, shoulders, back, and chest, and in individuals with fragile skin. The author has never seen a keloid forming after a papillary dermis or IRD-level peel. Race is a factor since the rate of keloid formation is much higher in Blacks and Asians (5% to 10%) than in Whites with light skin (1% to 2%). Those with fragile or thin skin, as well as those with a history of poor healing or keloid formation, are also more susceptible. Infection, cracking, or patient picking of scabs during the healing phase also increase the chance of keloid formation.

Treatment of keloids should begin as soon as possible and be very aggressive. Intralesional injection of steroid (Kenalog, 10 mg/cc) into the stroma of the thickened areas is the primary initial therapy, repeated every 3 to 4 weeks. The keloids should be covered with silicon gel sheeting as much as possible in the early stages. If keloid growth is not curbed with

Box 10-2

Any localized, persistent erythema should be considered a sign of keloid unless proven otherwise.

the first Kenalog injection, switch to Aristopan (triamcinolone) 20 mg/ml, diluted to 10 mg/ml or, in severe cases, undiluted. However, care must be taken when injecting Aristopan, for it is a very potent steroid that can cause skin atrophy. Injection of 0.5 ml to 1 ml in a lesion every 4 to 6 weeks is the maximum. Alternating Aristopan with Kenalog is helpful in cases of large keloids. Follow the patient at frequent intervals for injections. Assign a number to each keloid or segment of a keloid, and inject each one on alternate weeks. For example, inject keloids 1, 3, and 5 at one session and keloids 2, 4, and 6 at another session 1 week later. Do not inject more than 1 ml of Aristopan at 1 session.

Alternative Treatments: For early-growing keloids, Intron A (interferon alfa-2b recombinant), a water-soluble protein that exerts its activity by binding to specific receptors on the cell surface, is an alternative treatment. The intracellular events that follow binding include enzyme induction, suppression of cell proliferation, immunomodulating activities, and inhibition of virus replication in virus-infected cells. A dose of 1 million international units (IU) is to be injected intralesionally in 1 treatment, repeated 3 times weekly, not to exceed a total of 5 million IU per week. Both Intron and intralesional steroids can be used to treat the same keloids, with the steroid injected once every 3 to 6 weeks and Intron 3 times each week. However, based on the author's personal experience, Intron should not be injected 3 days before or 3 days after steroid injections.

Treatment with the FLDP laser at a frequency of once every 4 to 6 weeks is helpful in shrinking the keloid, eliminating the redness, and improving the surface texture. Compresses of silicon gel sheeting (topiGel or Sil-K), applied daily for 12 hours, can be helpful. This treatment is based on the assumption that occlusion suppresses the action of fibroblasts, but the exact mechanism has not been defined (Figure 10-9).

SCARS

Scarring (total thickness slough) is very rare, occurring only after deep, poorly controlled procedures, such as deep chemical peels, dermabrasion, or CO_2 laser resurfacing, or when such deep procedures are performed on the flap of a facelift at the same time. They can also occur after a severe infection during the healing stage. Some sloughing scars that appear as small indentations or shallow lines can be corrected after a few months by repeated resurfacing, a spot peel, or a repeat peel.

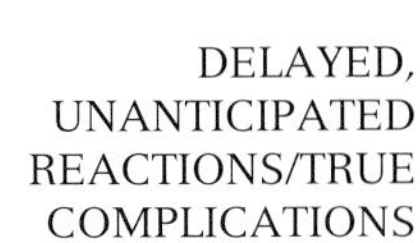

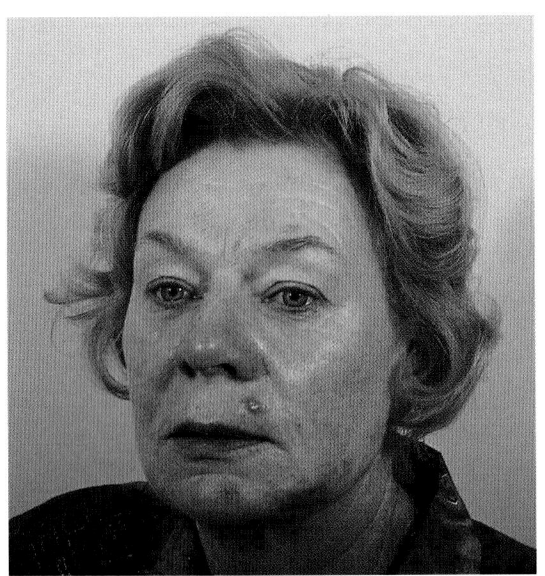

FIGURE 10-9. *Keloid on the upper lip, chin, and jawline after a medium Controlled-Depth TCA Peel that resolved after treatment with steroid injections and FLDP laser treatment.*

HYPOPIGMENTATION AND DEPIGMENTATION

Hypopigmentation is caused by dysfunction of or a reduced number of functioning melanocytes. The likelihood of occurrence is correlated with the type and depth of the procedure. For example, it is common after a phenol peel and deep procedures such as CO_2 laser resurfacing, dermabrasion, or medium to deep TCA peels. Patients with severe photodamage, thin or fragile skin, or skin that had previously been treated with dermabrasion or phenol peeling are more susceptible.

In the author's experience with medium-depth TCA peels, hypopigmentation improves with time before becoming permanent. Hypopigmentation can sometimes be treated successfully by early aggressive stimulation with tretinoin for 3 to 4 months or psoralen plus UVA light. If these fail, blending and feathering into untreated areas with a papillary dermis-level peel, such as the Blue Peel, may be effective.

Depigmentation (the complete loss of skin color) is caused by total destruction of melanocytes. Very white, sharply demarcated lines or patches, resembling islands surrounded by normally colored skin, appear following deep procedures performed in thin skin, skin poor in adnexal structures, or severely photodamaged skin. It may also appear as a result of infection complicating such procedures. The condition can be treated with epidermal grafts or epidermal and dermal punch grafts, along with aggressive stimulation with tretinoin. Depigmentation of the darker areas surrounding the white skin in order to produce more even coloration can be helpful. If loss of color is severe, Benequin cream (monobenzone 2%) can be used to depigment the dark areas of skin, but it is a cumbersome process, has toxic side effects, and takes a long time to work (Figures 10-10, 10-11, and 10-12).

Box 10-3

PERFORMING THE LID SNAP TEST

With your fingers, press the skin 4 inches below the lower lid and move it upward with a gentle pull in 1/2 inch increments. The point at which the lid margin is pulled down should be noted as the point at which an IRD-level peel should end and a papillary dermis level peel begin.

ECTROPION

Ectropion (eversion of the lower eyelid) is more likely to occur after procedures deeper than the papillary dermis performed on lower eyelids that are already lax (weak snap test). Unintentionally deeper peels or CO_2 laser resurfacing can cause full-thickness injury to the thin and lax skin of the eyelids, resulting in ectropion or scleral show. True ectropion should be distinguished from false ectropion that may appear due to retraction of the lower lid during the swelling and scabbing period after the peel or the early tightness after CO_2 laser resurfacing. To prevent ectropion, the lid snap test should be performed on every patient in order to tailor the depth of the procedure in the eyelid area. True ectropion can be corrected surgically with skin grafts. Mild conditions can be helped by massaging with vitamin E oil for 2 to 3 months (Figure 10-13).

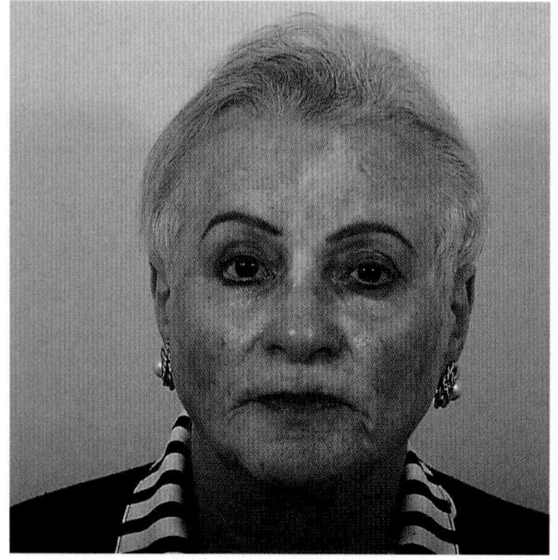

a

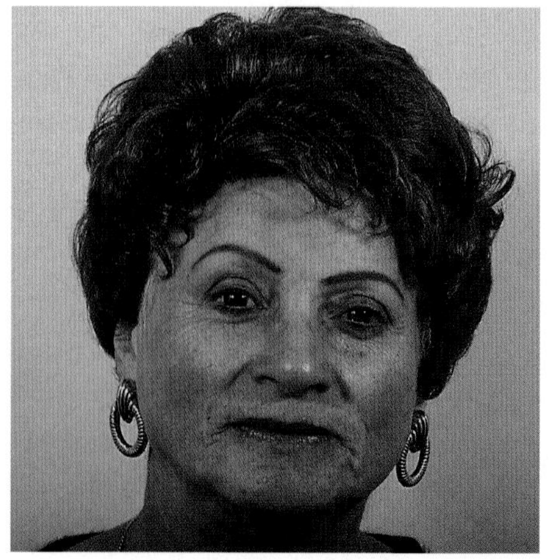

b

FIGURE 10-10. *(a) Hypopigmentation following a Controlled-Depth Peel. (b) Improvement in same patient at 1 year, treated with Skin Conditioning for correction and stimulation.*

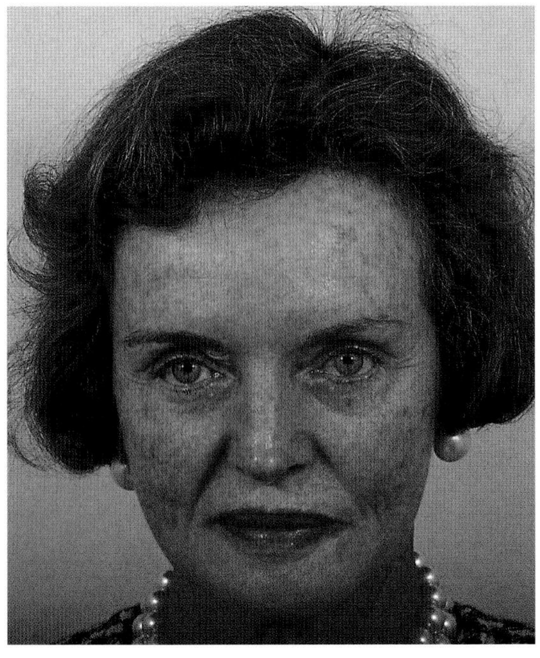

FIGURE 10-11. *Perioral depigmentation following a phenol peel.*

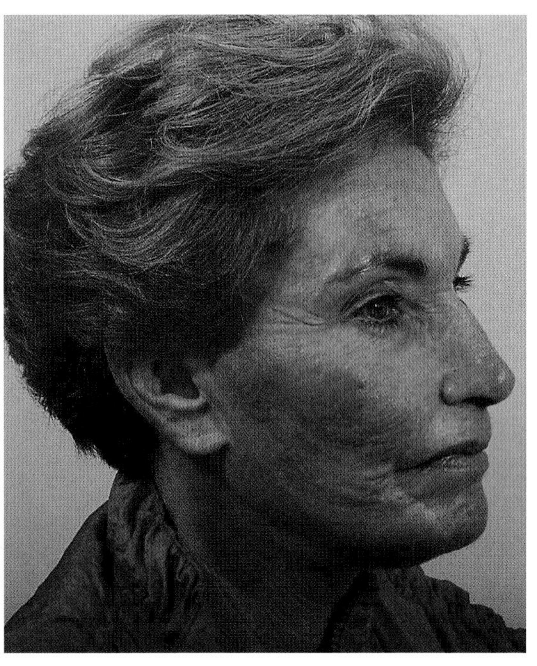

FIGURE 10-12. *Perioral depigmentation following a face-lift and dermabrasion.*

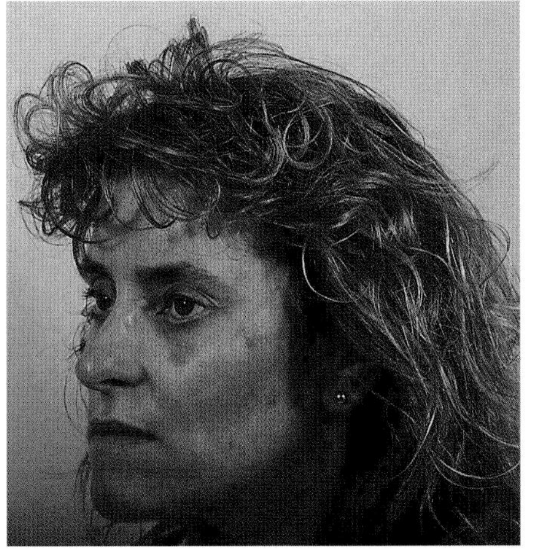

a

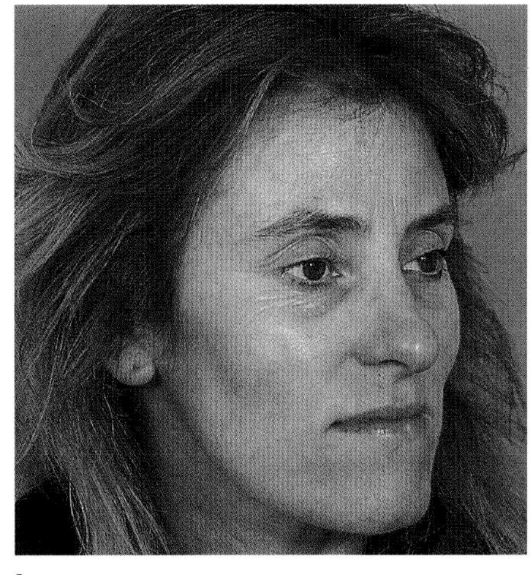

b

FIGURE 10-13. *(a) Hypertrophic reaction and mild ectropion on lower lid after a controlled medium-depth peel complicated by infection that responded to steroid injections. (b) Same patient showing resolution after treatment.*

CHAPTER

11

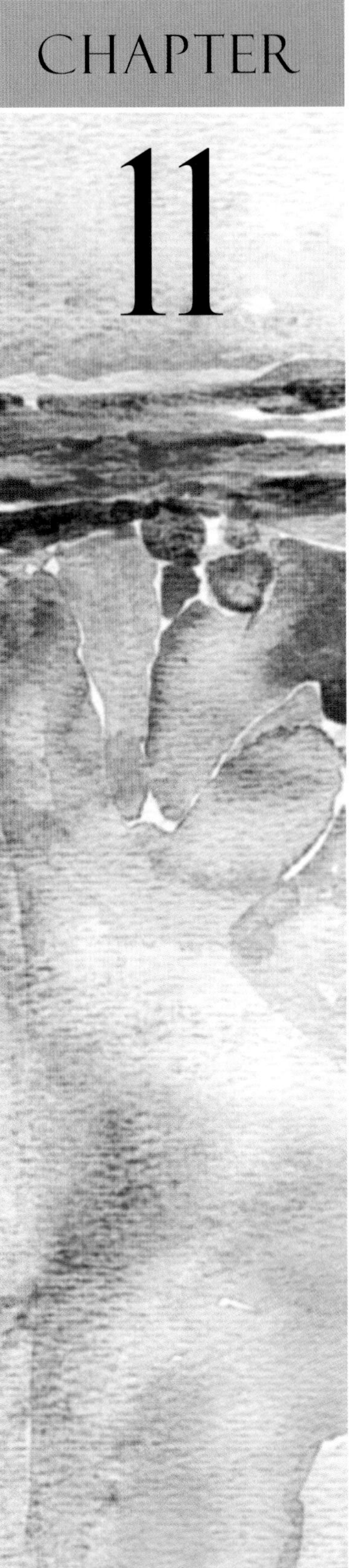

LASER SKIN RESURFACING AND COMBINED PROCEDURES

by Michael B. Stevens, M.D., Ph.D.
Aesthetic Plastic Surgery

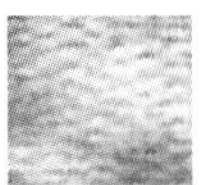

LASER PRINCIPLES

CONTINUOUS WAVE CO_2 LASERS

The carbon dioxide (CO_2) laser, emitting light as a continuous wave, has had a broad range of applications in dermatology and cosmetic surgery due to its ability to vaporize, coagulate, or cut tissue. Used in the focused mode (small spot size), the continuous wave laser delivers a large amount of energy to a small area, allowing it to be used as a cutting tool. The focused beam can incise tissue, coagulate bleeding from small blood vessels, and seal small nerve endings and lymphatics and is particularly useful for incisional surgeries, such as facelifts and blepharoplasties. In the defocused mode, the spot size is larger and power density is decreased, allowing tissue to be ablated and excised without damaging deeper structures. The bloodless field also gives the surgeon better visualization and produces less postoperative bruising and swelling.

Despite the effectiveness of the continuous wave laser for these applications, it has been less than ideal for resurfacing skin to treat acne scarring, actinic keratoses, small skin tumors, and photoaging. These lasers cannot deliver sufficient power density to vaporize target tissue in one pulse, so multiple pulses are needed. This, however, heats surrounding tissues as well as the target tissues and leads to thermal damage of collagen, a zone of tissue necrosis, and an unacceptable incidence of scarring. Thus, demabrasion and chemical peeling continued to be the procedures of choice for skin resurfacing until the development of high-energy, short-pulsed CO_2 lasers with the feature of selective photothermolysis.[1–16] Table 11-1 lists commonly used laser terms and Box 11-1 reviews laser physics fundamentals.

DERMABRASION AND CHEMICAL PEELING

Dermabrasion is a time-honored technique for mechanically removing the epidermis and dermis to improve the appearance of photoaged or acne-scarred skin.[17] In the hands of a skilled physician, the results attained through dermabrasion can match those attained with the new CO_2 lasers in the treatment of acne or traumatic scarring.[18] However, the disadvantages of dermabrasion are numerous, especially in comparison with new laser techniques.

Dermabrasion is highly operator dependent, and expertise is usually acquired only after a fairly long learning curve. Precise control of the der-

TABLE 11.1
LASER TERMINOLOGY

Term	*Definition*
joules (J)	the unit of measure for energy produced by the laser
power	the rate of laser energy delivery; measured in watts (W) (1 watt = 1 J/sec)
power density (irradiance)	power per unit area incident on the skin during a single pulse; expressed as W/cm^2
continuous wave	little variance of power over time
fluence	beam energy density; the energy delivered to the skin per unit area for a specific period of time; expressed as J/cm^2
hertz	delivery rate (pulses per second)

Box 11-1

LASER FUNDAMENTALS

Briefly, a laser functions as follows: The addition of a direct current electricity or radio frequency to the laser medium (CO_2, nitrogen, and helium in the case of the CO_2 laser) shifts atom electron orbits into a higher and less stable state known as an *excited state*. As the excited atoms spontaneously return to a stable state, photons of light are emitted. The reaction is contained within a mirrored tube that allows the photons to be reflected back, stimulating other atoms to a higher energy level. This chain reaction produces an enormous amounts of light energy in a short time. Upon achieving a critical amount of energy, the light is released from the tube as a laser light beam.

When a laser beam strikes tissue, light may be reflected, scattered, transmitted, or absorbed. Reflection is of significance for the patient and the operating room personnel and necessitates the use of protective eyewear, but is negligible regarding tissue effects. Transmission of the laser energy into tissue may occur, depending on the type of laser being used and the tissue upon which the laser is directed. With the CO_2 laser, however, transmission generally is not significant. Scattering also plays a minor role, since CO_2 laser light is highly absorbed by water.

The CO_2 laser's primary clinical effect on skin tissue is absorption. At the wavelength of 10,600 nm, which is in the far infrared region of the electromagnetic spectrum, tissue is rapidly heated, resulting in ablation (vaporization or cutting) and coagulation. The management of a balance between ablation and coagulation—achieved through selective photothermolysis—is the goal of cutaneous laser surgery.[1,2]

mabrasion handpiece can be difficult, and a great deal of skill is needed to achieve equal depth of penetration over the area to be treated. The tissue to be treated is usually made firm by freezing with a topical agent, which can produce cold injury. Lack of technical expertise or overzealous dermabrasion can lead to hypopigmentation and atrophic or hypertrophic scarring.[17,18]

Although some visualization of the desired endpoint (point at which the goal has been reached and the procedure should be terminated) is possible, dermabrasion produces bleeding that may make endpoint determination difficult. Bloodborne viruses, such as HIV, hepatitis B, and hepatitis C can be present in the aerosol formed during the procedure and, theoretically, can be transmitted to operating room personnel or other patients. The dermabrasion equipment should be fitted with splatter shields, and the staff must wear surgical gowns and face shields. Dermabrasion of the very fine lines and wrinkles commonly seen around the eyelids is considered risky and is not advised. Another modality, such as a chemical peel, is best used to treat these areas in conjunction with dermabrasion.

Successful facial peeling with a chemical, such as trichloroacetic acid (TCA), also depends highly on the peel type and the skill of the operator. Precise depth control, which is critical in any resurfacing procedure, may be difficult, and nonuniform depth of penetration, which can produce a poor outcome or complications, may result. Multiple variables may reduce the predictability and reproducibility of chemical peeling. Lack of standardization of chemical peeling is common, and results achieved depend greatly on variables such as patient skin type, skin conditioning, skin preparation, the type and concentration of the chemical used, postoperative care, presence or absence of occlusion, contact time, and possible associated systemic toxicity (phenol peel).

HIGH-ENERGY, SHORT-PULSED CO_2 LASERS

Many of the disadvantages of continuous wave lasers have been eliminated with the new high-energy, short-pulsed CO_2 lasers that have collimated handpieces and a variety of computer-generated scanned patterns. In just a few years, the CO_2 laser has become one of the most predictable and reproducible modalities for skin resurfacing. The advantages are based on the precise depth and spot control that allow the operator to carefully and precisely ablate small areas of tissue layer by layer to variable depths of injury. The modality is also bloodless, quick, and nontoxic. An immediate effect is seen and the endpoint is well defined.

The long- and short-term effects of laser skin resurfacing have been studied, and the modality appears to be safe. However, physicians are advised to follow published research findings carefully and to be alert to previously undetected effects. Laser manufacturers have at times positioned the CO_2 resurfacing modality as the best and safest technique. However, when chemical peeling and laser resurfacing techniques are compared based on the same depth of injury and skill of the operator for each procedure, the differences are probably insignificant with respect to swelling, healing time, pigmentation abnormalities, scarring, and results achieved. Understanding the theory and mastering the technical skills are overwhelmingly important for performing resurfacing safely and effectively with any modality. The physician is advised to master several different modalities and to use what appears to be most appropriate in a given situation.

LASER–SKIN INTERACTION

The desired ablation and vaporization of tissue (instead of coagulation) is achieved through the use of high-energy pulsed CO_2 lasers whose long wavelength targets intracellular water. The intracellular water absorbs the

Box 11-2

SELECTIVE PHOTOTHERMOLYSIS

- **Process of causing highly selective target damage**
- **The duration of laser energy exposure is shorter than the thermal relaxation time of the skin. Target tissue is vaporized so quickly that minimal heat is conducted to surrounding and deeper normal tissues.**
- **Achieved through the use of pulsed lasers or scanning lasers**

energy and is heated to a temperature of 100°C or higher. Ablation can then occur, leading to vaporization of the tissue and its water into the steam, smoke, and dehydrated superficial or surface eschar of a laser plume. Lasers with high peak power and rapid pulses deliver this energy very quickly—the pulse duration is shorter than the target tissue thermal relaxation time (the time that it takes for the tissue to cool 50%), which is approximately 700 μs for skin tissue.[19] As a result, the target skin tissue is vaporized with minimal diffusion of heat to adjacent tissues.

If, on the other hand, the pulse duration is longer than the thermal relaxation time (e.g., $>$700 μs), heat accumulates. In effect, a "heat sink" develops that allows diffusion of heat to tissue below the level of vaporization.[20] This increases depth of injury and prolongs wound healing and may result in scarring and other complications of laser skin resurfacing.

The other factor important in selective photothermolysis is the energy density level. For ablation of skin, the critical energy density level (fluence) for the CO_2 laser is 4 to 5 J/cm^2.[21] This corresponds approximately to 250 mJ per pulse with a 3-mm spot size (the vaporization threshold of skin). Resurfacing with an energy density below this threshold energy density level causes coagulation and heat conduction without complete tissue vaporization. A CO_2 laser with a fluence of 5 J/cm^2 in 1 ms or less vaporizes the intended tissue with a minimal risk of sequelae such as prolonged healing, scarring, hypopigmentation, and prolonged erythema.[13–15,20–24]

THE BASIS FOR CLINICAL IMPROVEMENT

After the first pass of high-energy, short-pulsed CO_2 laser light on the skin, tissue is vaporized through the epidermis up to the basal layer, and an eschar composed of desiccated epidermis is formed. A fluence of 4 to 5 J/cm^2 vaporizes tissue to the depth of approximately 100 μm, with collateral damage of 20 to 50 μm. No gross bleeding occurs because the laser energy coagulates smaller blood vessels and lymphatics. Subsequent passes produce less vaporization because the CO_2 laser acts on water and the first pass dessicated the upper skin layer and left less water to absorb the laser en-

Box 11-3

As a rejuvenation modality, CO_2 laser resurfacing offers precise incremental control of depth and a low incidence of scarring and other complications

ergy. Thus, each subsequent pass vaporizes less tissue than the one before, while the layer of thermal necrosis increases to some extent.[25] Minimal or no eschar is generally produced with subsequent passes.

Clinically, the results seen following laser skin resurfacing appear to arise from a combination of mechanisms.[26–28] Removal of the aged and/or photodamaged epidermis and upper papillary dermis and the formation of a more even skin surface results in immediate clinical improvement. However, this does not explain the clinical improvement that follows in deeper wrinkles and scars. The second mechanism appears to be a heat-mediated collagen effect. Type 1 collagen is exquisitely sensitive to temperatures of 50°C and above and responds to such increase in temperature by loss of its helical structure and contraction (shrinkage) of its fibrils. This shrinkage effect, however, does not completely persist and is partially lost with time.[28] Above 60°C, irreversible destruction of collagen occurs, and this damage to the collagen fibrils may produce additional collagen remodeling, which improves the appearance of wrinkles. This is mediated by the healing process and is maximally several weeks to months after the initial resurfacing procedure.

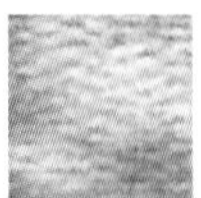

RESURFACING LASER SYSTEMS

PULSED AND SCANNING LASERS

The laser systems in use today for skin resurfacing fall into the broad categories of CO_2 lasers (either pulsed or scanned) and the erbium:YAG laser. No one system is clearly best, and in trained and skilled hands excellent results can be obtained with any system. All useful systems have the characteristic of selectivity. This means that the laser possesses a high peak power above the vaporization threshold and a pulse duration shorter than the thermal relaxation time to allow selective epidermal and dermal injury with minimal residual thermal damage.

Modern high-energy CO_2 resurfacing lasers are broadly classified as pulsed or scanning. Pulsed lasers have intermittent outputs of the laser beam, and the tissue dwell time is determined by pulse duration. In the pulsed CO_2 laser, the individual pulses have a Gaussian-shaped energy density curve (highest intensity centrally and decreasing energy toward the edges or tails of the curve). Because of the decay of the pulse energy in the periphery of the spot, slight overlap of spots is necessary to achieve uniform vaporization. Ultrapulsed lasers have a single pulse that exceeds the vaporization threshold. Superpulsed lasers stack multiple pulses in order to achieve a total energy level that exceeds the vaporization threshold. This results in a high peak power with a rapid decay of pulse energy. The long low-energy tail on the pulse power curve of superpulsed lasers may allow tissue heating.

By contrast, scanning lasers have a continuous laser output and a tissue dwell time limited by a mechanical scanning device that moves the beam continuously so that contact time is less than the thermal relaxation time. Because the pulse energy curve in a scanned laser is in the shape of a "top hat," any overlap of pulses results in additive tissue effects and may produce increased depth of injury to the skin. It is therefore important to avoid overlap of pulses when using scanned lasers. Increasing wattage in pulsed lasers increases speed, but not depth of penetration. In a scanned laser, on the other hand, increasing wattage increases depth. The clinical end results of pulsed and scanned CO_2 lasers in skilled hands are probably the same.

THE ERBIUM:YAG LASER

The erbium:YAG laser has a wavelength of 2,940 nm, which is 10 to 18 times more absorbed by water than the CO_2 laser. This increased absorption results in less depth of penetration per pulse and more superficial ablation with each pulse of laser energy. The thermal effect is lower, and more passes are required to achieve a depth similar to that obtained with a CO_2 laser. In fact, 5 to 10 passes may be required to fully ablate the epidermis. This may be a disadvantage if dermal resurfacing is required, because as the number of passes required increases, the variability of spot placement and overlap increases and the technique becomes less precise and reproducible.

With its more superficial depth of penetration, the erbium laser may be used in combination with CO_2 lasers and appears to be more useful in areas of nonfacial skin, such as the neck and hands. But, because thermal effects are minimal, collagen shrinkage seen with the CO_2 resurfacing lasers is not seen with the erbium:YAG lasers. Punctuate bleeding is more frequently encountered with the erbium laser. Claims of faster healing, less pain, less erythema, and reduced complications after treatment with the erbium:YAG laser are probably unfounded if laser systems are compared for equivalent depths of resurfacing.

MECHANISM OF RESURFACING WITH THE CO_2 LASER

CO_2 laser skin resurfacing works primarily by leveling and vaporization of skin textural abnormalities. Secondary effects include firming and tightening resulting from heat-mediated collagen contraction and new collagen formation.

A recent histological study[29] clearly demonstrated rejuvenation of the epidermis and the dermis following CO_2 laser resurfacing. Epidermal atrophy was reversed and orderly epidermal maturation was reestablished with healthy keratinocytes. Melanocyte hypertrophy and hyperplasia were corrected. In the dermis, large clumps of abnormal elastic tissue were eliminated and replaced by a proliferation of normal, thin elastic fibers. The thin subepidermal Grenz collagen zone was replaced with a much thicker band of new collagen.

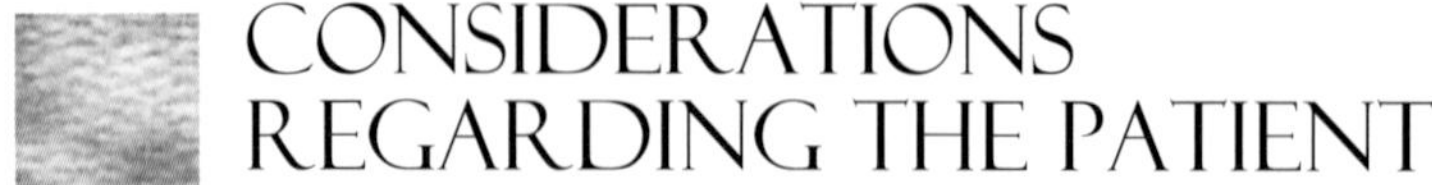

CONSIDERATIONS REGARDING THE PATIENT

INDICATIONS FOR CO_2 LASER RESURFACING

Primary indications for laser skin resurfacing include textural abnormalities of the facial skin. These include facial rhytides, actinic damage and solar elastosis, and scars. Facial scarring resulting from trauma, surgery, acne, and chicken pox may be treated. Other secondary conditions, such as actinic chelitis, rhinophyma, keratoses, epidermal pigmentation abnormalities, and benign skin growths, may also be amenable to laser skin resurfacing techniques. In general, dermal pigmentation is not responsive to skin resurfacing.

PATIENT SELECTION

With aging, the skin of the face develops textural changes and laxity. Laser skin resurfacing is not a substitute for surgical treatment of skin laxity; however, dermal resurfacing does produce some visible skin tightening, as suggested years ago by Obagi.[30]

Resurfacing is ideal for the patient who primarily has textural changes in the skin. This patient may still be young and not ready for a facelift but may want some textural improvement and tightening. Such a patient may also be an excellent candidate for a light chemical peel. In choosing a resurfacing procedure for this patient, the physician must take into consideration whether leveling (best with laser resurfacing) or tightening (best with chemical peeling) is needed.

Laser skin resurfacing is ideal for the patient who does not want or is not a candidate for a surgical procedure. Also, patients who have had a previous facelift often have superb results following laser resurfacing. The textural problems that remain after a facelift subtract from the overall result; such problems can be improved very nicely by laser skin resurfacing.

Many patients will benefit from a combination of resurfacing and surgical procedures. With careful patient selection, preconditioning, and precise depth control, these procedures can be performed simultaneously to give the patient maximal improvement in texture and laxity with a low risk of complications and a single recovery period.

Classification of the patient's skin preoperatively is very important. A simplified approach is to assess the patient's skin for color, thickness, and oiliness. Patients with darker skin types have a greater tendency for postin-

Box 11-4

With careful patient selection, preconditioning, and precise depth control, cosmetic surgical procedures can be performed simultaneously with CO_2 laser resurfacing, giving the patient maximal improvement in texture and laxity with a low risk of complications and a single recovery period.

flammatory hyperpigmentation (PIH) and need to have preprocedure skin conditioning and melanocyte function control to prevent this problem. Light-colored skin types exhibit more erythema following resurfacing and need to be told of this possibility. Patients with thinner skin seem to have the best results following laser resurfacing but also have a smaller margin for error in depth of resurfacing and a greater risk of delayed healing should resurfacing go too deep. Patients with thick, oily skin have a higher population of skin appendages and a larger safety margin but exhibit less contraction of the skin, a greater risk of PIH, and more difficulty in conditioning, as the oiliness can interfere with the absorption of topical medications.

Classification of wrinkles may be useful for the surgeon's personal follow-up of results. A variety of wrinkle classification systems exist which grade rhytides on a continuum, from superficial, fine lines to deep lines and elastosis.

RELATIVE RESPONSES TO RESURFACING

Superficial textural abnormalities respond better to laser skin resurfacing than do deeper problems. However, many problems that are of concern to patients reside deeper in the dermis. Resurfacing to at least the depth of the papillary or upper reticular dermis is required for significant reduction of facial rhytides. Patients with thin, crepey skin respond relatively better than patients with thicker, oily skin.

Actinic damage responds better than wrinkles, which generally respond better than elastosis. Fine wrinkles respond better than deeper wrinkles. Scars respond less well to resurfacing than do wrinkles. Rolling-type scars do better than ice-pick scars, which often require additional techniques such as punch excision and punch grafting to improve results.

Regional resurfacing alone is usually not as effective as full-face resurfacing because of the additive effect of tightening from collagen contraction from surrounding areas. Regional laser skin resurfacing can be combined with a light chemical peel of the non-laser-treated areas of the face to reduce demarcation lines and improve skin tightness without the need for full-face laser resurfacing. Static lines in the cheeks and periorbital areas respond better than lines in the nasolabial fold, lips, and forehead. Static wrinkles also respond better than dynamic, muscle-driven creases and lines. Dynamic lines are the most frequent cause of early recurrence of wrinkles after resurfacing.

CONTRAINDICATIONS TO LASER SKIN RESURFACING

Recent use of high dose (40 mg/day and greater) oral isotretinoin (Accutane) is a contraindication to laser skin resurfacing, as it is for other resurfacing procedures. Increased incidence of delayed healing and scarring has been reported in laser resurfacing and chemical peeling in patients who took Accutane. While more superficial procedures can be performed in patients with recent Accutane use, deeper resurfacing procedures should be postponed for 6 to 12 months or until the oiliness has returned to the patient's skin.[31–33]

Laser skin resurfacing in the presence of other conditions in which healing problems may be expected or in which skin adnexal structure may be compromised must be approached cautiously. These include patients with a history of keloid scarring, collagen vascular disease, facial radiation, a previous deep phenol peel, or a skin graft. It is interesting to note, however, that successful CO_2 laser resurfacing of perioral rhytides in patients with scleroderma was recently reported.[34]

Patients with active or frequently recurring infections are also poor candidates for laser skin resurfacing. Patients with active acne or other inflammatory conditions should have these conditions controlled prior to resurfacing. Patients undergoing an outbreak of Herpes labialis should not have laser resurfacing. In addition, antibody titers remain high for several weeks, and the optimal time for resurfacing in these patients would be approximately 2 weeks after the last lesion is completely healed. Because of the risk of infection, immunocompromised patients are not considered good candidates for laser skin resurfacing.

Patients who describe their skin as "very sensitive" should be informed that resurfacing may increase the sensitivity of the skin after the procedure. These patients may benefit from a longer, slow course of skin preconditioning to build skin tolerance prior to resurfacing. Patients with psychiatric problems or those who are unwilling to cooperate fully with the doctor may present problems with postresurfacing management. It may be prudent to not accept such persons as resurfacing patients.

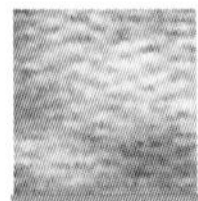

PREOPERATIVE CONSIDERATIONS

TRAINING IN THE USE OF THE CO_2 LASER FOR SKIN RESURFACING

Mastery of laser skin resurfacing is associated with a significant learning curve. The beginner should receive substantial hands-on training and supplemented with an ongoing review of pertinent medical and surgical literature and attendance at laser seminars and meetings. Study under the direction of an experienced preceptor is also helpful for refining laser resurfacing technique.

To gain insight into the healing process and possible development of complications, a surgeon should follow patients very closely following the resurfacing procedure. Confidence in the safe and effective application of this technique may require the sucessful treatment of 25 to 50 patients.

CO_2 LASER SAFETY PRECAUTIONS

Most laser-related injuries to the patient, operator, or other personnel can be prevented by continuous diligence by the laser operator. Laser goggles or eyeglasses adequately protect the operator's eyes, since the CO_2 laser beam does not penetrate glass or plastic upon incidental contact. To protect the patient's eyes, use well-lubricated metallic corneal protectors. Any instruments on the operative field that could come into contact with the laser beam should have a dull surface to reduce reflection of the laser beam. To prevent darkening of the patient's tooth enamel, protect the patient's teeth from contact with the laser beam. Use moistened drapes to reduce the risk of fire, and discontinue any supplemental oxygen from the nasal cannula.

The laser smoke evacuator draws up the laser plume produced from ablation of the skin. A face mask specifically designed to filter the laser plume can be used. Intranasal transmission of papilloma virus from the laser plume has been reported.[35] Thus the presence and possible transmission of biologically active agents within the CO_2 laser plume should be assumed and precautions taken to avoid exposure.

A frank preprocedure discussion with the candidate for laser skin resurfacing is mandatory. Patients must understand that the laser is not the "magic wand" that the media has led them to believe. Showing prospective patients a series of before and after photographs that represent the entire spectrum of outcomes is recommended. Pictures of patients in various phases of healing are also helpful to let the patient know what to expect postoperatively and will enhance the informed consent process. Baseline photographs of the patient should be taken for documentation and because patients often forget their presurgery appearance.

Skin conditioning should be started. The need for and benefit of skin conditioning in conjunction with CO_2 laser resurfacing is somewhat controversial, but there is no doubt that epidermal eschar can be removed more easily with less rubbing and perhaps with less dermal damage in patients who have had good preconditioning. Studies in patients who have undergone chemical peeling and dermabrasion suggest that healing and collagen reformation are better in patients who have had pretreatment.[36] Detailed pre- and postprocedure instructions should be provided. These will cut down on "panic calls." Post-operative medications should also be picked up before the procedure day.

PREPROCEDURE EVALUATION

The physician should evaluate the patient and decide whether he or she is a good candidate for laser resurfacing. The ideal patient has realistic expectations and has a lifestyle congruous with maintenance of improvements after laser skin resurfacing. If the patient is not willing to use sunscreen and avoid prolonged sun exposure, resurfacing should be reconsidered. A history should be obtained for previous skin treatments and for occurrence of Herpes simplex labialis, allergies, and keloids.

PREPROCEDURE SKIN CONDITIONING

The goals of skin conditioning are to control skin cell function, develop and restore normal skin tolerance, and put patients in the "compliance mode" of taking responsibility for their own care. Some practitioners suggest that skin preconditioning before laser resurfacing is of no value because the laser burns off the surface of the skin. However, unconditioned skin may be rough and irregular, with lentigo, pigmentary problems, acne, and other inflammatory conditions, which can all be improved with preconditioning. The major advantage of not conditioning seems to be to allow the patient into the operating theater sooner than if time is taken (6 weeks or more) to condition the skin.

With a balanced skin conditioning program, it is possible to make the epidermis thinner and more even, stimulate the dermal fibroblasts, improve dermal hydration, and suppress the production of melanin by the melanocyte. This results in an even, compact, gelatinous-appearing stratum corneum, dermal thickening and organization with stimulation of dermal fibroblasts, increased glycosaminoglycan and growth factor production, and deactivated melanocytes. It follows that pretreated skin responds better to laser skin resurfacing because the thin epidermis and improved hydration allow for fewer passes with the laser than untreated skin. Quicker healing and less PIH are also to be expected.[37–40] While all skin types benefit from conditioning, patients with darker skin types, very oily skin, pigmentation problems, and inflammatory conditions, such as acne, are particularly in need of preconditioning.

The primary components of a balanced preconditioning program are tretinoin, alpha-hydroxy acids, hydroquinone, and sunscreens.[36–39] Other agents, such as topical vitamin C and kojic acid, may be used in selected cases. Our usual preconditioning program involves 4 to 6 weeks of once-to-twice daily use of these products in a dose of 1 g per application.

PREPARATION FOR THE LASER RESURFACING PROCEDURE

Since a negative previous history of Herpes simplex labialis does not predict lack of an eruption following laser skin resurfacing, all patients receive prophylaxis with antiherpes medications, such as Zovirax, Valtrex, and Famvir. These drugs differ primarily in their pharmacokinetics and less so in their efficacy. Instruct the patient to shampoo and wash the face with antibacterial soap the evening before and the morning of the laser treatment.

Telephone the patient the evening before surgery to review the procedures and give instructions on use of medications. If general anesthesia is to be used, the anesthesiologist will often call the patient to explain anesthesia techniques. To reduce the risk of nausea, emesis, and potential pulmonary aspiration, the patient is asked not to eat or drink anything after 12 midnight on the evening prior to surgery. This is particularly important when sedatives or intravenous or general anesthesia are used.

Photograph the patient before the procedure and have him/her wash the face with an antibacterial soap. With the patient sitting up, mark the location of wrinkles or lesions, because the appearance of these may change when the patient lies down. A line drawn at the angle of the jaw from one ear to the other serves as the border between facial and neck skin and indicates where the edge of the laser-treated area is to be feathered. Bring the patient into the operating room and position him/her comfortably on the operating table. Insert an intravenous catheter for administration of an intravenous antibiotic, usually a cephalosporin. Clean the area to be resurfaced with a nonflammable antiseptic solution, such as Zepharin or chlorhexidine. Flammable cleansing liquids are a fire hazard and should be avoided.

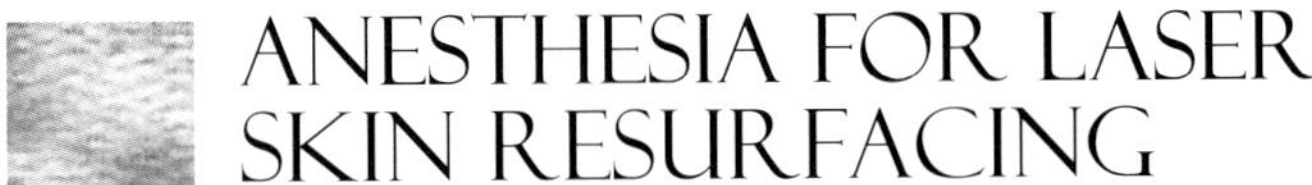

ANESTHESIA FOR LASER SKIN RESURFACING

Laser skin resurfacing is painful, especially if performed to the level of the papillary and upper reticular dermis, and the adequacy of anesthesia should be tested before beginning the procedure.

Laser skin resurfacing may be performed with local anesthesia, with or without intravenous sedation, or under general anesthesia. Smaller and more superficial areas may be treated with topical agents such as EMLA cream, which provides epidermal anesthesia. This is rarely sufficient, however, for deeper resurfacing.

Regional facial nerve blocks consisting of lidocaine or bupivacaine reduce the need for intravenous agents and are used routinely. Along with some supplemental local infiltration, regional blocks are usually sufficient for performing laser facial resurfacing. The regional facial nerves to be blocked are:

1. supraorbital and nasociliary nerves
2. infraorbital nerve
3. auriculotemporal nerve
4. zygomaticofacial nerve
5. mental nerve
6. inferior alveolar nerve
7. greater auricular nerve

In placing these blocks, start at the top of the face and work down. This allows the resurfacing procedure to be started in the region first blocked immediately after completion of the last injection. Anesthesia will be maximal approximately 15 to 30 minutes after injection. Administer approximately 3 cc of injection with a small-gauge needle at each site, injecting just above the periosteum where the nerves exit their bony foramina. Bicarbonate can be added to reduce discomfort with injection. Hyaluronidase (Wydase) can also be added to enhance diffusion of the injections through the tissue planes.

Supplementation of facial nerve blocks with subcutaneous infiltration may be required, especially at the periphery of the treated areas, such as at the jawline and the preauricular region, in a "horseshoe" pattern. If subcutaneous infiltration is used, epinephrine can be deleted because the blanching from the epinephrine solution may interfere with endpoint visualization. Tumescent anesthesia for laser skin resurfacing has been described, but if infiltration is carried out to the endpoint of tissue tumescence, many of the target lines and wrinkles may be ablated. Nerve block and infiltration anesthesia can be supplemented with intravenous sedation.

Intravenous administration of sedatives and analgesics increases patient comfort and provides amnesia for the procedure, but additional monitoring is mandatory. After establishing cardiovascular and oximetry monitoring, a small dose of intravenous sedative and analgesic can be administered to reduce anxiety and discomfort from further preparations and injections. The agents most commonly used are propofol (Diprivan); hypnotics such as midazolam (Versed) or diazepam (Valium); and analgesics such as alfenta, fentanyl, mepridine (Demerol), and morphine.

In California and other states, it is now illegal to administer intravenous sedation in a sufficient amount to potentially result in the loss of the patient's "life-preserving reflexes" in an unaccredited setting (AB 595), and any facility where such anesthesia is used must be accredited or licensed. Check with your local regulatory agencies to see whether similar restrictions apply in your area. Supplementary oxygen delivered through nasal cannulae presents a fire risk; thus, oxygen should be discontinued while laser energy is being applied to the patient's facial skin.

I have been using general anesthesia more often because of improved patient comfort, monitoring by an anesthesiologist, and more efficient use of my time. However, oxygen-enriched anesthetic gases can be ignited by the laser and cause tracheobronchial burns. A laser-resistant endotracheal tube can be used during general anesthesia procedures. Metallic foil can also be used to wrap the endotracheal tube to reduce the possibility of contact with the laser beam.

Potent analgesics or anesthetics often cause postoperative nausea and vomiting. This should be anticipated and treated with antiemetic medications.

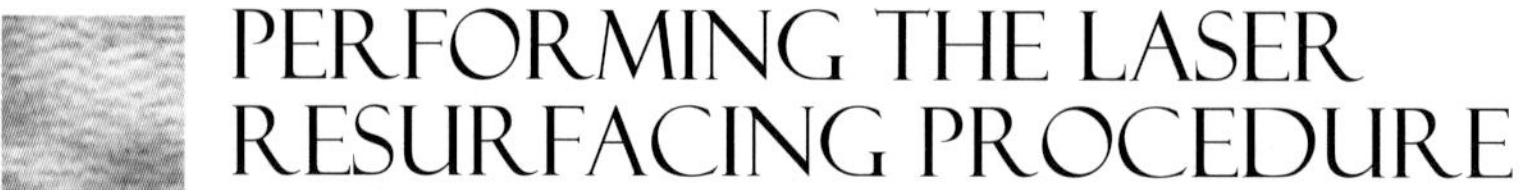

PERFORMING THE LASER RESURFACING PROCEDURE

INSTRUMENTATION

The laser should be set up and tested on a wooden tongue blade prior to applying laser energy to the patient's skin. Laser power settings (fluence and density) should be individualized for each patient. There are no binding rules for laser parameters, and it is always wise to begin cautiously. More important than the energy applied is the appreciation of having reached the appropriate endpoints. Remember that complications with any resurfacing procedure are related to the depth of injury of the skin, so care is advised, especially early in the learning process. While variations in skin thickness, adnexal structure population, laser energy, and power density are important in the conduct of a laser skin resurfacing procedure, the most important variable is the skill and experience of the person operating the laser.

As a general guideline (to be individualized for each patient), the Coherent Ultrapulse laser with the computerized pattern generator (CPG) handpiece can be set at 300 mJ and the first pass performed on the face, cheek, and brow with a large square pattern at a setting of 3-9–6. The second pass is then performed at 300 mJ and a lower pattern density of 3-9–5. Histologically, there appears to be no difference between 250 and 300 mJ with the CPG. The eyelids are then treated at 250 to 300 mJ with a smaller hexagonal pattern at a setting of 1-4-5. A second, nonconfluent pass with no overlap can be performed on the eyelids, if indicated, at the same settings. Additional selective focal treatments can be performed with the single 3-mm spot handpiece at 350 to 450 mJ and 5 to 10 watts.

Begin slowly with application of the laser light to the skin and move your hand at a uniform speed. Despite collimation in pulsed lasers, hold the handpieces perpendicular to the skin. Loupe magnification will allow you to see the skin surface better to detect the endpoint and will protect your eyes from the laser as well.

Two handpieces are usually available with skin resurfacing laser systems: 1) a scanning or patterned handpiece, and 2) a single-spot handpiece for precise resurfacing of smaller areas and for filling of any areas not covered by the other handpiece. Use of the smaller handpiece can be quite tedious for covering larger areas. With the advent of computerized pattern generators and scanners, larger surface areas can now be uniformly covered in a shorter time, thus increasing the efficiency of these procedures. Also, more precise overlap with the pattern generators may be reducing postprocedure erythema. Various power densities are available on these pattern generators, which depend on overlap of nearby pulses. The computer-generated patterns are also available in a variety of shapes.

DEPTH AND ENDPOINTS

Control of the depth of resurfacing is critical for obtaining the best results and limiting the potential complications. Penetration must be sufficiently deep into the dermis to affect the target chromophores, yet sufficiently superficial to avoid delayed healing or a scar. Keep in mind that skin adnexal structures are primarily responsible for healing after laser skin resurfacing, and the depth of ablation should not go below the level of adnexal structures. Also, as depth of penetration increases, the risk of skin textural changes and hypopigmentation from melanocyte injury increases.

Box 11-5

Skin adnexal structures are primarily responsible for healing after laser skin resurfacing. Ablation depth should therefore not go below the level of adnexal structures.

Box 11-6

The endpoints of laser skin resurfacing are:

- **the cosmetic endpoint: flattening or ablation of the target lesion or wrinkle with no further tissue shrinkage**
- **the safety endpoint: appearance of the "chamois" yellow skin color that persists after wiping with a saline-soaked gauze (even if the lesion or wrinkle is still present)**

The endpoints of laser skin resurfacing are either 1) flattening or ablation of the target lesion or wrinkle with no further tissue shrinkage (cosmetic endpoint), or 2) the appearance of the "chamois" yellow skin color, which persists after wiping with a saline-soaked gauze, even if the lesion or wrinkle is still present (safety endpoint). The chamois yellow color appears to be subject to a fading phenomenon similar to the defrosting phenomenon seen with a TCA peel. Wiping with saline-soaked gauze causes the color to fade, and rapid fading may be an indication for an additional pass as the desired depth has not been achieved. Do not go to the point of a solid, confluent, and persistent chamois yellow coloration.

Application of laser energy to the skin must be even, with minimal or no operator overlap of pulses. This is particularly important with scanned CO_2 lasers, which, because of their "top hat"-shaped energy application curves, will cause deeper injury in any area of overlap. This phenomenon may lead to small hypopigmented scars that appear like white lines or spots. Pulsed lasers, by the Gaussian nature of their beam have a density-dependent overlap. Any additional overlap by the operator may result in char formation.

Laser resurfacing is usually done in a systematic fashion, beginning on the forehead and proceeding down the remainder of the face. The eyelids are often done last because they are treated at lower power settings and densities and require additional care to avoid burning the eyelashes.

REGIONAL RESURFACING

If regional resurfacing is performed, entire facial subunits should be treated. The patient should be advised that regional resurfacing might temporarily lead to more uneven coloration postoperatively that may be difficult to cover completely with make-up. This contrast between resurfaced and nonresurfaced areas can be improved if a different resurfacing technique is used in the non-laser-treated areas, such as a low-concentration TCA peel like the Blue Peel. In men, camouflage make-up is usually not acceptable, and full-face laser skin resurfacing is recommended. In both men and women, full-face laser skin resurfacing is most frequently performed. It creates fewer demarcation lines and allows for better blending of treated areas. Better tightening is also seen following tissue shrinkage in a larger surface area.

LASER PASSES

The even application of laser energy to a given surface area of skin is defined as a laser "pass." The first pass predominately results in water vaporization and tissue ablation. With a CO_2 laser, the first pass produces a whitish-yellow, dry eschar. Occasionally some contracture of the skin may be seen, especially in thinner skinned areas of the face, such as the eyelids. The endpoint for the first pass is the production of an even, homogeneously colored eschar. In areas of overlap, a yellow-brown char may be evident. This represents a double-pulsed area and is at increased risk for skin texture changes. Char should be avoided, as "char may become scar."

If the eschar is not removed prior to a second laser pass, charring and thermal damage are possible. Selectively, the eschar may be left in place and the resurfacing procedure terminated at this point. The dry eschar can be treated with ointment without a dressing and will subsequently slough during the reepithelialization process, similar to the sloughing of the eschar following a chemical peel. This will obviously result in a more superficial depth of resurfacing but will produce less pain and erythema and is well tolerated by patients. Theoretically, residual coagulated tissue may increase the risk of infection, but this has not been seen clinically. This technique may be useful when regional laser skin resurfacing is performed or when laser skin resurfacing is combined with other procedures, such as chemical peels or surgery.

The dry eschar of dehydrated epidermis is usually removed and the dermis rehydrated by gentle rubbing with a saline-soaked gauze pad. Care should be taken to avoid aggressive rubbing that may increase depth of injury and lead to prolonged erythema or delayed healing. Removal of residual eschar after the first laser pass seems to be easier in patients whose skin has been well conditioned prior to the resurfacing procedure.

After the first pass, the debrided skin will appear smooth and whitish-pink, with a glistening surface. This appearance usually signifies ablation to the basal layer of the epidermis or upper papillary dermis, depending on skin thickness. Any residual epidermis missed with the first pass may be treated precisely with the single-spot handpiece. Tissue fluid may now accumulate on the resurfaced area and should be blotted prior to performing a second pass. Failure to blot this fluid will result in an audible "sizzle" and absorption of the laser energy by the fluid with inadequate penetration of the laser energy into the skin.

The second pass with the laser usually results in immediate visible shrinkage and often a dramatic (20% to 40%) tightening of the resurfaced skin with production of a chamois yellow color and a rougher surface texture. This usually signifies ablation into the papillary or upper reticular dermis. The depth of laser passes is not linear. While the penetration of the second pass is significantly less deep than the first pass, it is more effective in tightening and leveling than the first.

Shrinkage of the resurfaced skin is thought to represent reversible collagen contraction, but it is not well understood.[13,41,42] Other theories to explain contracture include denaturation or cross-linking of collagen, dehydration of the dermis, or evaporation of dermal ground substance. Contracture clearly represents a desirable endpoint of resurfacing with the CO_2 laser and is thought to be a special effect associated with this resurfacing technique. Whether collagen contraction is a permanent phenomenon following CO_2 laser resurfacing is not known.

A third and subsequent passes may be indicated to reach the desired endpoint. These passes should be used selectively on the shoulders and on furrows of persistent wrinkles and to accomplish selective tightening of malar bags and perioral rhytides, and to selectively increase skin shrinkage of the upper and lower eyelids. Each pass penetrates less deeply than the one before, and residual thermal damage increases. It may be advisable to reduce the pattern density if more passes are used. Among experienced laser surgeons, the growing trend has been to use fewer passes.

FEATHERING

Feathering of the margin between the resurfaced and nonresurfaced skin edges is next performed to reduce demarcation lines. This can be accomplished by any technique that will create a gradient of depth of penetration between these 2 areas. A band of skin between the resurfaced and nonresurfaced skin is usually treated with either the spot handpiece or a pattern at lower fluences to accomplish the desired blending. Demarcation lines are more obvious if deeper resurfacing is performed and hypopigmentation occurs. Demarcation lines can also be reduced by carrying the resurfaced areas up to the mandibular hollow (as marked before the procedure with the patient upright), into the hairline and onto the ear. Skin

Box 11-7

The depth of laser passes is not linear. While the second pass penetrates significantly less deeply than the first pass, the second pass is more effective in tightening and leveling than the first.

preconditioning and a superficial-depth TCA peel of the nonresurfaced skin, especially the neck area, may be helpful to reduce demarcation lines, especially if the neck skin is hyperpigmented from tanning or photoaging.

An advanced technique of multipulse vaporization may be used to specifically treat deeper lines and lesions. In this technique, laser pulses from a spot handpiece are "stacked" atop one another to allow deeper penetration and ablation resulting from the accumulation of thermal damage. This technique is very effective but risky, and it is not appropriate for the inexperienced operator.

RESURFACING SKIN WITH SPECIFIC CONDITIONS

Actinic damage is generally uniform and is well treated with uniform passes with the laser. Focal dermal abnormalities, such as scars and wrinkles, require additional focal treatments. A selective third pass with a spot handpiece is often indicated for localized deeper ablation of persistent lines, wrinkles, or scars. Generally this is performed with subsequent passes on the raised shoulders of these focal abnormalities. Care must be taken, as increased passes result in increased depth of penetration and raise the risk of depth-related complications, such as delayed healing, hypopigmentation, or scarring.

Acne scars signify a focal dermal collagen abnormality and may appear as a rolling, irregular-type scar or as an "ice-pick" scar. Initially, the entire region is usually treated with 2 passes of the laser. Then the shoulders of the scar are treated with additional passes until they are smoothed out or until a darker chamois yellow color is achieved. The elevated shoulder of an acne scar can be double-pulsed in an attempt to push the laser energy deeper into the fibrotic area. Firm, fibrotic scars may benefit from punch excision or grafting as a separate procedure. The laser can then be used to resurface the "pin-cushion" appearance of the healed punch graft.

Laser resurfacing of surgical and posttraumatic hypertrophic scars can improve the scar's appearance. The optimum timing for treatment is 6 to 8 weeks postinjury to take advantage of the active collagen and scar remodeling process. The shoulder of the hypertrophic scar is treated to a solid chamois yellow color, and the surrounding nonscarred areas are treated lightly to blend and prevent sharp demarcation lines around the treated areas.

Patients with rhinophyma also benefit from laser resurfacing. Multiple passes may be required, but the nose with rhinophyma changes is quite tolerant of laser resurfacing. Alternatively, the laser may be used in the cutting mode with the laser slightly defocused to achieve a slightly more rapid tissue ablation.

Actinic chelitis responds well to laser skin resurfacing. Because this is primarily a superficial epidermal process, deep resurfacing is not needed. Usually 1 pass is sufficient, and the lip vermilion is treated in a similar fashion as the lower eyelid. Protection of the teeth from the laser beam is also important to prevent fracturing and darkening of the tooth enamel.

A variety of other superficial epidermal and dermal lesions can be treated successfully with the laser, including skin tags, seborrheic keratoses, dermatosis pupulosa nigrans, epidermal nevi, epidermal inclusion cysts, and others. Laser skin resurfacing may also lighten epidermal and superficial dermal tattoos if the pigment resides in a treated tissue plane.

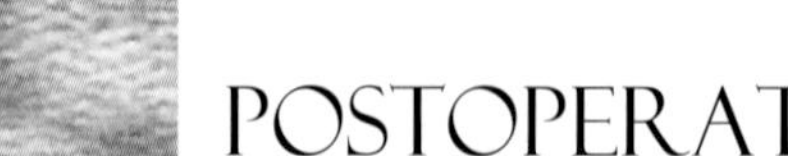

POSTOPERATIVE CONSIDERATIONS

Laser skin resurfacing is almost always done on an outpatient basis. After the patient has awakened and stabilized in the recovery area, she or he is allowed to return home or to go to a care facility. The postprocedure instructions and medications are discussed with the patient's caretaker after the procedure but prior to discharge. Oral analgesics, anti-inflammatory medications, antibiotics, and antiviral prophylaxis are routinely prescribed. Oral anxiolytics, such as diazepam (Valium), may be helpful to reduce patient anxiety and to improve sleep patterns in the early period after resurfacing. Oral steroids are not usually used. Antiemetics and antipruritics are prescribed for use on an as-needed basis if the patient experiences nausea or vomiting, or itching, respectively.

Laser skin resurfacing results in a skin injury somewhat like a superficial thermal or chemical burn with loss of the epidermis and a denuded and thermally damaged dermis. However, unlike chemical peeling or a thermal burn, laser skin resurfacing does not result in formation of an overlying eschar. Principles learned in the care of patients with thermal injury can be applied to patients with laser skin resurfacing. Because the dermis is "raw," a dressing is required to protect it and prevent drying and extension of the depth of injury. Reepithelialization occurs more rapidly if the healing surface is kept moist by occlusion.[13,20,43–45] Dressings such as ointments or masks are commonly used.

POSTOPERATIVE DRESSINGS

After completion of laser skin resurfacing, unless otherwise contaminated, the patient's skin can be assumed to be nearly sterile. No cleansing or other preparation is needed prior to application of dressings. The dressings, if used, are applied immediately after completion of the procedure to reduce drying of the open treated areas and to reduce contamination.

Some controversy exists with regard to dressings. Some operators elect to use an "open" technique in which an occlusive ointment is applied several times daily until reepithelialization is complete. This technique is more painful to the patient than a "closed," or mask, technique and is messier and more time consuming because of the need for cleansing and application of the ointment. It does have the theoretical advantage of a decreased rate of and earlier detection of infection, but the incidence of milia and acne flare-up in patients treated with occlusive ointments is higher. The open technique is also more useful in treatment of patients with localized and regional resurfacing.

The closed technique is only semiocclusive, as exchange of gases and vapor occurs across most mask materials. This technique is very "user friendly" and is becoming standard since it results in less pain, quicker reepithelialization, and less erythema compared to the open technique. Patients are not required to participate directly in their wound care, but some may find the mask makes them feel claustrophobic. There is less need for potentially sensitizing ointments. The risk of infection can be maintained at a lower rate by frequent observation of the patient's skin and early removal or changing of the mask at the first sign of infection, loosening, or contamination. In patients with a mask dressing, resurfaced areas not covered by the mask should be treated with a semiocclusive ointment until healed.

A variety of mask materials are available, which vary in composition, adherence, and other properties. The mask may adhere or may need to be held in place with tape or an elastic net dressing. No one material has yet proven to be superior to the others. The expense of a procedure is increased when a semiocclusive mask is used because of the cost of the mask material and the increased staff time devoted to mask care (these patients must be seen frequently and the mask changed if it becomes loose or displaced).

PROGRESS DURING RECOVERY

The recovery period must be clearly discussed with patients preoperatively so they know what to expect and are not surprised during the healing phase. At least 7 to 14 days are needed for recovery after the usual full-face laser skin resurfacing procedure. During the first week, the patient will experience variable degrees of oozing, crusting, and swelling. After the second week, tightness will be felt and the skin will appear pink. Swelling will be nearly completely resolved, but scabs may occasionally persist up to this point. Make-up can be worn after healing is complete and all scabs have healed. By 3 to 4 weeks after resurfacing, fine lanugo hairs will return and the face will have a more natural appearance. Skin reconditioning will be reintroduced, and an improved skin texture will be noted at this time. Gradual improvement will continue over the next few months.

The time course of healing and reepithelialization is depth dependent and varies among individuals, but generally 7 to 14 days are required. Collagen deposition and maturation and remodeling begin during reepithelialization but are not complete for 6 to 12 weeks postprocedure. The effects of laser-induced leveling of wrinkles, lines, scars, and lesions will be noticed immediately upon completion of healing. The effects may lessen some with resolution of edema, and the patient may be concerned that the problem is "coming back." Firming and tightening depend on collagen maturation and will be maximal after 6 to 12 weeks. Patients should understand this time course and its implications regarding their recovery, time of return to usual activities, and the results of their procedure.

POSTPROCEDURE SKIN RECONDITIONING

Skin reconditioning is begun early during the healing process. After removal of the semiocclusive mask, the patient is routinely treated with moisturizers. Trauma to the resurfaced area, induced by activities such as scrubbing or having the shower directly hit the resurfaced skin, is to be avoided since epidermal adherence is not complete. Sunblocks are to be used as soon as tolerated instead of sunscreens, which may not prevent sun-related development of hyperpigmentation. In patients prone to hyperpigmentation, hydroquinone can be introduced early (at 2 to 3 weeks) after healing as it is generally less irritating. Tretinoin is usually reintroduced in low dosages by 1 month after resurfacing. Alphahydroxy acids are best avoided in the postresurfacing period, as the epidermis is already very thin and easily stripped by these substances. Occasionally, high-potency topical steroids are used.

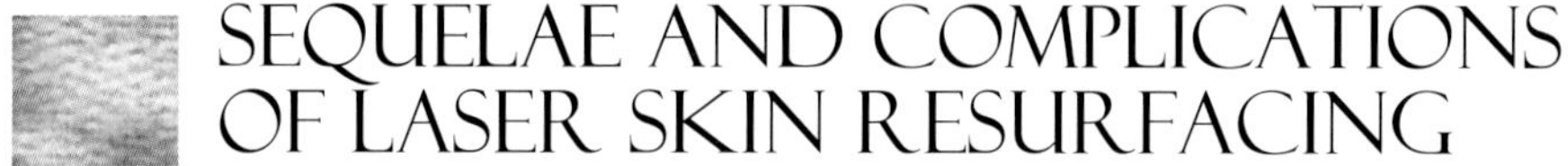

SEQUELAE AND COMPLICATIONS OF LASER SKIN RESURFACING

SEQUELAE

Expected sequelae are not complications and must be clearly differentiated in the patient's mind. Common sequelae include discomfort, inconvenience, erythema, hyperpigmentation, and milia and acne.

Discomfort is reduced by use of a semiocclusive mask dressing and oral analgesics. Often a synthetic opiate is combined with a nonsteroidal anti-inflammatory agent to achieve a synergistic effect on pain reduction. Most patients treated with a mask dressing will have minimal discomfort. Ice compresses can be helpful for the first 24 hours to reduce discomfort, but precautions must be taken to avoid adding cold injury to the existing thermal injury by prolonged direct contact with ice. Any patient who describes the new onset of pain during the first few days after resurfacing needs to be seen by the physician to rule out the development of an infection or other problem.

Following resurfacing, patients may describe "cabin fever" because of the time spent in semiseclusion. Support and reassurance can usually help them through this temporary inconvenience.

Erythema to some degree is seen in every patient resurfaced into the dermis with the CO_2 laser. Erythema may be more obvious in patients with lighter skin types, those of northern European descent, and those with a history of easy blushing or flushing or of rosacea who were not preconditioned and who had aggressive resurfacing and "open" postprocedure treatment. Erythema is always transient but may persist for weeks to months. Erythema may be covered somewhat by a green or yellow-tinted camouflage make-up, and this should be offered to treated patients. Topical steroids are not routinely used to reduce erythema because these agents

Box 11-8

Erythema after laser resurfacing is not the enemy.

- **Patients with the greatest degree and duration of erythema often have the best response.**
- **Lasers that do not produce erythema are too superficial to affect collagen remodeling.**

reduce collagen synthesis. Erythema is a marker for metabolic activity, inflammation, collagen remodeling, and increased skin blood flow. Patients with the greatest degree and duration of erythema often have the best response to laser skin resurfacing. Lasers that do not produce erythema are too superficial to affect collagen remodeling. Not all erythema is the same, however, and diffuse erythema must be differentiated from focal, itchy, palpable, or raised spots of erythema, which may be a sign of a developing hypertrophic scar and require early treatment.

Hyperpigmentation may initially be seen around 14 to 21 days after resurfacing as a "dirty" or "bronzed" appearance to the treated skin. It appears to be postinflammatory in etiology and may be anticipated in patients of darker skin color, especially if preconditioning failed to suppress melanocyte function. Patients with a prior history of postinflammatory hyperpigmentation, melasma, or estrogen use, and patients with darkening of the knuckles, knees, and elbows are also more susceptible. While hyperpigmentation may resolve without treatment in 6 to 12 months, early reconditioning and use of sunblocks and hydroquinone can result in improvement within 2 weeks. Occasionally, superficial chemical peels may be required to completely clear residual hyperpigmentation.

Milia and acne are relatively common following resurfacing and appear after completion of reepithelialization at 2 to 4 weeks as small, isolated "pearls" or inflamed cysts just below the skin surface on the forehead and cheeks. Occasionally milia may appear disseminated over the entire face. Milia and acne seem to be more common with the use of occlusive ointments. Reconditioning with introduction of topical antibiotics may be helpful in treating an acne flare-up. Occasionally a short course of low-dose oral isotretinoin (Accutane) may be required to suppress the temporary inflammation-mediated increase in sebum production following laser skin resurfacing. Milia usually respond to reconditioning (especially exfoliation) but may require manual removal with a comedone extractor or a superficial chemical peel.

COMPLICATIONS OF LASER SKIN RESURFACING

Complications of laser skin resurfacing are fortunately not common. Many can be controlled and treated successfully with minimal adverse outcome by early detection and aggressive intervention. Strict adherence to laser safety rules can prevent laser injuries from inadvertent contact with the laser beam and ignition of a fire.

Corneal Injury

Corneal injuries, including perforation of the cornea by the laser beam, have been reported but can be prevented by the routine use of metallic corneal shields. Retinal damage does not result from exposure to CO_2 laser light, since the laser light is absorbed completely by the cornea. Irritation and abrasion of the cornea by the corneal shield can be reduced by application of an ophthalmic lubricating ointment prior to placement of the shield and by gentle handling. Should a corneal injury accidentally occur, ophthalmologic consultation is indicated.

Irritation Reactions

Because the skin is vaporized during laser skin resurfacing, the normal signs of skin irritation or infection are absent. Vesiculation and erythema are not reliable markers for these conditions after laser resurfacing. Thus, if an otherwise normal postprocedure healing process is interrupted by breakdown of the skin, a high index of suspicion for sensitization, infection, or pending scar formation is warranted. Skin tolerance following laser skin resurfacing is normally diminished by loss of the stratum corneum and barrier function, and this may lead to increased skin sensitivity. Skin sensitization may appear as itching, erythema, and vesicles outside of the resurfaced area. It is usually caused by a reaction to a new topical antibiotic or ointment and may even occur from soaps, make-up, hairspray, or other cosmetics that were well tolerated by the patient before the resurfacing procedure. Treatment involves withdrawal of any potentially irritating agent or a change of antibiotics, as well as use of topical steroids, oral antihistamines, and antipruritics. If necessary, potentially offending substances can then be reintroduced one by one, while observing for development of a skin reaction. Sensitization may be seen more frequently in individuals with a history of atopy.

Infection

Infection in the postresurfacing patient, whether bacterial, viral, or fungal, may be heralded by the late onset of pain or skin deterioration. The incidence is higher in patients with undetected preexisting immunosuppression or anergy. Erythema is not a good marker for infection because it is normally present. Also, because the epidermis is absent, pustules may not be seen. A high index of suspicion is important. If one suspects the development of an infection, appropriate histologic stains for bacterial, viral (Herpes), and fungal agents should be obtained, as well as cultures and sensitivity tests. Appropriate antimicrobial agents should be administered prior to the return of culture results and should be based on specific stains and tests.

Laser skin resurfacing appears to be a potent stimulus for activation of the Herpes virus. While a history of chicken pox may be predictive, a history of cold sores, previous Herpes labialis, or a history of shingles is not necessarily predictive of increased risk of recurrent Herpes. Universal prophylaxis is recommended. While the sequelae of recurrent Herpes are limited and scarring unusual, there is a risk of dissemination and postherpetic neuralgia.

Scarring

The incidence of scarring following laser skin resurfacing is less than 1%, but it appears to be increasing as laser resurfacing is performed by inexperienced occasional operators on poorly selected patients. There is a fine line between spectacular results and spectacular complications. Taking a conservative approach to resurfacing can minimize scarring. It is safer to come back and do a "touch-up" in 6 months than to run the risk of complications by performing a "one-shot," overly aggressive resurfacing procedure. Scarring can be manifested in a continuum of alterations from minimal skin texture changes to overt hypertrophic scarring. The deeper the injury, the more coarse is the regenerated collagen, and the greater the risk of skin textural change.

The regions of the face most prone to scarring include the lips, eyelids, crow's-feet areas, and the border of the mandible. Scar formation is depth related and may result from a variety of causes, including too-low (below vaporization threshold) or too-high applied power, too many passes, double pulses, infection, desiccation, and disorders of reepithelialization caused by abnormal skin adnexal structures (such as might be seen following Accutane treatment).

The key to successful limitation of pending scarring is early recognition and treatment. A developing hypertrophic scar is never asymptotic, and 2 to 4 weeks after treatment it may present as persistent focal erythema, especially if palpable or itchy. It is important to feel the skin for induration to detect early scar formation. High-potency topical corticosteroids are the first line of treatment, and early use may prevent the development of a hypertrophic scar. These are of little use, however, for an established hypertrophic scar. Steroid ointments have a lower alcohol content than steroid creams and are preferable. Intralesional steroid injections are the primary treatment for an established hypertrophic scar. Other treatment options may include steroid-impregnated tapes, fluorouracil injections, topical silicone gel sheeting, and pulsed-dye laser treatments. Scar revision is rarely necessary, since resultant scars tend to be small and localized.

Hypopigmentation

Hypopigmentation is the result of injury to melanocytes in the skin with loss of normal skin coloration. Laser skin resurfacing generally results in minimal or no change in skin color, but it may lighten the appearance of the facial skin, especially in darker skin types and in tanned or photoaged skin. Often patients consider hypopigmentation an acceptable trade-off for improvement of their skin. Hypopigmentation may appear several months after resurfacing as whitening of the resurfaced area or as a demarcation line. It is usually seen following resolution of erythema and may be permanent. It appears to be related to increasing depths of resurfacing. No reliable treatment is known, though some improvement occasionally may be seen with return to sun exposure. It is best prevented by feathering of demarcation lines and limiting resurfacing to 2 passes with the laser with the pattern density kept on the low side.

Scleral Show and Ectropion

Postresurfacing scleral show and ectropion formation can occur if resurfacing is performed on a lax lower eyelid or on a patient who has a previous blepharoplasty with skin excision. Before eyelid resurfacing, a lower lid traction test and snap test are indicated. If lower lid laxity is demonstrated, the risk can be reduced by performing a prophylactic lateral canthopexy and lid-tightening procedure simultaneously with the resurfacing procedure. Resurfacing of the eyelids should generally be conservative. The medial canthal area should be avoided to reduce the possibility of webbing after laser resurfacing. Usually a mild degree of postprocedure scleral show and lagophthalmos (inability to completely close the eyelids) is present early after resurfacing prior to healing while the lids are swollen. These are best managed with eye lubrication and usually resolve with progression of healing. Occasionally upward massage of the lid may help speed resolution of these problems. Rarely are surgical release or skin grafts needed.

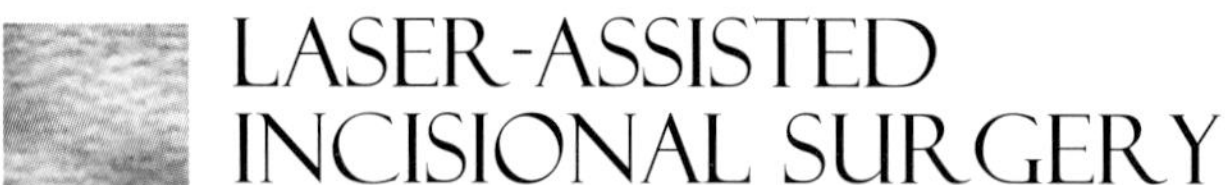

LASER-ASSISTED INCISIONAL SURGERY

Most CO_2 lasers have an additional incisional mode that allows their use as a cutting instrument or "laser scalpel." Compared to the cold steel scalpel, the incisional mode of the laser has the benefits of simultaneous coagulation of small blood vessels and lymphatics, which improves hemostasis and allows better visualization.

Additional hemostasis can be achieved if the laser is used in a slightly defocused mode. Precise and excellent hemostasis with coagulation of blood vessels of up to 0.5 mm can be accomplished in vascular areas, such as the eyelids. Clinically there appears to be less bruising, swelling, and pain, leading to quicker recovery and return to usual activities. Patient acceptance has been high, and no increase in complications has been seen.

The disadvantages of laser incisional surgery compared to scalpel incisional surgery include the risk of laser-related injury to associated structures. Corneal protection is as important as it is in laser resurfacing procedures, especially during incisional procedures around the eyes. The special equipment required for performing laser incisional surgery is more costly and cumbersome than that used in traditional techniques. Back-up of laser incisional techniques by traditional techniques is also necessary in case of laser malfunction or failure.

Laser incisional surgery has been applied to facial cosmetic surgical procedures such as blepharoplasty, facelift, brow-lift, and others. Laser skin resurfacing can also be combined with laser incisional surgery, especially in the case of the lower transconjunctival blepharoplasty with combined skin resurfacing of the lower eyelids for simultaneous improvement of "fat bags" and lower eyelid textural abnormalities.

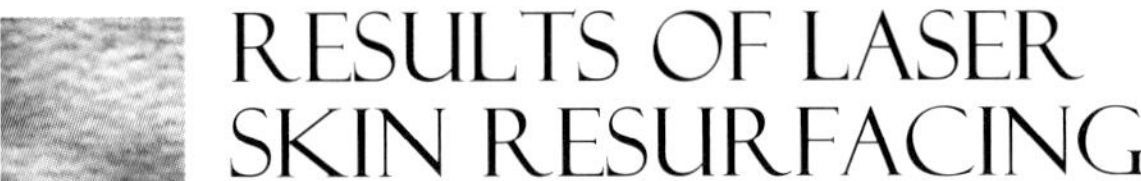

RESULTS OF LASER SKIN RESURFACING

The results of laser skin resurfacing have been good to excellent, depending on the indication for which the procedure was performed, and patient satisfaction overall has been high. Patients have a softer, rejuvenated appearance and a significant smoothing of skin textural abnormalities resulting from the combined leveling and tightening effects of the procedure.

Actinic changes are improved to the greatest degree. Wrinkles typically are improved by 60% to 80%, while scars are improved to a lesser degree. These results depend on the type and extent of the wrinkles and scars. Improvement may be seen in deeper skin folds of the cheek, forehead, and neck, in malar bags, and even in the excess skin of the upper eyelid (pseudoblepharoplasty effect), but these improvements are less predictable. Static lines are improved to a greater degree than dynamic lines. Dynamic lines should be discussed with the patient prior to treatment, since combined use of botulinum toxin (Botox, Allergan, Inc.) may be indicated.

Improvement continues for several months after treatment as collagen remodeling progresses. To best estimate the degree of improvement after healing is complete, results should be assessed 6 months after resurfacing. Some loss of early improvement and recurrence of wrinkles and lines can be expected as edema resolves. Multiple repeat treatments are possible and should be spaced approximately 6 months apart. Because laser resurfacing has been available for only a limited time, there are no long-term follow-up studies comparing it to other resurfacing techniques.

Patient satisfaction is based on the delivery of natural results with minimal downtime and a low incidence of complications. The most frequent cause of patient dissatisfaction is unmet expectations. Some patients expect laser skin resurfacing to have the same effect as a surgical lifting procedure, such as a facelift. Some patients unrealistically expect every line and wrinkle to be entirely eliminated.

Other factors in patient dissatisfaction include erythema, pigmentation abnormalities, lack of improvement, early recurrence, and failure to improve dynamic expression lines and preexisting laxity. Patients sometimes behave as if they have forgotten how they looked prior to the procedure. Good preoperative photographs are very helpful in these situations. Expectations of postprocedure appearance are best discussed and resolved prior to the procedure. If the discussion occurs prior to performing the procedure, it is considered full disclosure. If a similar discussion occurs after completion of the procedure and the patient is dissatisfied, it is considered an excuse.

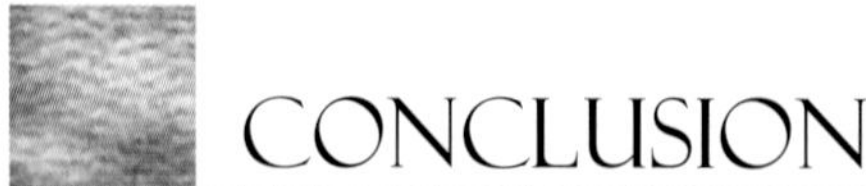

CONCLUSION

Based on its record of safety and effectiveness, CO_2 laser skin resurfacing has advanced to a competitive position among the modalities available for improving skin textural abnormalities. Spectacular results can be achieved; however, the possibility of morbidity should limit the overly aggressive application of the procedure, as it should with any other resurfacing modality.

Patient dissatisfaction with results is most often caused by unrealistic expectations that were not realized; thus, patients with conditions suitable to laser resurfacing who also have realistic expectations must be selected. They should be made aware of the fact that the laser is not a "magic wand" but a tool that will be used to make certain changes. The laser operator must take responsibility for being adequately trained and for the safe application of this tool. The greatest variable in the laser resurfacing equation is the person performing the procedure. Should complications occur, it is inappropriate to blame the laser.

The key to success in laser skin resurfacing lies in attentive patient selection, diligent pre- and postprocedure care, and, very importantly, in the recognition of the endpoint for application of the laser energy that maximizes results while limiting potential complications.

With further study, we will be better able to determine long-term results and to position laser skin resurfacing among the different resurfacing modalities. To date, no study has demonstrated clinical superiority of one resurfacing modality over any other. Also unknown is whether results differ among the modalities when resurfacing is performed to equivalent depths. Each resurfacing technique has its own advantages and disadvantages, and it is our responsibility to choose the modality that provides the best result for each of our patients without outside considerations influencing this decision.

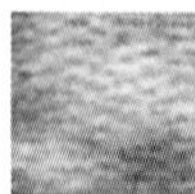

COMBINED PROCEDURES

Many aesthetic surgery patients have combinations of laxity and skin texture abnormalities that cannot be treated with a single modality. Also, the depth of such skin texture abnormalities varies. Available modalities for resurfacing have an optimal depth for their action, and no single modality is ideal for all textural problems. Furthermore, not all areas of the face age at the same rate and need the same depth of resurfacing, and there may be a predominant need for regional leveling or regional firming in an aging face. While a single procedure cannot address all of these concerns, there has been disagreement over whether combined procedures should be performed on the same surgical date.[46–50]

When resurfacing procedures are combined, laxity and skin texture problems can be treated simultaneously and demarcation lines can be made less obvious. No additional anesthesia is required, and there is a single period of healing. This is quite important for our busy patients, who demand a quick return to their usual activities as well as a natural postoperative appearance and minimal complications. Additive and continued firming of the skin flaps and continued improvement over time is also noted. All of these add up to a more complete rejuvenation process.

Whether a TCA-based Blue Peel or CO_2 laser skin resurfacing is better is often debated. The real question should be which region and which patient will benefit from CO_2 laser resurfacing and which ones would benefit more from the Blue Peel. The advantages of the laser skin resurfacing and the Blue Peel have been discussed in detail in this and previous chapters. Briefly, CO_2 laser skin resurfacing is used predominantly in areas requiring leveling, whereas the Blue Peel is better in areas requiring firming.

Indications for combined procedures are similar to those for laser resurfacing or the Blue Peel alone. These include facial rhytidosis, photoaging, mild laxity, superficial scars, and hyperpigmentation problems.

The Blue Peel is a light TCA peel that works well in combination with a variety of resurfacing modalities, including laser skin resurfacing as well as laser incisional surgery. The Blue Peel can also be performed as a superficial peel over skin flaps and over composite flaps of skin and muscle.

PERFORMING THE BLUE PEEL TOGETHER WITH LASER RESURFACING

In performing an Obagi Blue Peel combined with laser skin resurfacing, the preoperative markings are made initially. These outline the jawline and follow the aesthetic subunit approach to the face. Full-face nerve block anesthesia is usually administered, although some patients benefit from general anesthesia.

The Blue Peel is performed first because less anesthesia is required and this allows time for the onset of the nerve blocks. There is also less risk of TCA inadvertently getting onto freshly resurfaced skin, and the edges can be feathered better around the Blue Peel. After completion of the Blue Peel, the CO_2 laser skin resurfacing is performed. Immediate postprocedure care is similar to the care of the patient with laser resurfacing alone. Because resurfaced areas are smaller, the face is washed several times a day and a light ointment is applied to prevent drying. A full-face CO_2 laser resurfacing can be combined with a Blue Peel of the neck, or a regional laser resurfacing can be combined with a Blue Peel of the non-laser-resurfaced areas.

PERFORMING THE BLUE PEEL TOGETHER WITH INCISONAL SURGERY

When combining the Blue Peel with incisional surgery, perform the sterile procedure first, followed by the Blue Peel. Frequently, the combination is a lower laser transconjunctival blepharoplasty followed by a full-face Blue Peel.

The Blue Peel can also be performed over skin flaps. The ideal candidate is one who would otherwise undergo a facelift and neck-lift and wishes to have light superficial resurfacing over the facelift flaps to treat keratoses or pigmentation abnormalities. When applying a Blue Peel over an undermined skin flap, it is important to remember that the margin for error is thin. Patient selection is very important. Unsatisfactory candidates are patients who are smokers, have active facial infections, or are questionable regarding postprocedure compliance. A history of previous Accutane use or previous radiation therapy to the face would also preclude this procedure. In the setting of collagen vascular disease or a previous deep chemical peel, reepithelialization may be limited.

Key to performing a Blue Peel over undermined skin is to maintain circulation to the skin flaps. The usual surgical techniques are used, and the skin flaps are kept thick. Handle the flap gently. Use normal skin flap tension and suture placement during closure.

It is important to design variable peel depths on the flaps. The peel can be deeper in the nonundermined skin of the central face, but it must become more superficial on the periphery of the undermined flap. The upper papillary dermis is the maximum depth on the periphery of the undermined skin flap. Sharp transitions between the zones of the variable depth of the peel must be avoided, and the incisions must be protected from the TCA solution.

Intravenous steroids are not routinely used; however, oral steroids may be helpful in the postoperative period to reduce swelling. Postoperative care is the same as if the patient had not had an additional peel. The blue coloration may be expected to last from 2 to 7 days, depending upon the vigor with which the face is cleansed in the postoperative period. Sutures are usually removed between the fifth and the seventh day.

Recognizing the endpoints for the Blue Peel on the undermined skin flaps is very important. In the central face, the maximum depth is the lower papillary or upper reticular dermis, indicated by an even blue coloration with frost and with less pink background. In the proximal aspect of the flap, a prominent pink background to the frost must be observed. In the periphery of the flap, an even blue coloration is more important than frosting, and a solid frost should not be achieved there because of the risk of excessively deep penetration with the peel.

The Blue Peel can also be performed over skin-muscle and composite flaps. Candidates include patients undergoing deep-plane facelifts and endoscopic or open brow-lifts. In these situations, skin-muscle flaps and composite flaps normally have circulation comparable to that of nonundermined skin.

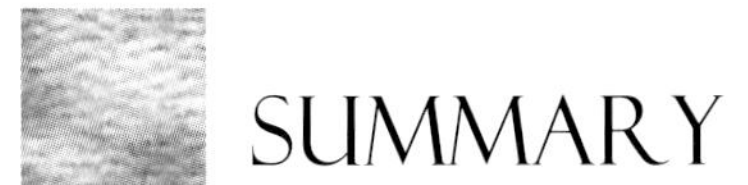

SUMMARY

Results of rejuvenation procedures can be enhanced with combined procedures. Healing time does not appear to depend upon which procedures are combined, but instead to depend on the maximum depth of injury. The addition of the Blue Peel does not appear to delay healing time in resurfacing procedures, since skin generally heals faster after this peel than after either laser or surgical procedures.

Potential complications, including hypertrophic scars or keloids, overtightening, delayed healing, milia, persistent erythema, hyperpigmentation, and hypopigmentation, have not been seen.

Excellent results have been achieved by combining resurfacing procedures. Skin texture can be improved very effectively and demarcation lines can be reduced. These procedures can be performed safely without increased complications. There appears to be no delay in healing or recovery and there is a very high patient satisfaction rate.

The keys to successfully combining resurfacing procedures are

1. careful patient selection
2. preprocedure skin preparation and conditioning

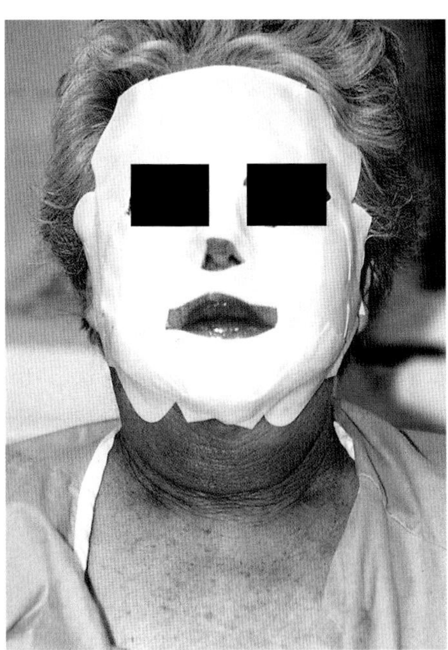

FIGURE 11-1. *Appearance immediately following combined upper and lower laser blepharoplasty, full-face CO_2 laser skin resurfacing (with semiocclusive dressing), and Blue Peel of the neck and chest.*

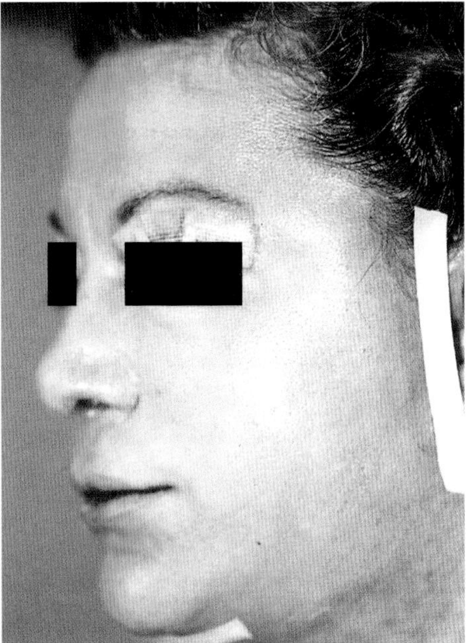

FIGURE 11-2. *Combined standard SMAS facelift with upper and lower blepharoplasty and full-face Blue Peel. Note transition in Blue Peel depth without sharp demarcation lines.*

3. precise depth control, and
4. careful postoperative care and follow-up.

Patients undergoing or having undergone procedures combining CO_2 laser resurfacing along with other cosmetic procedures are shown in Figures 11-1 to 11-6.

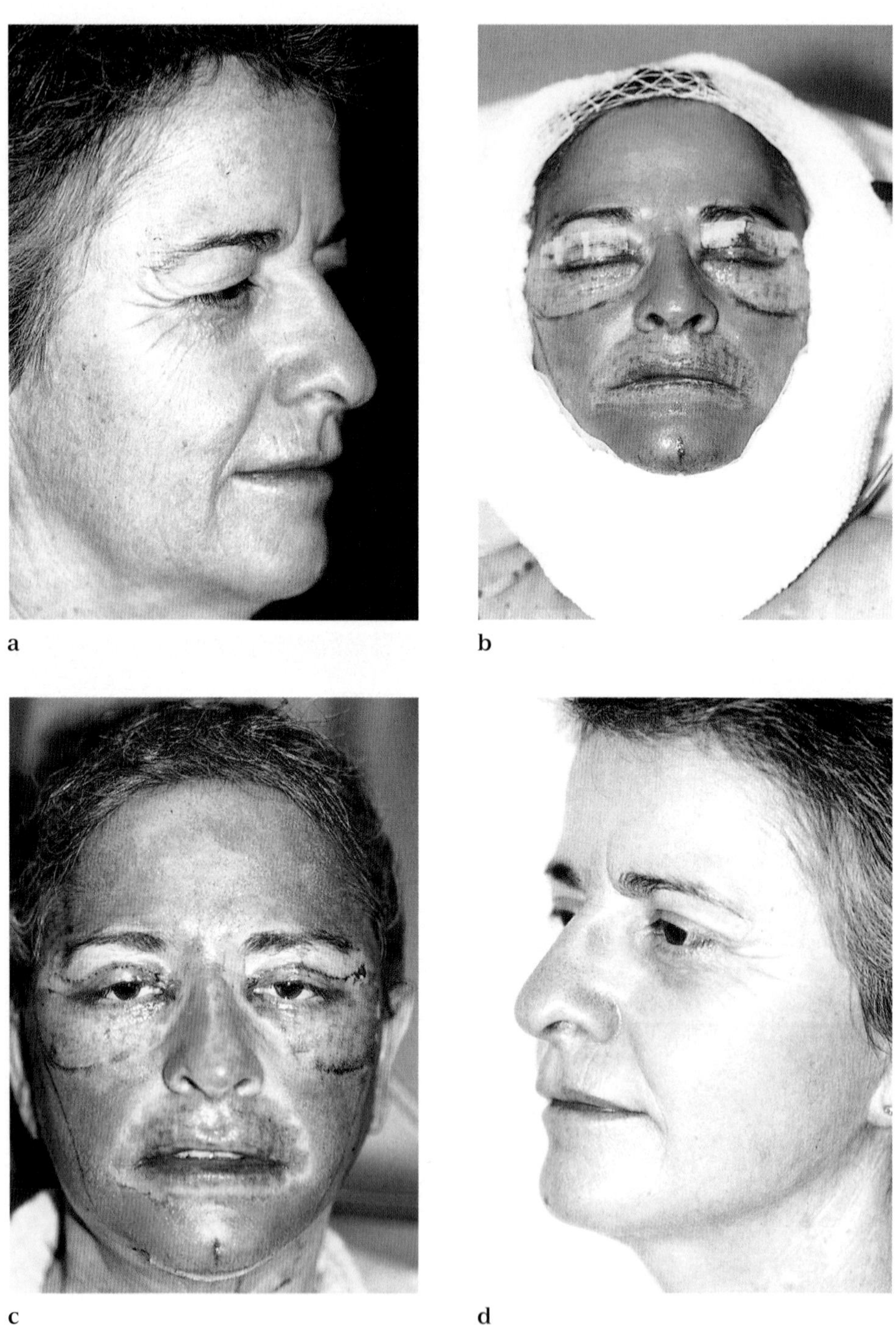

FIGURE 11-3. *(a) Before procedures. (b) Immediately after combined upper and lower laser blepharoplasty, perioral and periorbital CO_2 laser skin resurfacing, SMAS facelift, and full-face Blue Peel. (c) 2 days postoperatively. (d) After, 6 months. Note simultaneous improvement in laxity, skin texture, and pigmentation.*

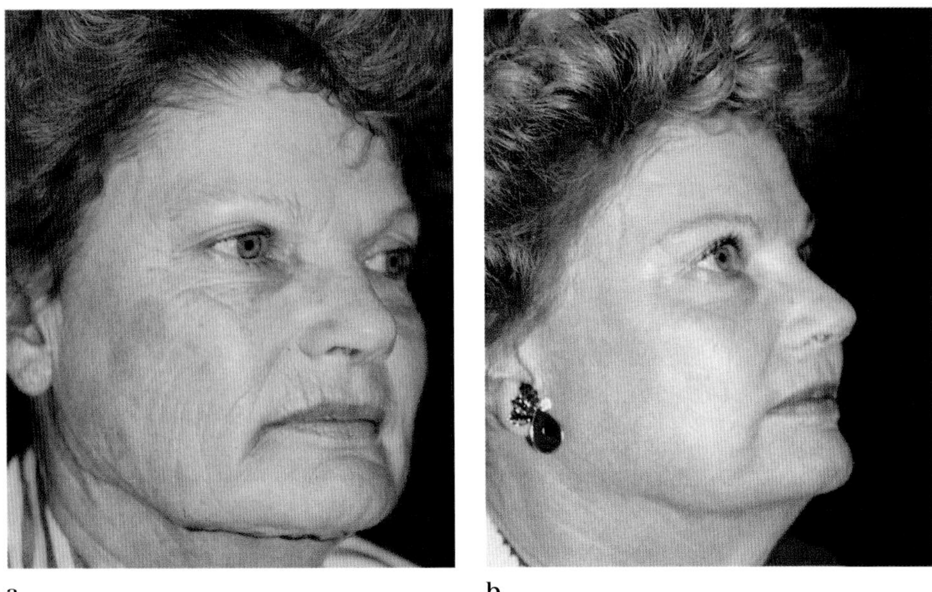

a b

FIGURE 11-4. *(a) Before procedure. (b) After, 6 months. Full-face laser skin resurfacing with the UltraPulse CO_2 laser (CPG 300 mJ, density 5, 2 confluent passes, 1 selective pass with 3-mm spot 350 mJ).*

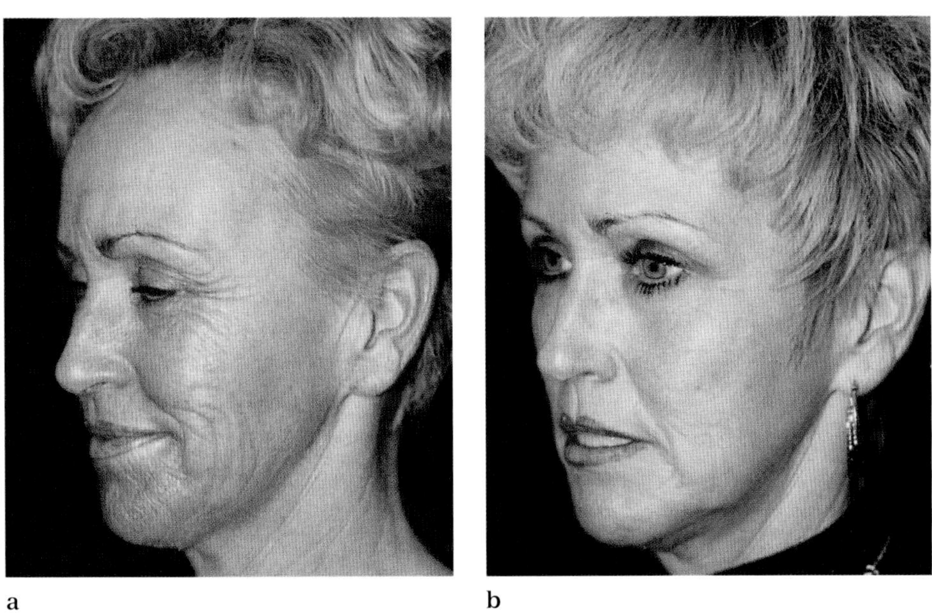

a b

FIGURE 11-5. *(a) Before procedures. (b) After, 6 months. Full-face laser resurfacing with the UltraPulse CO_2 laser (CPG 300 mJ, density 5 and 6, 2 confluent passes, 1 selective pass with 3-mm spot 350 mJ).*

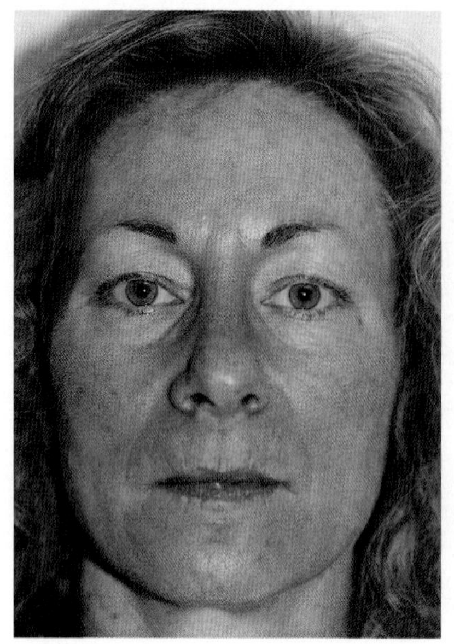

a

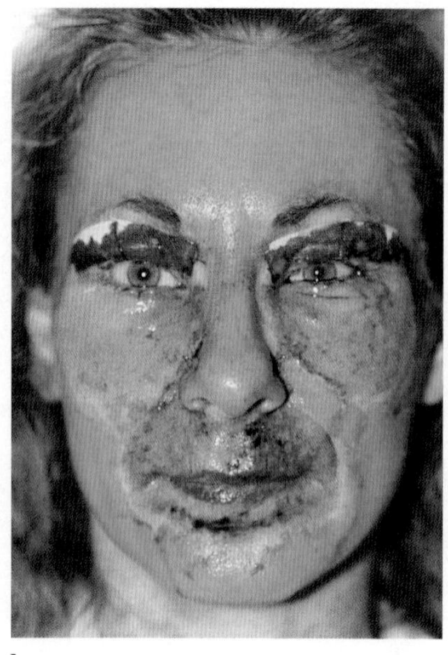

b

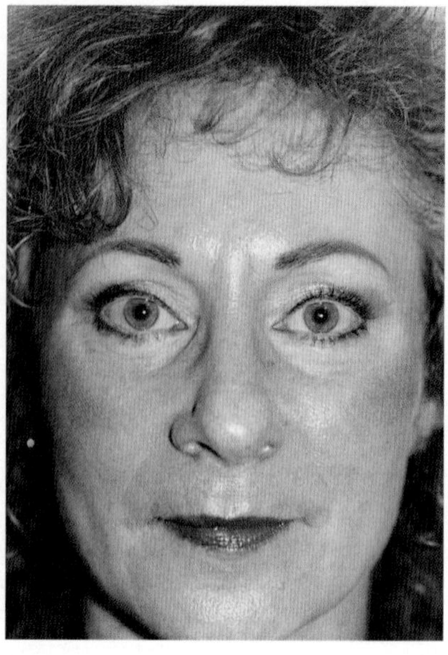

c

FIGURE 11-6. *(a) Before procedures. (b) Immediately after combined upper and lower laser blepharoplasty, perioral and periorbital CO_2 laser skin resurfacing, and regional Blue Peel. (c) After, 6 months.*

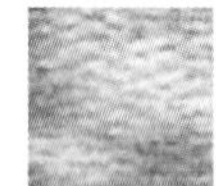

REFERENCES

1. Anderson RR, Parrish JA. Selective photothermolysis: precise microsurgery by selective absorption of pulsed radiation. *Science.* 1983;220: 524–527.
2. Hobbs ER, Bailing PL, Wheeland RG, Ratz JL. Superpulsed lasers: minimizing thermal damage with short duration, high irradiance pulses. *J Dermatol Surg Oncol.* 1987;13:955–964.
3. Fitzpatrick RE, Ruiz-Esparza J, Goldman MP. The depth of thermal necrosis using the CO_2 laser: a comparison of the superpulsed mode and the conventional mode. *J Dermatol Surg Oncol.* 1991;17:340–344.
4. Nelson JS. Lasers: state of the art in dermatology. *Dermatol Clin.* 1993;11: 15–25.
5. Wheeland RG. Clinical uses of lasers in dermatology. *Lasers Surg Med.* 1995;16:2–23.
6. Lowe NJ, Lask G, Griffin ME, et al. Skin resurfacing with the ultrapulse carbon dioxide laser: observations on 100 patients. *Dermatol Surg.* 1995;21:1025–1029.
7. Lask G, Keller G, Lowe N, et al. Laser skin resurfacing with the silktouch flashscanner for facial rhytides. *Dermatol Surg.* 1995;21:1021–1024.
8. Waldorf HA, Kauvar A, Geronemus RG. Skin resurfacing of fine to deep rhytides using a char-free carbon dioxide laser in 47 patients. *Dermatol Surg.* 1995;21:940–946.
9. Hruza GJ. Skin resurfacing with lasers. *Fitzpatrick's J of Clin Dermatol.* 1995;3:38–41.

10. Schoenrock LD, Chernoff WG, Rubach BW. Cutaneous ultrapulse laser resurfacing of the eyelids. *Int J Aesthetic Restor Surg.* 1995;3:31–36.

11. Alster TS, West TB. Resurfacing of atrophic facial acne scars with a high-energy, pulsed carbon dioxide laser. *Dermatol Surg.* 1996;22:151–155.

12. Fulton JE Jr. Skin resurfacing and lesion ablation with the ultrapulse CO_2 laser. *Am J Cosmet Surg.* 1996;13:323–336.

13. Fitzpatrick RE, Goldman MP, Satur NM, et al. Pulsed carbon dioxide laser resurfacing of photoaged facial skin. *Arch Dermatol.* 1996;132:395–402.

14. Biesman BS. Cutaneous facial resurfacing with the carbon dioxide laser. *Ophthalmic Surg Lasers.* 1996;27:685–698.

15. Spicer MS, Goldberg DJ. Lasers in dermatology. *J Am Acad Dermatol.* 1996;34:1–25.

16. Weinstein C, Alster TS. Skin resurfacing with high energy, pulsed carbon dioxide lasers. In: Alster TS, Apfelberg DB, eds. *Cosmetic Laser Surgery.* New York, NY: Wiley-Liss; 1996:9–27.

17. Yarborough JM. Dermabrasive surgery. *Clin Dermatol.* 1987;5:75–78.

18. Fulton JE. Dermabrasion, chemabrasion, and laserabrasion: historical perspectives, modern dermabrasion techniques, and future trends. *Dermatol Surg.* 1996;22:619–628.

19. Walsh JT, Florre TJ, Anderson RR, Deutsch TF. Pulsed CO_2 laser tissue ablation: effect of tissue type and pulse duration on thermal damage. *Lasers Surg Med.* 1988;8:108–118.

20. Weinstein C. Carbon dioxide laser resurfacing. In: Coleman WP, et al., eds. *Cosmetic Surgery of the Skin.* St Louis, Mo: CV Mosby; 1997:152–177.

21. Tang SV, Kamat B, Arndt KA, et al. Low energy density CO_2 laser irradiation causes intraepidermal damage. *Lasers Surg Med.* 1984;3:329–335.

22. Rosenberg GJ, Gregory RO. Lasers in aesthetic surgery. *Clin Plast Surg.* 1996;23:29–48.

23. Reid R. Physical and surgical principles governing carbon dioxide laser surgery of the skin. *Dermatol Clin.* 1991;9:297–315.

24. Anderson RR. Laser tissue interactions. In: Goldman MP, Fitzpatrick RE, eds. *Cutaneous Laser Surgery.* St. Louis, Mo: Mosby; 1995:53–72.

25. Fitzpatrick RF, Tope WD, Goldma MP, et al. Pulsed carbon dioxide laser, trichloroacetic acid, Baker-Gordon phenol, and dermabrasion: a comparative clinical and histologic study of cutaneous resurfacing in a porcine model. *Arch Dermatol.* 1996;132:469–471.

26. Nelson BR, Fader DJ, Gillard M, et al. Pilot histologic and ultrastructural study of the effects of medium-depth chemical facial peels on dermal collagen in patients with actinically damaged skin. *J Am Acad Dermatol.* 1995;32:472–480.

27. Ross EV, Naseef M, Skrobal M, et al. In vivo dermal collagen shrinkage and remodeling following CO_2 laser resurfacing. *Lasers Surg Med.* 1996;19(suppl):38–42.

28. Gardner ES, Reinisch L, Stricklin GP. Dermal changes following cutaneous laser resurfacing. *Lasers Surg Med.* 1996;19(suppl):33–37.

29. Stuzin JM, Baker TJ, Baker TM, Kligman AM. Histologic effects of the high-energy pulsed CO_2 laser on photoaged facial skin. *Plast Reconstr Surg.* 1997;99:2036–2055.

30. Obagi ZE, Mazen M, Sawof M, Johnson JB, Laub DR, Stevens MB. The controlled depth trichloroacetic acid peel: methodology, outcome, and complication rate. *Int J Aesthetic Restor Surg.* 1996;4:81–94.

31. Abergel RP, Meeker CA, Oikarinen H., et al. Retinoid modulation of connective tissue metabolism in keloid fibroblast cultures. *Arch Dermatol.* 1985;121:632–635.

32. Rubenstein R, Roenigk HH, Stegman SJ, et al. Atypical keloids after dermabrasion of patients taking isotretinoin. *J Am Acad Dermatol.* 1986;15:280–285.

33. Moy RL, Moy LS, Bennett RG., et al. Systemic isotretinoin: effects on dermal wound healing in a rabbit ear model in vivo. *J Dermatol Surg Oncol.* 1990;16:1142–1146.

34. Apfelberg DB, Varga J, Greenbaum SS. Carbon dioxide laser resurfacing of peri-oral rhytids in scleroderma patients. *Dermatol Surg.* 1998; 24:517–519.

35. Gloster HM, Roenigk RK. Risk of acquiring human papillomavirus from the plume produced by the carbon dioxide laser in the treatment of warts. *J Am Acad Dermatol.* 1995;32:436–441.

36. Hevia O, Nemeth AJ, Taylor R. Tretinoin accelerates healing after trichloroacetic acid peel. *Arch Dermatol.* 1991;127:40–48.

37. Beasley D, Jones C, McDonald WS. Effect of pretreated skin on laser resurfacing. *Lasers Surg Med.* 1997;5(suppl):43.

38. Vagotis FL, Brundage SR. Histologic study of dermabrasion and chemical peel in an animal model after treatment with Retin-A. *Aesthetic Plast Surg.* 1995;19:243–246.

39. Lowe NJ, Lask G, Griffin ME, Maxwell A. Laser skin resurfacing, pre and post treatment guidelines. *Dermatol Surg.* 1995;21:1017–1019.

40. Duke D, Grevelink JM. Care before and after laser skin resurfacing: a survey and review of the literature. *Dermatol Surg.* 1998;24:201–206.

41. Thompson VM, Seiler T, Durrie DS, Cavanaugh TB. Holmium:YAG laser thermokeratoplasty for hyperopia and astigmatism: an overview. *Refract Corneal Surg.* 1993;9:S134–S147.

42. Allain JC, Lous LE, Cohen-Solan L, et al. Isometric tension lines developed during the hydrothermal swelling of rat skin. *Connect Tissue Res.* 1980;7:127–133.

43. Winter GD. Formation of the scab and rate of epithelialization of superficial wounds. *Nature.* 1962;193:293–294.

44. Fulton JE Jr. Complications of laser resurfacing: methods of prevention and management. *Dermatol Surg.* 1998;24:91–99.

45. Suarez M, Fulton JE Jr. A novel occlusive dressing for skin resurfacing. *Dermatol Surg.* 1998;24:567–570.

46. Davies B, Guyuron B, Husami T. The role of lidocaine, epinephrine, and flap elevation in wound healing after chemical peel. *Ann Plast Surg.* 1991;26:273–278.

47. Guyuron B, Michelow B, Schmelzer R, et al. Delayed healing of rhytidectomy flap resurfaced with CO_2 laser. *Plast Reconstr Surg.* 1998;101:816–819.

48. Dingman DL, Hartog J, Siemionow M. Simultaneous deep-plane face lift and trichloroacetic acid peel. *Plast Reconstr Surg.* 1994;93:86–93.

49. Ramirez OM, Pozner JM. Laser resurfacing as an adjunct to endoforehead lift, endofacelift, and biplanar facelift. *Ann Plast Surg.* 1997;4:315–321.

50. Bisaccia E, Sequeira M, Magidson J, Scarborough D. Surgical intervention of the aging face: combination of mini facelifting and superficial carbon dioxide laser resurfacing. *Dermatol Drug.* 1998;24:821–826.

INDEX

Note: Page numbers followed by *f* or *t* indicate figures or tables, respectively.

B

C

E

F

I

J

K

L

P

R

S

T